RARE DISEASES AND ORPHAN PRODUCTS

Accelerating Research and Development

Committee on Accelerating Rare Diseases Research and
Orphan Product Development

Board on Health Sciences Policy

Marilyn J. Field and Thomas F. Boat, *Editors*

INSTITUTE OF MEDICINE
OF THE NATIONAL ACADEMIES

THE NATIONAL ACADEMIES PRESS
Washington, D.C.
www.nap.edu

THE NATIONAL ACADEMIES PRESS • 500 Fifth Street, N.W. • Washington, DC 20001

NOTICE: The project that is the subject of this report was approved by the Governing Board of the National Research Council, whose members are drawn from the councils of the National Academy of Sciences, the National Academy of Engineering, and the Institute of Medicine. The members of the committee responsible for the report were chosen for their special competences and with regard for appropriate balance.

This study was supported by Contract No. N01-OD-4-2139, TO # 215 between the National Academy of Sciences and the National Institutes of Health. Additional support was provided by the Food and Drug Administration. Any opinions, findings, conclusions, or recommendations expressed in this publication are those of the authors and do not necessarily reflect the view of the organizations or agencies that provided support for the project.

International Standard Book Number-13: 978-0-309-15806-0
International Standard Book Number-10: 0-309-15806-0

Additional copies of this report are available from the National Academies Press, 500 Fifth Street, N.W., Lockbox 285, Washington, DC 20055; (800) 624-6242 or (202) 334-3313 (in the Washington metropolitan area); Internet, http://www.nap.edu.

For more information about the Institute of Medicine, visit the IOM home page at: **www.iom.edu.**

Printed in the United States of America

The serpent has been a symbol of long life, healing, and knowledge among almost all cultures and religions since the beginning of recorded history. The serpent adopted as a logotype by the Institute of Medicine is a relief carving from ancient Greece, now held by the Staatliche Museen in Berlin.

Front cover photographs (top to bottom):

Using electropheresis apparatus to separate proteins by molecular weight.
Photo courtesy of National Institute of Arthritis and Musculoskeletal and Skin Diseases.

96-well, 384-well, and 1,536-well plates used in pharmaceutical and life science research. Photo courtesy of National Human Genome Research Institute.

Children with ectodermal dysplasia. Used with permission. Photo courtesy of the National Foundation for Ectodermal Dysplasias.

Image of chromosomal abnormalities in mouse cells from a study of leukemia-promoting effects of tumor necrosis factor-alpha in Fanconi anemia group C stem cells. Photo courtesy of the laboratory of Dr. Qishen Pang at Cincinnati Children's Hospital Medical Center. U.S.A. Copyright 2007, American Society for Clinical Investigation. Used with permission.

Friedreich's ataxia patient and Friedreich's Ataxia Research Alliance (FARA) spokeperson, Kyle Bryant, on his recumbent trike during the cycling competition Race Across America. Copyright 2010, www.SLOtography.com. Used with permission.

Children with sickle cell disease. Used with permission. Photo courtesy of Cincinnati Children's Hospital Medical Center.

Suggested citation: IOM (Institute of Medicine). 2010. *Rare Diseases and Orphan Products: Accelerating Research and Development.* Washington, DC: The National Academies Press.

"Knowing is not enough; we must apply.
Willing is not enough; we must do."
—Goethe

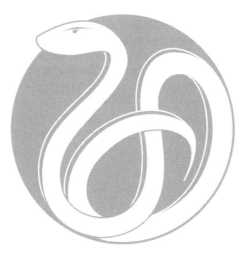

INSTITUTE OF MEDICINE

OF THE NATIONAL ACADEMIES

Advising the Nation. Improving Health.

THE NATIONAL ACADEMIES
Advisers to the Nation on Science, Engineering, and Medicine

The **National Academy of Sciences** is a private, nonprofit, self-perpetuating society of distinguished scholars engaged in scientific and engineering research, dedicated to the furtherance of science and technology and to their use for the general welfare. Upon the authority of the charter granted to it by the Congress in 1863, the Academy has a mandate that requires it to advise the federal government on scientific and technical matters. Dr. Ralph J. Cicerone is president of the National Academy of Sciences.

The **National Academy of Engineering** was established in 1964, under the charter of the National Academy of Sciences, as a parallel organization of outstanding engineers. It is autonomous in its administration and in the selection of its members, sharing with the National Academy of Sciences the responsibility for advising the federal government. The National Academy of Engineering also sponsors engineering programs aimed at meeting national needs, encourages education and research, and recognizes the superior achievements of engineers. Dr. Charles M. Vest is president of the National Academy of Engineering.

The **Institute of Medicine** was established in 1970 by the National Academy of Sciences to secure the services of eminent members of appropriate professions in the examination of policy matters pertaining to the health of the public. The Institute acts under the responsibility given to the National Academy of Sciences by its congressional charter to be an adviser to the federal government and, upon its own initiative, to identify issues of medical care, research, and education. Dr. Harvey V. Fineberg is president of the Institute of Medicine.

The **National Research Council** was organized by the National Academy of Sciences in 1916 to associate the broad community of science and technology with the Academy's purposes of furthering knowledge and advising the federal government. Functioning in accordance with general policies determined by the Academy, the Council has become the principal operating agency of both the National Academy of Sciences and the National Academy of Engineering in providing services to the government, the public, and the scientific and engineering communities. The Council is administered jointly by both Academies and the Institute of Medicine. Dr. Ralph J. Cicerone and Dr. Charles M. Vest are chair and vice chair, respectively, of the National Research Council.

www.national-academies.org

AARON SETH KESSELHEIM, Instructor in Medicine, Harvard Medical School; Division of Pharmacoepidemiology and Pharmacoeconomics, Brigham and Women's Hospital
ALISON MACK, Independent Consultant

IOM Staff

MARILYN J. FIELD, Senior Program Officer
CLAIRE GIAMMARIA, Research Associate (from August 2010)
ERIN S. HAMMERS, Research Associate (until May 2010)
ROBIN E. PARSELL, Senior Program Assistant
ANDREW M. POPE, Director, Board on Health Sciences Policy

Acknowledgments

In preparing this report, the committee and project staff benefited greatly from the assistance and expertise of many individuals and groups. Important information and insights came from three public meetings that the committee organized to collect information and perspectives from a range of academic, professional, consumer, patient, and other organizations and individuals. A number of speakers at these meetings also shared their knowledge at other times during the course of the study. Appendix A includes the agendas of the public meetings and a list of organizations that submitted written statements of views. The committee appreciates the contributions of Aaron Kesselheim, author of Appendix B, and Laura Brooks Faden, coauthor of Appendix C.

Our project officer at the National Institutes of Health (NIH), Stephen Groft, was an invaluable resource and unfailingly helpful. We also were advised by others at NIH including Stephen Hirschfield (National Institute for Child Health and Human Development) and Jeffrey Abrams and Isis Mikhail (National Cancer Institute). Our project officer at the Food and Drug Administration (FDA), Timothy Coté, likewise was a great help, patiently answering questions about the workings of the Orphan Drug Act and its results. We also were assisted by other FDA staff, particularly Debra Lewis and Anne Pariser as well as Kui Xu, Menfo Imoisili, and Katherine Needleman. Joan Sokolovsky at the Medicare Payment Advisory Commission helped with questions about drug coverage under Medicare Parts B and D. Scott Grosse at the Centers for Disease Control and Prevention offered useful insights into the complexities of epidemiologic research on rare conditions.

Sharon Terry and colleagues at the Genetic Alliance and Peter Saltonstall, Mary Dunkle, and colleagues at the National Organization for Rare Diseases worked with the committee on an invitation for their members to submit statements of views on issues before the committee. At Orphanet, Seygolene Ayme provided important information and guidance about their information resources. A number of individuals in other organizations were also helpful in a variety of ways. In addition to those who made presentations during committee meetings and with whom we talked at other meetings, among those we consulted were Stephen Bajardi and Anthony Horton (International Rett Syndrome Foundation), Ron Bartek (Freidriech's Ataxia Research Alliance), Robert Beall (Cystic Fibrosis Foundation), Wendy Book (American Partnership for Eosinophilic Disorders), Amy Hewitt (Scleroderma Research Foundation), Cynthia Joyce (Spinal Muscular Atrophy Association), Jill Raleigh (LAM [Lymphangioleiomyomatosis] Foundation), Jodi Edgar Reinhardt (National Foundation for Ectodermal Dysplasias), and John Walsh (Alpha-1 Foundation). We also called on Carl Whalen at the National Disease Research Interchange; Yann Le Cam (Eurodis); Marty Liggett, Ulvana Desiderio, and Stephanie Kart (American Society of Hematology); Qishen Pang, Vicky Klensch, and Kori Siroky (Cincinnati Children's Hospital Medical Center); and Enrique Seoane-Vazquez (Ohio State University).

In addition, the committee and project staff appreciate the work of copy editor Florence Poillon; Debra Gilliam, Chanda Chay, and John Bowers of Caset Associates; and temporary research assistant Cassandra Fletcher. Within the National Academies, we particularly acknowledge the assistance of Clyde Behney, Adam Berger, Robert Giffin (now at the Center for Medical Technology Policy), Greta Gorman, Christine Micheel, Amy Packman, Donna Randall, and Vilija Teel.

Reviewers

This report has been reviewed in draft form by individuals chosen for their diverse perspectives and technical expertise, in accordance with procedures approved by the National Research Council's Report Review Committee. The purpose of this independent review is to provide candid and critical comments that will assist the institution in making its published reports as sound as possible and to ensure that the report meets institutional standards for objectivity, evidence, and responsiveness to the study charge. The review comments and draft manuscript remain confidential to protect the integrity of the deliberative process. We wish to thank the following individuals for their review of this report:

Ronald J. Bartek, Friedreich's Ataxia Research Alliance
Edward M. Basile, King & Spalding
Jim Burns, Genzyme Corporation
David Frohnmayer, Fanconi Anemia Research Fund
Elaine Gallin, Doris Duke Charitable Foundation
Robert C. Griggs, University of Rochester School of Medicine
Susan Kelley, Multiple Myeloma Research Consortium
Chaitan Khosla, Stanford University
Michael Knowles, University of North Carolina at Chapel Hill
Roger J. Lewis, University of California, Los Angeles
John Linehan, Stanford University
Dawn S. Milliner, Mayo Clinic
Carol Mimura, University of California, Berkeley
John A. Parrish, Massachusetts General Hospital

Reed E. Pyeritz, University of Pennsylvania
Joan Sokolovsky, Medicare Payment Advisory Committee
Jess G. Thoene, University of Michigan

Although the reviewers listed above have provided many constructive comments and suggestions, they were not asked to endorse the conclusions or recommendations, nor did they see the final draft of the report before its release. The review of this report was overseen by **Neal A. Vanselow** and **Floyd E. Bloom,** Scripps Research Institute. Appointed by the National Research Council and the Institute of Medicine, these individuals were responsible for making certain that an independent examination of this report was carried out in accordance with the institutional procedures and that all review comments were carefully considered. Responsibility for the final content of this report rests entirely with the authoring committee and the institution.

Preface

Rare diseases are not rare, at least in aggregate. Approximately 7,000 rare diseases afflict millions of individuals in the United States and are responsible for untold losses in terms of physical health, behavioral health, and socioeconomic condition. Physicians, nurses, and others who care for this group of patients recognize the huge burden on patients, families, communities, the health care system, and the health care financing system. All too frequently, providers are reminded of the gap between patient needs and our inability individually and collectively to meet those needs.

Although rare diseases taken together have an enormous impact, there has been no "war on rare diseases" and no designation of a National Institutes of Health (NIH) institute (as for cancer) to address research on rare diseases, even though some U.S. prevalence figures for all rare diseases fall in the range of estimates of those with a history of a cancer diagnosis. Although neither of these cancer-specific responses to need may be suited to rare diseases, many patients with rare diseases today have difficulty in finding providers with the expertise and resources to diagnose and treat their conditions. In addition, research progress has suffered from segmented, disorder-specific approaches to projects and their funding.

The Institute of Medicine committee was asked to examine the current state of research on health care for rare diseases and products to better prevent, diagnose, and treat the large number of these diseases. The committee also was charged to consider how the development of research and therapeutics might be fostered. This task proved to be daunting in a number of respects. Each rare disease has its particular unmet needs, and these may not even have been documented for hundreds if not thousands of extremely rare conditions. Relatively few efforts have successfully addressed scientific or technical questions across a spectrum of rare diseases. Furthermore, incentives for pharmaceutical, biotechnology, and medical device companies, starting with the Orphan Drug Act in 1983, to invest in the development of new diagnostics, therapeutics, and preventive interventions for rare diseases have had a limited impact on the gap between needs and effective responses.

As documented in this report, opportunities now exist to accelerate progress toward understanding the basis for many more rare diseases and for developing innovative medical approaches. For example, the genomic era some 20 years ago promised when it was launched to unravel the mysteries of genetic contributions to disease. Estimates that 80 percent or more of rare diseases have a genetic cause provided hope for many that solutions to their health problems might be around the corner. However, much of the initial effort to understand the genetic basis of disease was understandably focused on more common problems. It has, however, become increasingly evident that many common diseases have a very complex genetic basis that is taking much longer to map than was originally expected. Because many rare conditions stem from defects in a single gene, they offer opportunities for faster progress, especially given scientific and technological advances that identify the genetic basis of rare diseases and find molecular targets for the development of new treatments for these diseases. Thus, we are poised to make rapid advances in the understanding and, in an increasing number of cases, the treatment of rare diseases. As past research has demonstrated, some of these advances will undoubtedly illuminate disease mechanisms and treatment avenues for more common conditions.

At the same time, many obstacles still complicate efforts to accelerate rare diseases research and product development. Regulatory efforts to ensure the safety and efficacy of new products for rare diseases need attention so that they do not impose avoidable delays or apply inappropriate standards in the evaluation of products for rare conditions. Funding for research for many rare diseases has lagged and lacked coordination, and investigators interested in pursuing research on rare diseases face many obstacles related not just to the availability of funding but to the mechanisms under which research grants are awarded. Furthermore, the cost of drug development under current models and the high costs of new drugs for rare conditions raise questions about whether it is time to create alternative pathways for drug development, including public-private partnerships.

For these reasons, the committee came to the conclusion that a more coordinated national, and ideally global, effort to plan and begin systematically to implement new strategies for addressing the needs of patients with rare diseases is a timely consideration. Leadership of this planning and implementation effort, as well as mechanisms to sustain the effort over time, present formidable challenges but are not insurmountable with the commitment of patients and families, advocacy groups, policy makers, companies, investigators, and others. The committee is hopeful that its efforts will catalyze thought and action that will benefit millions of our citizens with rare diseases and thereby contribute to the overall health of the nation.

As chair of the committee, I acknowledge the strong contributions of two groups. The committee members quickly created an effective team and gave generously of their time and expertise for committee meetings, phone calls, and writing and review assignments. The Institute of Medicine staff brought together the myriad and disparate inputs and assembled them in a lengthy and complex report. The report would not have materialized without the persistent gentle prodding and guidance of our study director, Dr. Marilyn Field. Without her insistence on documentation of report elements to ensure that the report's content and presentation met the highest standards under a very ambitious time line, the multifaceted and interdependent dimensions of the committee's charge could not have been so thoughtfully addressed.

Thomas F. Boat, *Chair*
Committee on Accelerating
Rare Diseases Research and
Orphan Product Development

Contents

Boxes, Figures, and Tables

BOXES

FIGURES

TABLES

Summary

In aggregate, rare diseases affect millions of Americans of all ages and additional millions of people globally. Most of these conditions are serious and life-altering. Many are life-threatening or fatal.

Some rare conditions are extremely rare, with the number of reported cases in the single or low double digits. Others occur in hundreds, thousands, or tens of thousands of people. Many of the estimated 5,000 to 8,000 rare conditions are genetic or have a genetic component. Others arise from exposure to infectious agents or toxins and, occasionally, from adverse responses to therapeutic interventions. Although prevalence information is incomplete and often unsatisfactory and frequently consists only of case reports, it appears that the distribution of rare conditions is skewed to the rarest.

Because the number of people affected with any particular rare disease is relatively small and the number of rare diseases is so large, a host of challenges complicates the development of safe and effective drugs, biologics, and medical devices to prevent, diagnose, treat, or cure these conditions. These challenges include difficulties in attracting public and private funding for research and development, recruiting sufficient numbers of research participants for clinical studies, appropriately using clinical research designs for small populations, and securing adequate expertise at the government agencies that review rare diseases research applications or authorize the marketing of products for rare conditions.

In recent decades, scientists, advocates, policy makers, medical product companies, and others have done much to respond to these challenges. Innovative approaches to basic research are making the identification of

1

genetic causes of rare diseases easier, faster, and less expensive. Some of the same research approaches and technologies are also altering the processes and efficiency of therapeutic discovery and product development for rare conditions.

Political and social developments also have altered the environment of rare diseases research and product development. Nearly 30 years ago, Congress passed the Orphan Drug Act, which provided incentives for companies to develop drugs for rare diseases. The law defines a rare disease or condition as one affecting fewer than 200,000 people in the United States. Since 1983, the Food and Drug Administration (FDA) has approved orphan drugs for approximately 355 uses or indications, and orphan drugs account for a significant proportion of the innovative drugs recently approved by the agency. Devising effective incentives for medical device developers has been particularly difficult, but more than four dozen devices have been approved under policies to encourage the development of devices for small populations.

At the National Institutes of Health (NIH), the Office of Rare Diseases Research (ORDR) undertakes a range of activities to encourage and support research on rare conditions. The Rare Diseases Clinical Research Network funds consortia to study groups of related rare conditions. The new Therapeutics for Rare and Neglected Diseases program aims to bring promising compounds to the point of clinical testing and adoption for further development by commercial interests. In the private sector, several small pharmaceutical companies now focus on drugs for rare diseases, and some large companies are expressing increased interest in the incentives for orphan drug development.

In addition, the substantial physical, emotional, and financial impact of rare diseases on individuals and families has motivated many to join together to try to have an impact on these diseases through research that unravels their causes and yields effective therapies. An increasing number of advocacy groups not only promote and fund research but also initiate and organize research in partnership with academic researchers, industry, and government.

Notwithstanding the successes, many rare conditions still lack even a basic understanding of their cause or the mechanisms that underlie them. Effective products are now available for only a small fraction of rare diseases.

In response to the difficulties confronting rare diseases research and orphan product development, NIH with support from FDA approached the Institute of Medicine (IOM) about a study to examine the opportunities for and obstacles to the development of drugs and medical devices to treat rare diseases. They requested a report that would assess strategies and propose an integrated national policy to accelerate rare diseases research and orphan product development. Consistent with its charge, the study committee that prepared this report did not examine medical foods or dietary supplements. Although it did not investigate initiatives involving neglected tropical diseases that are rare in the United States but common in many less developed countries, it did consider the applicability of some of these initiatives to this country. The committee was not asked to examine strategies for moving scientific advances into clinical care, public health practice, and health-related personal behavior and ensuring that they actually benefit individual and public health. The challenges of doing so are many and will raise difficult questions of affordability and equitable access.

As envisioned by the committee, an integrated national strategy to promote rare diseases research and product development has several dimensions (Box S-1). Elements of each already exist but lack a coordinated focus. Collaboration and continuing evaluation, which are always challenges, are particularly difficult given the number and diversity of rare diseases and the limited and even undocumented resources devoted to them individually and collectively.

BOX S-1
Elements of an Integrated National Strategy to Accelerate Research and Product Development for Rare Diseases

- Active involvement and collaboration by a wide range of public and private interests, including government agencies, commercial companies, academic institutions and investigators, and advocacy groups

- Timely application of advances in science and technology that can make rare diseases research and product development faster, easier, and less expensive

- Creative strategies for sharing research resources and infrastructure to make good and efficient use of scarce funding, expertise, data, biological specimens, and participation in research by people with rare diseases

- Appropriate use and further development of trial design and analytic methods tailored to the special challenges of conducting research on small populations

- Reasonable rewards and incentives for private-sector innovation and prudent use of public resources for product development when the latter appears a faster or less costly way to respond to important unmet needs

- Adequate organizations and resources, including staff with expertise on rare diseases research and product development, for the public agencies that fund biomedical research and regulate drugs and medical devices

- Mechanisms for weighing priorities for rare diseases research and product development, establishing collaborative as well as organization-specific goals, and assessing progress toward these goals

REGULATION OF DRUGS AND BIOLOGICS FOR RARE DISEASES

The Orphan Drug Act and other policies provide incentives for the development of drugs and biologic products for rare diseases. The incentives include 7 years of marketing exclusivity (a period of protection from competition), tax credits for certain research expenses, exemption from certain FDA fees, and research grants. (Except for the grants program, the statute does not otherwise cover medical devices.) The marketing exclusivity provisions of the act are widely viewed as the most important incentive of the Orphan Drug Act. In common with other drugs, sponsors of orphan drugs secure approval of the product from the Center for Drug Evaluation and Research (CDER) based on "adequate and well-controlled" investigations supporting the drug's safety and efficacy. (Certain orphan biologic products are approved by the Center for Biologics Evaluation and Research.)

Criticisms of FDA procedures related to orphan drug development and approval tend to focus on three issues—insufficient resources for timely meetings and guidance for sponsors; inconsistency in reviews of applications for orphan drug approvals across CDER divisions; and inadequate resources for the orphan products grants program. In addition, it is sometimes stated that FDA inappropriately requires two phase III, randomized, placebo-controlled, double-blind trials to support orphan drug approvals. Analyses of recent approval records for orphan drugs, however, show that a substantial proportion did not require two phase III trials. Some have been approved on the basis of phase II trials, and at least one approval has been based on a small historical case series.

At the same time, agency staff have identified a number of problems with studies that sponsors have submitted. These include delayed toxicology studies; inadequate characterization of chemical compounds; lack of natural history studies to characterize the disease process; poor use of early-phase studies (e.g., safety, dosing) to guide the design of phase III studies; inadequate trial design (including lack of a formal protocol, well-defined question, adequate controls, validated biomarkers, and appropriate surrogate measures), and lack of advance communication with FDA about the adequacy of clinical trial plans. Given the scarce resources available for rare diseases research and orphan product development, it is particularly unfortunate for these resources to be used ineffectively.

The recent creation by FDA of the new position of Associate Director for Rare Diseases within CDER is a positive step; it underscores that the review of drugs and biologics intended for rare diseases requires special scientific and methodological attention and expertise. In general, this new emphasis in CDER should find reinforcement in FDA's increasing efforts to strengthen regulatory science. One broad goal should be to achieve reasonable consistency in the review of similarly situated products (e.g., products for diseases with reasonably similar prevalence and time frames or magnitudes of product effects) and to justify reasoned flexibility in expectations for differently situated products.

RECOMMENDATION 3-1: The Center for Drug Evaluation and Research should undertake an assessment of staff reviews of applications for the approval of orphan drugs to identify problems and areas for further attention, including inconsistencies across CDER divisions in the evaluations of applications that appear to present similar issues for review. Based on this assessment, CDER should

• develop guidelines for CDER reviewers to promote appropriate consistency and reasoned flexibility in the review of orphan drugs, taking into account such considerations as the prevalence of the disease, its course and severity, and the characteristics of the drug; and
• use the analysis and the review guidelines to inform the advice and formal guidance provided to sponsors on the evidence needed to support orphan drug approvals.

The proposed analysis should help CDER develop a better overall understanding of the adequacy of the evidence submitted and the appropriateness of clinical trial designs. This understanding may suggest modifications in educational programs and guidance on trial design.

RECOMMENDATION 3-2: The Center for Drug Evaluation and Research should evaluate the extent to which studies submitted in support of orphan drugs are consistent with advances in the science of small clinical trials and associated analytic methods. Based on its findings, CDER should work with others at FDA, NIH, and outside organizations and experts, as appropriate, to

• adjust and expand existing educational programs on the design and conduct of small clinical trials;
• specify which CDER and NIH personnel should complete these educational programs;
• revise guidance for sponsors on trial design and analysis and on safety and efficacy reviews of products for rare diseases; and
• support further work to develop and test clinical research and data analysis strategies for small populations.

The identification of possible problem areas in drug approval reviews may guide the efforts of FDA and NIH to work collaboratively on mechanisms to ensure that all phases of NIH-funded product development studies are designed to be consistent with the requirements for FDA approval. Provision of communications and assistance to sponsors should reduce the likelihood that the investments of sponsors, funders, and research participants will be used unproductively or even wasted.

> RECOMMENDATION 3-3: To ensure that NIH-funded product development studies involving rare diseases are designed to fulfill requirements for FDA approval, NIH and FDA should develop a procedure for NIH grantees undertaking such studies to receive assistance from appropriate CDER drug review divisions that is similar to the assistance provided to investigators who receive orphan products grants. NIH study section review of rare diseases clinical trial applications should involve reviewers who are knowledgeable about clinical trial methods for small populations. For all sponsors of drugs for rare diseases, CDER should have resources to support sufficient and adequate meetings and discussions with sponsors from the earliest stages of the development process.

The committee concluded that funding for the orphan products grants program has lagged far behind inflation and seriously undermined an important resource. An increase would allow more qualified researchers to benefit from this focused product development program.

OPPORTUNITIES TO ACCELERATE DISCOVERY RESEARCH

Basic and then therapeutic discovery research is the foundation for the development of new preventive, diagnostic, and therapeutic products for patients with rare diseases. It identifies the causes and delineates the molecular mechanisms of these diseases as a basis for discovering therapeutic targets. The basic research tools available to biomedical investigators have changed dramatically over the past 20 years, with technological advances generating new knowledge at an unprecedented pace and, often, at lower cost for a given task. Some tools hold particular promise for rare diseases research. Also promising is the growth of innovative public-private partnerships and other collaborations to bridge the gulf between basic research findings and beneficial products.

Making the best use possible of research resources calls for arrangements that make existing knowledge and resources more accessible to rare diseases researchers and that also discourage a duplicative infrastructure of, for example, natural history data, animal models of disease, biorepositories, and chemical compound libraries. Although many barriers will have to be overcome, a "rare diseases research commons" with several unlinked or loosely linked elements should yield significant benefits.

RECOMMENDATION 4-1: NIH should initiate a collaborative effort involving government, industry, academia, and voluntary organizations to develop a comprehensive system of shared resources for discovery research on rare diseases and to facilitate communication and cooperation for such research.

This research resource would include, among other features, a repository of publicly available animal models for rare disorders and a publicly accessible database that includes mechanistic biological data on rare diseases generated by investigators funded by NIH, private foundations, and industry. It would develop model arrangements and agreements (e.g., template language on intellectual property) for making relevant portions of compound libraries available to researchers investigating rare disease.

Given the important role that NIH plays in supporting rare diseases research, a comprehensive NIH action plan on rare diseases would be useful to better integrate and expand existing work and attract new resources and investigators to the field. The following recommendation spans all phases of research on rare diseases and orphan products, including research on medical devices for people with rare diseases.

RECOMMENDATION 4-2: NIH should develop a comprehensive action plan for rare diseases research that covers all institutes and centers and that also defines and integrates goals and strategies across units. This plan should cover research program planning, grant review, training, and coordination of all phases of research on rare diseases.

DEVELOPMENT OF NEW DRUGS AND BIOLOGICS FOR RARE DISEASES

Once a potential therapeutic drug or biologic has been discovered, the process of developing the therapeutic for a particular disease, whether rare or not, begins with preclinical development and continues through increasingly complex and demanding phases of clinical testing. Much of this work has traditionally been done within companies and is expensive and risky, so companies usually choose to develop therapies with the greatest promise to generate a good financial return. As a result, potential therapies for rare diseases have often languished, even with the incentives of the Orphan Drug Act.

For product development as for basic research, a stronger infrastructure is again critically important. A major need is for innovative collaborative strategies to share and leverage resources to decrease research and development costs without sacrificing product safety or efficacy. To this end, one priority is to expand resources and options at the preclinical stage of drug development.

RECOMMENDATION 5-1: NIH should create a centralized preclinical development service that is dedicated to rare diseases and available to all nonprofit entities.

An important strategy to reduce the time and costs for clinical studies of drugs for rare diseases involves the development and validation of biomarkers for use as surrogate endpoints in such studies. Validation is critical for FDA's acceptance of the use of such endpoints in studies submitted to support approval of an orphan drug.

RECOMMENDATION 5-2: In collaboration with industry, academic researchers, NIH and FDA scientists, and patient organizations, FDA should expand its Critical Path Initiative to define criteria for the evaluation of surrogate endpoints for use in trials of products for rare conditions.

The expansion and improvement of patient registries and biorepositories is another important element in a strategy to accelerate rare diseases research and product development. Today, an uncounted number of organizations and researchers in this country and around the world maintain rare diseases registries in some form, sometimes for the same condition. No uniform, accepted standards govern the collection, organization, or availability of these data. The result is sometimes wasteful duplication and sometimes underuse of information or samples contributed by patients or research participants. Although it would undoubtedly be a complicated undertaking, moving toward common standards, including protections for patients and research participants, and data sharing arrangements should help resolve many of these problems.

RECOMMENDATION 5-3: The NIH should support a collaborative public-private partnership to develop and manage a freely available platform for creating or restructuring patient registries and biorepositories for rare diseases and for sharing de-identified data. The platform should include mechanisms to create standards for data collection, specimen storage, and informed consent by patients or research participants.

The committee recognizes the value of the Rare Diseases Clinical Research Network but notes its relatively limited scope and thus its limited opportunities to take advantage of unanticipated scientific discoveries. In some cases, other NIH research networks may respond with more flexibility. These networks, however, lack a specific focus on rare diseases. Existing clinical research activities can be enhanced and expanded by a program or programs that are not strictly organized around specific disease areas but rather have the flexibility to partner with or recruit other existing networks or sites to rapidly capitalize upon research advances and achieve common and broadly defined goals in rare diseases research.

> **RECOMMENDATION 5-4: NIH should increase its capacity and flexibility to support all phases of clinical research related to rare diseases, including clinical trials of new and repurposed therapeutic agents. Opportunities to be explored include**
>
> • expanding the Rare Diseases Clinical Research Network to address opportunities for diagnostic and therapeutic advances for a greater number of rare diseases;
> • setting priorities for rare diseases research within other NIH clinical trials networks;
> • creating a study group approach to rare diseases, modeled after the Children's Oncology Group; and
> • building additional capability for rare diseases clinical research within the Clinical and Translational Science Awards program.

A new NIH program that is not restricted to rare diseases research but will likely benefit such research is the Cures Acceleration Network. This program will focus on significant unmet medical needs, particularly in areas that are not attractive to commercial interests. The network should supplement and build on the current infrastructure for rare diseases research.

> **RECOMMENDATION 5-5: NIH should establish procedures to ensure coordination of the activities of the Cures Acceleration Network with those of the Office of Rare Diseases Research, FDA's orphan products grants program, and other existing initiatives to promote and facilitate the translation of basic science discoveries into effective treatments for rare diseases. It should build on existing resources when appropriate, avoid creating duplicative research infrastructure, and engage advocacy groups in its work.**

COVERAGE AND REIMBURSEMENT

A small market is generally viewed as a disincentive for the development of pharmaceuticals. Many of the costs of developing a new drug are incurred regardless of the size of the potential market. If, however, a company can expect to set a price that is high enough to recover its costs and to generate profits because public and private health insurance plans and patients and families will pay that price, then a manufacturer may not be deterred by a small target market. Public and private health plans that cover orphan drugs generally lack leverage to negotiate prices in the absence of alternative brand-name or generic products. The most expensive orphan drugs cost more than $400,000 per year.

The committee's analysis focused on Medicare, which covers many individuals with severe, disabling rare conditions. Based on its examination of drug coverage under Medicare Part B (which covers drugs administered by physicians and outpatient facilities) and Medicare Part D (which covers prescription drugs in private plans administered according to government rules), the committee concluded that nearly all orphan drugs are, within a relatively short period following approval, covered either under Part B or by a majority of Part D plans. Part D plans often place orphan drugs in a "specialty" category of coverage that requires much higher out-of-pocket costs, and they often require prior authorization before a drug will be covered. Little is known about how such requirements are implemented and whether they may restrict access.

> **RECOMMENDATION 6-1:** The Centers for Medicare and Medicaid Services or the Medicare Payment Advisory Commission should study how the implementation of prior authorization requirements by Medicare Part D and state Medicaid plans affects beneficiary access to orphan drugs. The findings should guide recommendations and actions to improve policies and practices for the Part D program.

In addition, little is known about the application of coverage restrictions when orphan or nonorphan drugs are used off-label to treat people with rare conditions that may have few or no FDA-approved treatments. Medicare requires coverage for off-label uses that are described in certain compendia (comprehensive listings of drugs with descriptions of their recommended uses). The creation of an evidence-based compendium focused specifically on off-label uses of drugs for rare diseases could inform clinicians, health plans, and potentially patients and families. It could also suggest areas for future research or literature reviews.

> **RECOMMENDATION 6-2:** The Agency for Healthcare Research and Quality or a similar appropriate agency should undertake a pilot project to develop an evidence-based compendium to inform health plan decisions on both orphan and nonorphan drugs that may have indications for rare conditions that have not been evaluated or approved by FDA.

MEDICAL DEVICES FOR SMALL POPULATIONS

Compared to pharmaceuticals, medical devices are an extremely diverse group of products. Some are as simple as adhesive bandages and tongue depressors. Others are complex, for example, various implanted cardiac, neurological, and orthopedic devices. For rare diseases, efforts to accelerate research and development have clearly focused on drugs and biological products. Given the differing characteristics of the device development process and the device industry, the incentives designed to stimulate orphan drug development have not transferred neatly to this sector.

The law usually does not require submission of clinical data before FDA can authorize a device for marketing. However, for a small percentage of high-risk devices, manufacturers must submit a premarket approval application that includes safety and efficacy data from clinical trials. Securing FDA approval of such devices is usually complex, costly, and time-consuming, which may discourage companies from pursuing devices for small populations. Such populations also present the practical challenges of ensuring sufficient research participants for clinical trials to demonstrate safety and effectiveness.

Devising meaningful alternative incentives to encourage the development of medical devices for small populations has proved a persistent challenge. For example, because medical device companies often engage in a continuous process of product refinement and innovation, marketing exclusivity may be less important as a source of competitive advantage for device companies than for pharmaceutical and biotechnology companies.

In 1990, Congress authorized the Humanitarian Device Exemption (HDE) to encourage the development and introduction of needed device technologies for small populations. To be eligible for this exemption, a manufacturer must first have a device designated as a Humanitarian Use Device, which is a "medical device intended to benefit patients in the treatment or diagnosis of a disease or condition that affects or is manifested in fewer than 4,000 individuals in the United States per year."

An HDE application must include evidence that the device is safe but need not include evidence of effectiveness. The application must, however, contain sufficient information for FDA to judge whether the device presents an unreasonable or significant risk of illness or injury and whether its probable benefit to health outweighs the potential for harm. Sponsors of an HDE device are allowed to recover certain development costs but may not make a profit on the device. Congress recently relaxed the profit restriction for HDE devices for children.

One unique and sometimes confusing feature of the HDE policy is the requirement that use of a Humanitarian Use Device requires approval by an institutional review board (IRB). The primary responsibility of IRBs is to protect human research participants through review of proposed research.

The committee found it difficult to assess the possible extent of unmet device needs for adults with rare conditions and the extent to which changes in FDA policies might promote innovation to meet these needs. A first step in understanding the potential for device innovation for rare conditions is a needs assessment.

> **RECOMMENDATION 7-1: FDA and NIH should collaborate on an assessment of unmet device needs and priorities relevant to rare diseases. That assessment should focus on the most plausible areas of unmet need, identify impediments to meeting these needs, and examine options for overcoming impediments and stimulating high-priority innovations.**

The options examined might include the additional orphan products grants and NIH awards for the development of devices to meet priority needs; tax credits for certain research and development costs; and the creation of inducement prizes for the design and initial testing of novel devices in areas of unmet need. Changes in the HDE incentives for pediatric devices, including removal of the restriction on profits, may provide an opportunity to gauge whether similar changes could encourage innovative devices for conditions affecting small populations of adults.

> **RECOMMENDATION 7-2: Congress should consider whether the rationale for creating additional incentives for pediatric device development also supports the use of such incentives to promote the development of devices to meet the needs of adults with rare conditions.**

A modest step to encourage some additional company interest in devices for small populations would involve greater flexibility in the limits on annual shipments of HDE-covered devices. For devices covered by an HDE, information on the number of device units shipped is not readily available nor are the estimates submitted by companies of the number of affected individuals. An analysis of such data might help in assessing how often the 4,000-per-year shipment limit is approached and thus how often the limit might restrict access within the framework of HDE policy.

> **RECOMMENDATION 7-3: As a basis for possible congressional action, the Center for Devices and Radiological Health should analyze the supporting justifications offered in successful and unsuccessful Humanitarian Device Exemption applications related to the 4,000-person-per-**

year limit and should evaluate the subsequent experience with actual device shipments for approved applications, including any communications about projections that a company might exceed the limits. Taking the findings into account, Congress should consider authorizing FDA to permit a small, defined deviation from the yearly limit on shipments for a specific device when the agency determines that such a deviation would benefit patients with a rare disease.

The HDE process is generally viewed as confusing and burdensome. FDA could act, within existing law, to make the process less intimidating and potentially more attractive to device developers.

RECOMMENDATION 7-4: FDA should take steps to reduce the burdens on potential sponsors of Humanitarian Use Devices, including

• assigning an ombudsman to help sponsors navigate the regulatory process for these applications;
• providing more specific guidance and technical assistance on the documentation of the size of the patient population as required for humanitarian use designations; and
• developing better guidance (including step-by-step instructions and sample documents) for sponsors and IRBs on their roles and responsibilities related to IRB review of HDEs.

INTEGRATING STRATEGIES FOR RARE DISEASES RESEARCH AND ORPHAN PRODUCT DEVELOPMENT

An integrated national strategy for rare diseases research and orphan product development will have many elements. As outlined earlier, such a strategy will actively involve the many parties that play essential roles in the process—government, industry, academic investigators, advocacy groups, and others. In response to sometimes duplicative, competing, and uncoordinated efforts, it will promote collaboration and cooperation and the elimination of wasteful and costly duplication of research and development efforts. An integrated strategy will include an array of mechanisms at NIH and elsewhere for devising partnerships and sharing resources—including, for example, chemical compound libraries and biological specimens. An integrated strategy will also include focused investigations of possible areas of unmet needs (e.g., for medical devices). FDA will continue to play an essential role in ensuring that products are safe and effective, taking into account the special challenges of developing products for rare conditions and providing sponsor guidance and product reviews that combine reasonable consistency and reasoned flexibility based on expert knowledge.

To encourage more collaboration and more efficient use of resources and build on the initiatives and recommendations discussed in this report, the committee proposes the creation of a time-limited task force on accelerating rare diseases research and product development. Because mobilizing such a task force might be difficult in the private sector and because high-level backing is crucial, the responsibility for creating the task force should rest with the Secretary of Health and Human Services. This task force, which might operate for 4 to 8 years, would bring together leaders in rare diseases research and product development from government, industry, academic and other research institutions, and advocacy groups and would involve international entities as appropriate.

RECOMMENDATION 8-1: The Secretary of Health and Human Services should establish a national task force on accelerating rare diseases research and product development. The objectives of the task force would be to promote, coordinate, monitor, and assess the implementation of NIH, FDA, and other public- and private-sector initiatives on rare diseases and orphan products and to support additional opportunities for public-private collaboration.

A task force on rare diseases research and product development will not lessen the need for all participants to improve their individual efforts and relationships as outlined in this report. Individual improvement will strengthen the foundation for collaboration.

1

Introduction

*Nature is nowhere accustomed more openly to display her secret
mysteries than in cases where she shows tracings of her workings
apart from the beaten paths; nor is there any better way to advance
the proper practice of medicine than to give our minds to the discovery of the usual law of nature, by careful investigation of cases
of rarer forms of disease.*

William Harvey, 1657

William Harvey's observation, familiar to many who study rare diseases, is echoed today in explanations of the broader significance of research on diseases that affect small populations. For example, research
on Wilms tumor, a rare pediatric cancer, has been cited as a model for
understanding the genetics, epigenetics, and molecular biology of pediatric
cancers and cancers generally (see, e.g., Feinberg and Williams, 2003).
Studies of Tangier disease (an extremely rare condition in which a gene
associated with cholesterol processing does not function properly) have
illuminated a target for therapies to reduce the risk of heart disease and
have also provided insights into Alzheimer disease (Delude, 2009). Research
on Liddle syndrome (a rare inherited kidney disorder associated with early
and severe hypertension) has contributed to knowledge about the pathology of hypertension (Lifton et al., 2001), and studies of Fanconi anemia
have illuminated disease mechanisms of bone marrow failure, cancer, and
resistance to chemotherapy (D'Andrea, 2010). More generally, "patients
with rare genetic disorders have fueled progress in the fields of human genetics and molecular therapeutics through their enthusiastic participation

in research, often based on a remote promise of personal gain and at a very real personal expense" (Dietz, 2010, p. 862).

Delineating the general value or multiplier effect of research on specific rare diseases is important because such research may otherwise be under-valued when policy makers consider the absolute numbers of people likely to benefit from a particular public investment in research. Studies of rare diseases often meet other criteria that policy makers consider, for example, that the condition to be studied imposes a serious burden on the health and well-being of affected individuals.

Notwithstanding the label *rare disease*, most adults probably have known at least one person and possibly several people who have a rare condition. They may have grieved with a family that lost an infant to trisomy 13 or another rare chromosomal disorder. They may know a child or young adult who is living with sickle cell disease or Marfan syndrome. They may be offering support to a relative or friend who has been diagnosed with ovarian cancer or amyotrophic lateral sclerosis in mid- or late life.

Although most of the conditions just cited affect tens of thousands of Americans, each meets the definition of rare disease established in a 1984 amendment to the 1983 Orphan Drug Act (P.L. 97-414): a disease or condition that affects fewer than 200,000 people in the United States (21 USC 360bb). Less common is a large group of rare diseases that affect perhaps a few hundred to a few thousand individuals each but that are generally unknown to most people, including many physicians. In addition, the published literature includes hundreds of extremely rare conditions with reported numbers of affected individuals in the single or double digits, for example, atransferrinemia (a metabolic disorder affecting the transport of iron through the blood) (Beutler et al., 2000) and reticular dysgenesis (a severe immunodeficiency disorder) (Pannicke et al., 2009).

Various estimates place the number of rare conditions at 5,000 to 8,000, and newly identified disorders are reported almost weekly (see Chapter 2). Box 1-1 shows just a few examples of the variety of rare diseases. Most result from genetic mutations, often inherited. Others are caused by infectious or toxic agents. The cause of some is unknown.

In aggregate, rare diseases afflict millions of Americans of all ages and more millions globally. Most are serious and life-altering, and many are life-threatening or fatal. Because the number of people affected with any one specific rare disease is relatively small, a host of challenges complicates the development of effective drugs and medical devices to prevent, diagnose, treat, or cure these conditions. In recent decades, scientists, advocates, policy makers, and others have done much to try to address these challenges. Yet despite these efforts, only a small fraction of rare diseases currently have effective treatments.

BOX 1-1
Examples of Rare Diseases

Dystonia: a group of rare movement disorders that cause involuntary muscle spasms and contractions. Dystonias may be inherited, arise from other conditions (e.g., tumors, infections, stroke), or be of unknown origin. One literature review reported prevalence estimates for primary dystonia (not caused by other medical conditions) that ranged from 2 cases to 50 cases per million for early-onset primary dystonia and from 30 cases to 7,320 cases per million for late-onset primary dystonia (Defazio et al., 2004). Treatment is not curative. Depending on an individual's specific condition, options may include physical, speech, and other nonpharmaceutical therapies; oral medications; injection with botulinum toxin; and surgery, including surgery to implant a deep brain stimulation device.

Glioblastoma multiformae: a rare, highly malignant central nervous system tumor and the most aggressive type of astrocytoma (grade 4). It occurs most often in adults. The Cancer Brain Tumor Registry of the United States estimates its U.S. incidence to be 3 new cases per 100,000 population and estimates that it accounts for approximately 17 percent of all primary brain and central nervous system cancers (CBTRUS, 2010). Surgical removal of as much of the tumor as feasible followed by radiation and chemotherapy is standard treatment but is not curative (NCI, 2009a).

Holocarboxylase synthetase deficiency: an inherited disorder of the metabolism of the vitamin biotin (Wolf, 2008). If not treated, it causes neurological problems (e.g., seizures, movement disorders, intellectual disability, hearing loss), and it may be fatal. It is recommended for inclusion in newborn screening panels. One analysis estimated that newborn screening in 2006 detected 3 cases of the disorder in the United States (Therrell et al., 2008). Early and lifelong treatment with supplemental biotin can prevent symptoms, and those who have developed symptoms may show some improvement with treatment.

Nocardiosis: a rare bacterial infection that most often affects the lungs, the brain, and the skin. People with suppressed immune systems are at higher risk for the disease. The Centers for Disease Control and Prevention estimates that 500 to 1,000 new cases of the disease occur each year and that 10 percent of those with less complicated disease (e.g., uncomplicated pneumonia) may die, but fatality rates are higher for those with more severe disease (CDC, 2008b). Treatment with sulfa drugs generally must continue for several months.

Von Hippel-Lindau syndrome: a complex and variable disease that is caused by defects in a single gene that governs cell growth. It is associated with a range of tumors and cysts, including hemangioblastomas of the brain, spinal cord, and retina; renal cysts; clear cell renal cell carcinoma (the most common cause of premature death); tumors of the adrenal gland; and tumors of the inner ear (Schimke et al., 2009). Based on one study in an English district, it is estimated to affect 1 in 53,000 individuals (Maher et al., 1991). No drug has been approved specifically to treat or cure this disease. Different manifestations of the disease may be treated with surgery, radiation, chemotherapy, and symptom-directed therapies of various types.

This report describes how scientific and technological advances on many fronts—combined with supportive public policies and private initiative—offer opportunities to intensify research on the causes and mechanisms of rare diseases and to reduce the number of rare diseases with no or inadequate means of prevention or treatment. It proposes an integrated strategy for the United States to accelerate research on rare diseases and increase the options for diagnosing, treating, and preventing these diseases. Box 1-2 outlines the elements of an integrated strategy.

Components of each of these elements of an integrated strategy already exist, some more robust than others. It is, however, difficult to achieve coherence because so many participants with differing perspectives and priorities are necessarily involved. Collaboration and continuing evaluation, which are always challenges, are particularly difficult given the number and diversity of rare diseases and the limited and even undocumented resources devoted to them individually and collectively. Thus, this report proposes further steps to develop a more integrated approach to rare diseases research and product development.

BOX 1-2
Elements of an Integrated National Strategy to Accelerate Research and Product Development for Rare Diseases

- Active involvement and collaboration by a wide range of public and private interests, including government agencies, commercial companies, academic institutions and investigators, and advocacy groups

- Timely application of advances in science and technology that can make rare diseases research and product development faster, easier, and less expensive

- Creative strategies for sharing research resources and infrastructure to make good and efficient use of scarce funding, expertise, data, biological specimens, and participation in research by people with rare diseases

- Appropriate use and further development of trial design and analytic methods tailored to the special challenges of conducting research on small populations

- Reasonable rewards and incentives for private-sector innovation and prudent use of public resources for product development when the latter appears a faster or less costly way to respond to important unmet needs

- Adequate organizations and resources, including staff with expertise on rare diseases research and product development, for the public agencies that fund biomedical research and regulate drugs and medical devices

- Mechanisms for weighing priorities for rare diseases research and product development, establishing collaborative as well as organization-specific goals, and assessing progress toward these goals

---

The rest of this chapter provides an introduction to rare diseases and orphan products, including a policy overview and definitions of key terms. Chapter 2 presents a profile of rare diseases, including information about their epidemiology and causes; their prevention, diagnosis, and treatment; and their impact on individuals and families. Chapter 3 presents a brief overview of the regulation of pharmaceuticals and biological products in the United States before examining the Orphan Drug Act and other policies that establish incentives for the development of products for rare conditions. The chapter also provides summary information about drugs approved under the legislation; Appendix B provides more detailed information. Chapter 4 highlights some of the scientific and technological advances that are reshaping the study of rare diseases and the identification of promising therapies. In Chapter 5, the focus shifts to the complexities of moving from a promising therapy to an approved drug. Chapters 4 and 5 both discuss the infrastructure needed for the conduct of basic and clinical research on rare diseases and models of innovation to accelerate research and development. (Appendix E lists the consortia funded by the NIH Rare Diseases Clinical Research Network, and Appendix F presents illustrative examples of the research strategies of selected advocacy groups.)

Because the coverage and payment policies of Medicare, Medicaid, and private health plans may influence the product development decisions of pharmaceutical and biotechnology companies, Chapter 6 describes some key features of these policies. It also briefly reviews health plan coverage of certain clinical care expenses in clinical trials. (Appendix C analyzes the coverage of orphan drugs by private prescription drug plans for Medicare beneficiaries.)

The development and regulation of drugs and medical devices differ in significant respects. Chapter 7 consolidates much of the discussion of medical devices, including device regulation, incentives for the development of devices for small populations, and coverage and reimbursement. Chapter 8 recaps the elements of a more integrated approach to rare diseases research and product development and proposes a process to encourage the implementation of this approach.

OVERVIEW OF RARE DISEASES RESEARCH AND PRODUCT DEVELOPMENT: CHALLENGES AND OPPORTUNITIES

For some rare conditions, scientific progress has brought dramatic improvements in the length and quality of life for patients. The following are just a few examples.

• In the 1960s, children with cystic fibrosis faced an average life expectancy of less than 10 years; today, a cure remains elusive, but targeted treatments have helped increase average life expectancy to nearly 40 years (CFF, 2008).

- Research into the basic mechanisms of disease has laid the foundation for therapeutic advances that have transformed the lives of patients (and families) affected by such diverse conditions as phenylketonuria (an enzyme deficiency disorder) and chronic myeloid leukemia.

- Other research has contributed to progress in prevention, for example, by providing the knowledge that has allowed women to follow simple nutritional measures before and during pregnancy to reduce the incidence of birth defects such as spina bifida.

Notwithstanding the successes, many rare conditions still lack even basic understanding of the mechanisms that underlie them—much less effective treatments. In clinical practice, one of the complexities of rare diseases is that many are so rare that most physicians, even specialists, have never encountered a single patient with the condition. Diagnosis is often difficult and may take years as one diagnosis after another is considered and eventually ruled out. If an effective treatment is available, a patient with a delayed diagnosis may suffer preventable and irreparable harm.

In recent years, innovative approaches to basic research have made the identification of genetic causes of rare diseases easier, faster, and less expensive, although painstaking work may then be required to delineate how a genetic defect in combination with other factors leads to the physical or mental expressions of a disease. At the same time, the study of common conditions is subdividing many of them into smaller and smaller—even rare—molecularly defined subgroups with different therapeutic profiles and different product development requirements. These investigations offer the promise of personalized medicine with more targeted treatments, but researchers studying therapies for narrower and narrower disease subgroups of common conditions will also likely share with rare disease researchers the difficulties of conducting clinical studies on small patient populations.

Some of the same research approaches and technologies that contribute to the faster and more efficient identification of genes are also altering the processes of drug discovery and development and increasing the efficiency of procedures to identify and refine promising drug candidates to treat rare conditions. These strategies could reduce the time and cost of drug development for both common and rare conditions. Scientific advances have also revolutionized the development of medicines derived from biological sources. Such biological products are particularly prominent in treatments for a number of very rare conditions that arise from an array of different enzyme deficiencies. Advances in engineering and bioengineering are likewise contributing to the development of innovative medical devices to treat certain rare conditions. The National Institutes of Health (NIH) is allocating more resources to promote the translation of basic science discoveries into clinically significant products and is investing in sophisticated informatics and other tools to support the sharing of data, biological specimens, and other research resources.

In addition to the dramatically changing landscape of science and technology, other political and social developments have also altered the environment of rare diseases research and product development. As described further below, the Orphan Drug Act, enacted in 1983, provides incentives for companies to develop products for rare diseases. Since 1983, the Food and Drug Administration (FDA) has approved more than 350 orphan drug applications. Drugs for rare conditions accounted for more than 30 percent of the innovative drugs approved by FDA from 2004 to 2008 (Coté, 2009). NIH has created the Rare Diseases Clinical Research Network and other targeted programs of research for a number of rare diseases. Several small companies now focus on the development of drugs to treat rare diseases, and some large pharmaceutical companies are expressing increased interest in the incentives of the Orphan Drug Act. Moreover, patient advocacy groups have become increasingly active and have helped create innovative models for funding and organizing rare diseases research and product development, including various kinds of public-private partnerships as discussed in Chapter 5.

Certainly, daunting obstacles remain to continued advances in rare diseases research and product development. These obstacles range from attracting funding from public agencies for basic and translational research to securing commercial investments to develop products for very small markets. Even with funding, researchers often struggle to obtain enough biological specimens for critical preclinical studies or to identify and recruit enough research participants for clinical trials of a product's safety and efficacy. Difficulties and costs mount to the extent that a product under study has a subtle effect or one that emerges slowly. Identifying and winning acceptance of biological markers and surrogate measures of disease and treatment effects is challenging for researchers investigating common conditions and even more so when the condition is rare. Attracting trained investigators to the study of a rare disease is another challenge.

Despite the obstacles, with support from NIH, FDA, and a variety of philanthropic and industry sources, researchers are studying hundreds if not thousands of rare diseases, including some that are extremely rare. Box 1-3 highlights one example of research progress involving Hutchinson-Gilford progeria syndrome, an extremely rare condition that physicians have diagnosed in only a few dozen children worldwide. These and other examples of scientific progress with rare diseases offer encouragement and motivation for continuing efforts to bring the advances in science and technology more fully to bear on rare diseases and thereby accelerate the creation of

---

BOX 1-3
Organized Research on Exceptionally
Rare Diseases Is Possible

Hutchinson-Gilford progeria syndrome is a lethal condition caused by a mutation in a single gene. Children with the condition appear to age prematurely and
experience stiffness of joints, growth failures, hair loss, wrinkled skin, and cardiovascular disease among other problems. Most affected children die by their early
teens. In 1999, Dr. Leslie Gordon and Dr. Scott Berns, parents of a child diagnosed
with the condition, founded the Progeria Research Foundation, which has identified 54 children in 30 countries who are living with the condition. As described
by the foundation, the organization began by developing information for patients,
families, and researchers; lobbied successfully for legislation mandating that NIH
develop a research plan for progeria; organized with NIH the first workshop on the
disease in 2001; formed a consortium to identify the causal gene, which occurred
in 2002; established, also in 2002, a tissue bank and DNA repository to support
research; collaborated in the first study of the natural history of the disease beginning in 2004; and raised funds to help initiate the first clinical trial of a potential
treatment that began enrolling patients in 2007.

SOURCE: PRF, 2008.

---

knowledge that will lead to more and more effective means of prevention,
diagnosis, and treatment.

HISTORICAL AND POLICY CONTEXT

Creating Policy Incentives for Product Development

*The development of significant drugs of limited commercial value repre-
sents an activity in the public interest calling for the combined support of
government, industry, voluntary organizations, and others concerned with
health care. In our society, it should be possible to provide assistance to
small groups of patients as well as the general population, and to encourage research on medical problems of limited scope which may later have
great beneficial effect.*

Interagency Task Force, 1979, p. 1

More than 30 years ago and after years of discussion and concern, a
task force created by what is now the U.S. Department of Health and Human Services (DHHS) issued a call for action in a report on what might be
done to promote the development of drugs with limited commercial value.
Although a particular focus was drugs aimed at small groups of patients

affected by rare diseases, concern extended to drugs intended for larger populations that were, for various reasons (e.g., lack of patentability; need for long-term trials to demonstrate efficacy), not attractive development targets for pharmaceutical companies (see, e.g., Asbury, 1985). Creation of the interagency task force in 1978 came after hearings on the recommendations of a congressionally created Commission for the Control of Huntington's Disease and Its Consequences, calls for action from the Neurologic Drugs Advisory Committee of FDA, and pressure from other individuals and groups that were highlighting the barriers to the development of therapies for rare conditions and proposing government action to overcome these barriers (Asbury, 1985). (Table 1-1 highlights these and other significant events in the evolution of public policy on rare diseases and orphan products.)

The pharmaceutical industry reportedly declined to participate in the task force, but the Pharmaceutical Manufacturers Association (now the Pharmaceutical Research and Manufacturers of America) surveyed its member firms in 1978 and developed an inventory of company activities related to drugs for rare conditions (Asbury, 1985; Haffner, 1991). This survey reported that the association's member companies had marketed 34 drugs that were primarily for rare conditions. Of these, 28 targeted conditions that affected fewer than 100,000 people in the United States; 3 were for conditions affecting 100,000 to 500,000 people, and the other 3 were for conditions affecting 500,000 to 1 million people (Asbury, 1991). Of the 34 products, 24 benefited significantly from federal funding for research and development. In addition to marketed products, the survey reported another 24 experimental drugs that companies had made available to specialists treating patients with rare conditions. Other sources identified an additional 13 approved products for rare conditions that had federal agencies or academic scientists as sponsors (Asbury, 1991).

The 1979 interagency task force report proposed a voluntary program to encourage drug development by pharmaceutical companies, nonprofit organizations, or consortia. The federal government would act as a catalyst, for example, by providing some form of financial subsidy (e.g., loans, contracts, or purchase arrangements with individual companies) and by offering priority in the review of new drug approval applications. The report also mentioned the possibility of legislation creating tax and patent incentives. Although the subsidy concept was not particularly influential, the ideas for tax and patent-like incentives were featured in legislation that was adopted just a few years later.

Congressional hearings in the early 1980s focused public attention on rare diseases and laid the foundation for passage of the Orphan Drug Act. Signed into law in 1983, the legislation marked the first significant public commitment by any nation to promote the development of drugs for people with rare diseases. The legislation defined rare disease or condition to mean

TABLE 1-1 Time Line of Selected Events Relevant to Policies Promoting Research and Development for Rare Diseases and Orphan Products

Year	Event
1964	Committee of the Public Health Service examines the effect of 1962 changes to FDA drug approval requirements on the commercial availability of unpatentable drugs and drugs for rare diseases
1970s	Informal coalition of organizations focused on rare conditions promotes need for action to encourage development of drugs for these conditions
1975	Interagency federal government committee publishes an interim report that describes problems surrounding drugs of limited commercial value and recommends further study
1977	Congress creates Commission for the Control of Huntington's Disease and its Consequences, which called for more basic neurological research and product development for rare diseases
1979	Interagency Task Force on Drugs of Limited Commercial Value (created in 1978) issues its final report
1980-1982	Congress holds hearings to learn more about problems of drugs for rare diseases
1983	President signs Orphan Drug Act, which creates a range of incentives for pharmaceutical manufacturers to develop drugs for rare diseases
	National Organization for Rare Disorders, a federation of voluntary health organizations, is established by patients and families who worked together to get the Orphan Drug Act passed
	FDA approves first two orphan drugs
1984	Congress amends Orphan Drug Act to define a rare disease or condition as one that that (1) affects fewer than 200,000 persons in the United States or (2) affects "more than 200,000 persons in the United States, but for which there is no reasonable expectation that the sales of the drug treatment will recover the costs"
	Congress directs the creation of a National Commission on Orphan Diseases to assess the research activities of NIH and other public and private organizations in connection with drug development
1989	National Commission on Orphan Diseases issues report
1990	Congress passes legislation to differentiate incentives for orphan drug development depending on commercial value but the President vetoes it
	Congress passes Safe Medical Devices Act of 1990, which (among other provisions) establishes the basis for the Humanitarian Device Exemption for devices to treat or diagnose a disease or condition that affects fewer than 4,000 individuals and that meet certain other conditions
1992	Congress waives the payment of filing fees for drug and biologic product review for the sponsors of orphan drugs
1993	The Office of Rare Diseases is established within the Office of the NIH Director
1997	Congress permanently extends a tax credit of up to 50 percent for clinical research performed for designated orphan drugs and grants an exemption for

TABLE 1-1 Continued

Year	Event
	orphan drugs from the usual drug approval application fees charged by the Food and Drug Administration
2002	Rare Diseases Act and Rare Disease Orphan Product Development Act are signed into law. The former legislatively establishes the NIH Office of Rare Diseases (now the Office of Rare Diseases Research) and requires NIH to support regional centers of excellence for clinical research into, training in, and demonstration of diagnostic, prevention, control, and treatment methods for rare diseases
2003	NIH Office of Rare Diseases creates Rare Diseases Clinical Research Network beginning with seven research consortia
2007	FDA Amendments Act includes the Pediatric Medical Device Safety and Improvement Act, which provides incentives for industry and researchers to design devices for children
2008	Congress enacts the Genetic Nondiscrimination Act to prohibit discrimination in health insurance and employment based on genetic information.
2009	NIH announces Therapeutics for Rare and Neglected Diseases Program
	NIH announces expansion of Rare Diseases Clinical Research Network

SOURCES: Scheinberg and Walshe, 1986; Asbury, 1991; Haffner, 1991; Henkel, 1999; Villarreal, 2001; Iribarne, 2003; Meyers and DiPaola, 2003; Dorman, 2008; NIH, 2009a,b; Waxman, undated.

"any disease or condition which occurs so infrequently in the United States that there is no reasonable expectation that the cost of developing and making available in the United States a drug for such disease or condition will be recovered from sales in the United States of such drug" (21 USC 360bb(a)(2)). Reflecting difficulties in applying this definition to actual situations, Congress amended the law in 1984 to define a rare disease as a disease or condition that affected fewer than 200,000 people in the United States—without regard to the expected commercial value of a product to such a condition. Commercial value is, however, a consideration in a second provision that allows the law's incentives to apply to products affecting more than 200,000 people if there is no reasonable expectation that the sales of the drug will recover the costs of developing it. In regulations issued in 1992, FDA clarified that when a sponsor is seeking orphan designation for a drug to treat a subset of persons with a particular disease or condition, the sponsor must shown that the subset is medically plausible (57 FR 62076; 21 CFR 316.20(b)(6)).

As described in more detail in Chapter 3, the Orphan Drug Act and other policies provide several incentives for orphan drug development. They include

- seven years' protection from market competition for approved orphan drugs (market exclusivity);
- grants to support product development;
- tax credits for certain costs associated with clinical trials on orphan drugs;
- waiver of fees charged to those applying for FDA approval of a drug; and
- advice to product developers on the design of studies of safety and effectiveness to meet regulatory standards.

The first approvals of orphan drugs came the year the law was passed. Although the research supporting these drugs had to have been well under way or completed before 1983, the early applications for approval indicated industry's recognition of the incentives of the new law.

Also in 1983, several individuals who were active in pressing for legislation formed the National Organization for Rare Disorders (NORD). As an umbrella organization for groups supporting patients and families affected by rare conditions, NORD advocates for the identification, treatment, and cure of rare disorders through programs of education, advocacy, research, and service.[1]

In 1985 amendments to the Orphan Drug Act, Congress directed DHHS to create a new commission to take a broad look at orphan diseases. The National Commission on Orphan Diseases issued its report in 1989. It made a number of wide-ranging recommendations, including recommendations for the provision of better information for patients and physicians; increased funding of FDA product approval activities; and coverage by insurers for patients with rare diseases who are prescribed "off-label" use of drugs that were FDA approved only for nonorphan indications (NCOD, 1989). The report particularly focused on the need for expanded research on rare diseases and additional promotion of orphan product development.

The scientific context of rare diseases research and orphan product development has changed in many ways since the report was drafted. Nonetheless, the 1989 report sounds some of the same themes as this report, including the importance of public-private partnerships; mechanisms to

---

[1] Some of the groups involved in NORD's early years include the Cystinosis Foundation, Dystonia Medical Research Foundation, National Huntington's Disease Association, National Marfan Association, National Neurofibromatosis Foundation, Parkinson's Disease Foundation, Paget Disease Foundation, and Tourette Syndrome Association (Jean Campbell, Vice President of Membership Development, National Organization for Rare Disorders, December 16, 2009, personal communication). Some of these groups have since merged with similar groups or have changed their names. (Note: This report generally does not use the possessive form for eponymous disease names except when referring to organizations that use the possessive form.)

support sharing of data, biological specimens, and other resources (especially "precompetitively"); better tracking of NIH funding of rare diseases research; efforts to assure that drug development studies sponsored by NIH meet FDA criteria for marketing approval; and, generally, adequate resources and expertise to support FDA guidance for drug and device developers and review of marketing applications.

Although the 1989 report devoted relatively little attention to medical devices, it did recommend that Congress amend the Orphan Drug Act to provide incentives for the development of orphan medical devices and medical foods. As discussed in Chapter 7, developing equivalent incentives for medical devices has proved challenging, given that unlike an approved drug, a complex medical device typically is the object of ongoing refinements that make the marketing protections of the orphan drug much less meaningful as an incentive. In the Safe Medical Devices Act of 1990, Congress created the Humanitarian Device Exemption for devices to treat or diagnose a disease or condition that affects fewer than 4,000 individuals and that meet certain other conditions. This process allows FDA to approve a complex medical device based on evidence of safety and probable benefit without evidence of efficacy. This provision may reduce the time and costs required to develop evidence to support FDA approval, but an approval comes with significant restrictions, including a provision for cost recovery but not profits and limits on annual shipments of a device.

Periodically, legislators and others become concerned about reports citing the high price of some orphan drugs, including drugs that achieve blockbuster status (earning more than $1 billion a year). Several proposals have been introduced in response to such concerns. In 1990, Congress passed legislation that would have limited market exclusivity in some circumstances, but the President vetoed it (Schact and Thomas, 2009).

Promoting Research on Rare Diseases

In addition to promoting the creation of public policies to encourage industry to invest in product research and development, advocates also sought to establish a focus for rare disease research in the National Institutes of Health.[2] In 1993, the National Institutes of Health created the Office of Rare Diseases to promote research on rare conditions and help develop a more systematic strategy for such research. Congress provided statutory authorization for the office in 2002 and directed it, among other

---

[2] References to NIH in this report refer (unless otherwise specified) to all programs of the NIH, which is composed of 27 research institutes and centers. Medical research activities are supported and conducted by the Extramural Research Programs and the Intramural Research Scientific Programs, including the NIH Clinical Center hospital.

tasks, to recommend a research agenda, promote coordination within NIH, promote use of NIH resources for rare diseases research, and support the creation of a central clearinghouse of information on rare diseases. In 2000, an NIH panel produced a congressionally mandated report that led to the permanent establishment of the Office of Rare Diseases Research (ORDR) and the creation of a rare diseases clinical research initiative. By 2009, ORDR had designated as parts of a Rare Diseases Clinical Research Network nearly 20 research consortia, each involving a number of research institutions studying several related rare conditions (NIH, 2009a). (Appendix E lists the consortia and conditions.)

In addition, sometimes in coordination with ORDR but also independently, several NIH institutes fund research on rare diseases, for example, a number of rare cancers, sickle cell diseases and related blood disorders, and rare neurological disorders, such as various forms of muscular dystrophy.

The grants program of the FDA's Office of Orphan Products Development also supports clinical development of products for use in rare diseases or conditions. A number of grants have led to approved products.

Beyond DHHS, other federal agencies also have other research programs and activities that fund some research on rare conditions or orphan products. At the Department of Defense, the Congressionally Directed Medical Research Programs, which began with a directive for research on breast cancer, has also administered earmarked programs of research on other conditions, including several rare conditions—neurofibromatosis, ovarian cancer, tuberous sclerosis, and amyotrophic lateral sclerosis (CDMRP, 2008; see also Chapter 2).

Notwithstanding the visibility of the research programs of NIH, pharmaceutical, biotechnology, and medical device companies fund the major part of biomedical research in the United States (Table 1-2). Together, their spending accounted for nearly three-fifths (58 percent) of the total.

TABLE 1-2 Funding for Biomedical Research in the United States by Source, 2007

Funding Source	Spending in billions of dollars (% of total research funding)	
National Institutes of Health	27.8	(27.5)
Other federal	5.2	(5.1)
State and local government	5.2	(5.1)
Foundations, charities, and other private funds	4.3	(4.3)
Pharmaceutical firms	36.6	(36.2)
Biotechnology firms	15.3	(15.1)
Medical device firms	6.7	(6.7)
Total	101.1	(100.0)

SOURCE: Dorsey et al., 2010.

In addition to financing product development, commercial firms are almost always responsible for meeting the regulatory requirements necessary to obtain FDA approval to market drugs, biologics, and certain complex medical devices. They likewise manufacture and distribute products consistent with regulatory standards. Chapters 5 and 7 discuss the role of the private sector in product development in more depth.

Following the early initiatives of the Cystic Fibrosis Foundation and the Committee to Combat Huntington's Disease, an increasing number of patient advocacy groups have become active in research. They have helped create innovative models for funding and organizing research and product development. The emphases of advocacy groups vary, depending in part on the state of the science within different disease areas and in part on other factors that may include the number of affected individuals, the interests and skills of organizational founders and leaders, and the success of fundraising strategies. If researchers have not yet identified the genetic or other cause of a condition or delineated how the disease develops, a group may concentrate its grants and other activities on closing these gaps in knowledge.

Policies of Other Countries and International Initiatives

The policies of the United States on orphan drugs and pharmaceuticals do not exist in isolation. The United States was the earliest adopter of formal incentives for orphan drug development, but a number of other nations have followed with policies that are broadly similar, although differing in some details. The European Union has developed a common policy for its member states on some issues (e.g., length of market exclusivity period) but not all (e.g., the availability of grants). Table 1-3 summarizes selected policies.

FDA, regulatory agencies in other countries, industry, and advocacy groups have engaged in discussions to harmonize various aspects of orphan product policies (see, e.g., Wechsler, 2008). One result is that the European Medicines Agency (EMEA) and the FDA have adopted a joint application form for orphan product designation. Each agency still makes its own decisions, but the two regularly communicate about application reviews. Work to harmonize views on what constitutes acceptable clinical trial design and analytic strategies is particularly important when patient populations are small, multi-nation studies are essential, and confirmatory trials are difficult or impossible.

TABLE 1-3 Comparison of Selected National Policy Incentives for Orphan Drug Development

	United States	Japan	Australia	European Union (EU)
Original policy (date)	Legislation (1983)	Regulation (1993)	Regulation (1997)	Regulation (2000)
Years of market exclusivity	7	10	5 (same as for other drugs)	10
Grants program	Yes	Yes	No	Not at EU level
Tax credits for clinical research	Yes (50% for clinical costs)	Yes (6% of both clinical/ nonclinical costs)	No	Not at EU level (managed by member states)
Assistance with trial design	Yes	Yes	Yes	Yes (partial)
Application fee waivers	Yes	No	Yes	Reduced fees

SOURCES: Rinaldi, 2005; Shah, 2006; EMEA, 2007; Haffner et al., 2008; Villa et al., 2008.

STUDY ORIGINS AND FOCUS

This Institute of Medicine (IOM) study grew out of discussions with the NIH Office of Rare Diseases Research and the FDA Office of Orphan Products Development about opportunities to accelerate rare diseases research and orphan product development. As discussions progressed, the focus expanded from drugs and biologics to include medical devices. In 2009, the IOM appointed a 14-person committee to oversee the study. Consistent with its charge (which is presented in full in Appendix A), the committee

- examined the epidemiology, impact, and treatment of rare diseases as context for an assessment of research and development;
- investigated the strengths and limitations of the current development pathways for new drugs, medical devices, and biologics for rare diseases;
- assessed public policies that may influence research and development decisions involving rare diseases and orphan products; and
- developed recommendations for an integrated national policy on rare diseases research and orphan product development.

This report presents the committee's conclusions and recommendations.

It is written for a broad and diverse audience, including public officials in research and regulatory agencies; advocacy and philanthropic groups that support rare diseases research and orphan product development; companies that develop pharmaceutical, medical device, and biologic products; academic medical centers, research institutes, and researchers engaged in basic and clinical research; and the interested general public.

In developing its conclusions and recommendations, the committee reviewed the literature on rare diseases and orphan product development and also examined the broader literature on scientific and policy issues related to medical product discovery and development. The literature review was complicated by both the very large number of diseases categorized as rare and the limited base of knowledge about most of these conditions. The committee also solicited information and perspectives from a range of individuals and organizations, including voluntary organizations that promote research on specific conditions or rare conditions more generally, companies that develop drugs and medical devices, and researchers engaged in various aspects of basic, translational, and clinical research. (Committee activities are summarized in Appendix A.)

Given the very broad scope of its task, the committee did not investigate international strategies to promote research and product development for diseases that are rare in the United States but common in less developed countries. Thus, this report does not examine in depth the various initiatives related to neglected tropical diseases such as Chagas disease, onchocerciasis (river blindness), and trypanosomiasis or sleeping sickness.

In addition, some issues were outside the committee's task, for example, research and development related to medical foods.[3] Also, consistent with its statement of task, the committee largely limited its investigations to rare diseases research and orphan product development *through the stage of FDA approval* of a product for marketing. Many products for rare diseases are approved with requirements for postmarket studies, but the committee did not examine the conduct, outcomes, or FDA review of these studies. It also did not review health services research on the translation of research findings and achievements into clinical practice.

Notwithstanding its focus on research and development, the committee recognized the crucial importance of applying preventive, diagnostic, and therapeutic advances in clinical care, public health practice, and personal behavior. Without this further effort, scientific advances will not benefit

---

[3] FDA says that to be considered a medical food, a product generally "must, at a minimum, meet the following criteria: the product must be a food for oral or tube feeding; the product must be labeled for the dietary management of a specific medical disorder, disease, or condition for which there are distinctive nutritional requirements; and the product must be intended to be used under medical supervision" (CFSAN, 2007). FDA does not review or approve medical foods before they are marketed.

individual and public health. Also, it is often in clinical practice that the limitations of products are revealed when drugs or devices that were studied under highly controlled conditions with carefully selected populations are used in real-world conditions with broader populations.

CONCEPTS AND DEFINITIONS

This section discusses a number of key concepts and definitions. Appendix D includes a glossary that defines additional terms.

Disease, Condition, and Disorder

Consistent with the preamble of the Orphan Drug Act, this report generally uses the terms *disease, condition, and disorder* interchangeably. The term condition is useful in describing injuries and entities such as hemochromatosis and sickle cell trait that do not cause symptoms or distress in the majority of people who have them.

Defining and Tabulating Rare Diseases

This report follows the statutory definition of a *rare disease or condition* as one that affects fewer than 200,000 people in the United States. As is true of many qualitative descriptions or definitions of magnitude, any operational definition of a term such as "rare" is subjective. That subjectivity is reflected in the variations in definitions adopted by different national policymakers as shown in Table 1-4. Some definitions specify absolute numbers of affected people whereas others specify rates. Japan and, in particular, Australia define "rare" more conservatively than the United States or the European Union. In contrast to the policy of the European Union, the U.S. definition does not specify that a disease condition must be chronically debilitating or life-threatening. In general, however, the committee found that public programs and industry activities tended to concentrate on serious conditions.

Because the U.S. figure as defined in 1984 amendments to the Orphan Product Act is an absolute number—200,000—and because the U.S. population has grown since 1984, the prevalence threshold expressed as a rate has dropped in the United States from 85 per 100,000 population in 1984 to 66 per 100,000 population in 2008. It is thus coming nearer to the European rate of 50/100,000. If the legislative definition of rare disease had been expressed as the 1984 rate, a rare disease could have affected nearly 258,000 people in the United States as of 2008.

Overall, the committee views the choice of a number rather than a rate to be reasonable. It is consistent with the rationale that conditions affecting

TABLE 1-4 Prevalence Criteria for the Definition of Rare Disease in Selected Countries

Country	Prevalence Criterion	Prevalence Expressed as Rate for Year of Policy Adoption
United States	200,000 people	1984: 85/100,000 2008: 66/100,000
Australia	2,000 people	1998: 11/100,000 2008: 9/100,000
European Union	5/10,000 population (~250,000 people, 27 EU nations)	[Not applicable]
Japan	50,000 people	1993: 40/100,000 2008: 39/100,000

SOURCES: For policies, United States: Orphan Drug Act of 1983; European Union: Regulation (EC) No. 141/2000; Australia: Therapeutic Goods Act of 1989; Japan: Pharmaceutical Affairs Law (JPMA, 2008). For population data: Library of Congress (U.S.), 1994; U.S. Census Bureau, 2001, 2009; Australian Bureau of Statistics, 2008; Statistics Bureau (Japan), 2008; Eurostat, 2010.

small numbers of people may create particular problems for research and product development that may require special responses, including incentives of the kind adopted by Congress in 1983.

Estimates of the number of rare diseases in the United States and Europe range from approximately 5,000 conditions to approximately 8,000 (see, e.g., European Commission, 2007; FDA, 2009c; NIH, 2009a). The Office of Rare Diseases Research at the National Institutes of Health includes more than 6,800 conditions in its list of rare diseases, which is available online (http://rarediseases.info.nih.gov/RareDiseaseList.aspx?PageID=1). The preface to the list states that it is based on "either (1) terms for which information requests have been made to the Office of Rare Diseases Research, the Genetic and Rare Diseases Information Center, or the National Human Genome Research Institute; or (2) diseases that have been suggested as being rare." It acknowledges that inclusion in the list does not guarantee that a condition is rare.

A European organization, Orphanet,[4] has been working more system-

---

[4] On its website, Orphanet describes its mission as follows: "Orphanet is a database of information on rare diseases and orphan drugs for all publics. Its aim is to contribute to the improvement of the diagnosis, care and treatment of patients with rare diseases. Orphanet includes a Professional Encyclopaedia, which is expert-authored and peer-reviewed, a Patient Encyclopaedia and a Directory of Expert Services. This Directory includes information on relevant clinics, clinical laboratories, research activities and patient organisations" (Orphanet, undateda).

atically to identify and classify rare conditions along several dimensions. These include prevalence, age at onset, pattern of inheritance, prevalence, clinical category (e.g., neurological), and identifier in the Online Mendelian Inheritance in Man (OMIM) database.

Although the committee concluded that the Orphanet database was not yet sufficiently developed to use for a comprehensive quantitative categorization of rare diseases, it proved a useful resource (see Chapter 2). The OMIM database, which is not limited to rare conditions, likewise was a useful resource that the committee consulted for its relatively extensive summaries of information on a great many rare diseases.[5] The committee also consulted the *NORD Guide to Rare Disorders* (NORD, 2003), which summarizes information (e.g., differential diagnosis, signs and symptoms, etiology/epidemiology, and treatment) on 800 conditions. The emphasis in the guide is on conditions that are not adequately described in medical texts or are frequently misdiagnosed.[6]

The NIH and the Orphanet lists of rare diseases are similar but not entirely consistent. For example, the latter includes familial breast cancer, whereas the NIH list does not. Conversely, only the NIH list includes inflammatory breast cancer and childhood breast cancer. The discussion at the Orphanet website observes that "whether a single pattern is considered unique depends on the state of our knowledge, on the accuracy of clinical and investigative analysis and on the way we choose to classify diseases in general" (Orphanet, undatedb). Factors that are likely to contribute to inconsistencies in the two lists include differences in

- prevalence thresholds for labeling a condition as rare in the United States compared to the European Union (see Table 1.3 above);
- actual frequency of certain conditions in the United States compared to Europe;
- decisions about listing subsets of common conditions that are defined by clinical features such as age, magnitude of an anatomical defect, or injury or failures to respond to conventional treatment;

---

[5] OMIM is a catalog of human genes and genetic disorders that emphasizes inherited conditions. For a particular genetic disorder, it will summarize and cite literature about the clinical features of a genetic disorder, its diagnosis, and its pattern of inheritance, molecular genetics, prevalence data, and other features.

[6] NORD also has an online index of more than 1,100 conditions on which it has reports for sale. Some of the conditions, for example, sleep apnea and tinnitus, are not rare.

- names used for the same condition;[7] and
- criteria and procedures for tracking and evaluating newly identified
conditions or other information and for reviewing and updating lists.

When newly reported syndromes or genetic anomalies should be categorized as a rare disease is, to some degree, a matter of judgment as is the determination that certain genetic or other variations within a common condition warrant designation as a rare disease. Reports of new diseases

---

[7] One useful feature of the OMIM and Orphanet listings is that they include alternative names for conditions—although they may differ in the alternatives offered. For example, for familial Mediterranean fever, the OMIM entry lists "polyserositis, recurrent" and "polyserositis, familial paroxysmal" whereas the alternative in the Orphanet entry is "periodic disease."

BOX 1-4
Examples of Ongoing Reporting of New Rare
Syndromes in Orphanet Newsletter

Combined immunodeficiency, facial dysmorphism, optic nerve atrophy, skeletal anomalies and developmental delay: Combined immunodeficiency can be isolated or associated with abnormalities affecting other organs, mainly the skeletal and neurological systems The authors report a new syndrome in sisters born to consanguineous parents, presenting with combined immunodeficiency, facial dysmorphism, developmental delay, optic atrophy, myoclonic seizures, and skeletal anomalies.

Spinocerebellar ataxia type 31: a new disease form associated with inserted penta-nucleotide repeats containing (TGGAA)n. The authors describe a new spinocerebellar ataxia disease entity. Spinocerebellar ataxia type 31 is an adult-onset autosomal-dominant neurodegenerative disorder showing progressive cerebellar ataxia mainly affecting Purkinje cells and caused by the insertion of a microsatellite sequence (TGGAA)n between the genes TK2 and BEAN.

Confetti-like macular atrophy: a new entity. The authors describe two female patients with diffuse, hypopigmented, atrophic, shiny macules on the upper limbs and upper trunk. Histopathological examination revealed an atrophic epidermis with disorganised, hyalinised and coarse collagen bundles in the middle and lower dermis. Elastic fiber loss and fragmentation were detected. Histopathological findings in these cases showed features of both atrophoderma and anetoderma. These two cases are interesting because they may represent a clinicopathological entity which has not been described before.

SOURCE: Orphanet November 2009 newsletter.

BOX 1-5
Rare by Genotype or Rare by Phenotype:
The Example of Hemochromatosis

Hemochromatosis is a disorder of iron metabolism. In 2001, analysts estimated that 718,000 individuals in the United States were homozygous for the C282Y mutation, which is associated with an estimated 50 percent to 100 percent of hereditary hemochromatosis in the U.S. population of European descent (Steinberg et al., 2001 based on sample data from 1992-1994). According to a Centers for Disease Control and Prevention (CDC) review (2007b), estimates of the percentage of homozygous individuals who have clinically defined disease range from less than 1 percent to 50 percent. Depending on how this range of estimates is evaluated and whether genotype or phenotype is stressed, people in this group might or might not be counted as having a rare disease. For example, if about 27 percent or less of the homozygous group, in fact, has clinically evident disease, then the number of people affected using this categorization would fall under the 200,000 person threshold specified in Orphan Drug Act.

and syndromes are frequent. In 2009, the monthly Orphanet newsletters announced 48 newly reported syndromes, most of which involved very small numbers of individuals (see Box 1-4 for examples).

Another complexity in categorizing a condition as rare involves conditions that are common when defined by genotype (the number of people who have a genetic mutation) but not common if defined by phenotype (the number of people who have clinically evident disease as determined by symptoms and tests). Box 1-5 summarizes the issue as presented by hemochromatosis, a disorder of iron metabolism. Classic hemochromatosis is not listed among rare diseases by ORDR. Orphanet lists the condition but describes the major form as not rare based on genotype alone.

Medical Products, Drugs, Biologics, Medical Devices, Orphan Products

This report uses the term *medical product* to cover drugs, biologic products, and medical devices. The legal definition of *drugs* includes products "intended for use in the diagnosis, cure, mitigation, treatment, or prevention of disease" and (except for foods) "intended to affect the structure or any function of the body of man or other animals" (21 USC 321(g)(1)). FDA includes *biological products* in this definition, although drugs are chemically based and biologics are derived from natural sources such as human cells or microorganisms (see Chapter 3 and Appendix D for fuller definitions). A *medical device* is a product that is intended for diagnostic, preventive, or therapeutic use that does not achieve its primary effect through chemical action on the body or through metabolic processes (see the more detailed legal definition in Chapter 7 and Appendix D).

As defined by statute, *orphan drugs* are, in general, medicines (including biological products) intended for people with rare diseases, that is, diseases affecting fewer than 200,000 people in the United States. If, however, the drug is a vaccine, diagnostic drug, or preventive drug, then orphan designation is possible if the drug would be administered in the United States to fewer than 200,000 per year. Moreover, if it is to treat a disease that affects a larger number of people, then a drug may be still designated as an orphan in certain situations in which there is no reasonable expectation that costs of research and development of the drug for a particular medical indication can be recovered by sales in the United States.

No law creates a category of orphan medical devices, but policymakers have created some incentives to encourage the development of devices for small populations with unmet needs. For example, clinical studies involving medical devices are eligible for the research grants program created by the Orphan Drug Act. Devices targeted by these incentives may be included under the general label of *orphan medical products* or *orphan products*.

Drugs, including orphan drugs, are designated and approved for specific indications. An *indication* describes a particular use of a drug or device. That use may involve a disease generally. The approved indication may also be limited to a medically plausible subset of people with a disease or condition, for example, those with advanced disease that is not responsive to commonly used treatments. As a case in point, FDA recently approved collagenase clostridium histolyticum (Xiaflex) for treatment of advanced Dupuytren contracture, a condition that can severely limit hand functioning (Rosebraugh, 2010). Physicians may legally use drugs *off-label* for unapproved indications, but companies may not promote such uses.

Neglected Diseases

As noted above, the committee did not examine research and drug development for diseases that are rare in the United States and other wealthy countries but common in many developing nations. The term *neglected disease* is applied, in particular, to certain tropical infections that are overwhelmingly concentrated in the world's poorest countries and that still lack adequate incentives for drug development or mechanisms to make existing treatments available. Examples include

• leishmaniases, a parasitic disease that has several forms (most commonly affecting the skin or the internal organs). It is estimated to infect an estimated 12 million people worldwide (WHO, 2009b) but is reported only occasionally in the United States in people who are thought to have acquired the disease outside the country (CDC, 2008a);

• dengue fever, which is caused by one of four viruses transmitted by mosquitoes, is rare in the continental United States (and generally is acquired during travel elsewhere). It has emerged as a significant health concern in the past half century and now affects an estimated 50 to 100 million people each year worldwide (CDC, 2009a); and

• schistosomiasis, a multi-organ disease caused by parasitic worms that infects approximately 200 million people worldwide but is not present in the United States (CDC, 2008c).

For some diseases such as tuberculosis and malaria, cost and other factors have limited the use of existing treatments and preventive strategies in poor countries.[8] Beyond humanitarian considerations, the increase in drug-resistant strains of infectious diseases that are now rare in developed countries has added to interest in the development of innovative preventive and therapeutic approaches to such diseases.

Research and Product Development

Broadly defined, *basic research* in medicine involves systematic study intended to build fundamental knowledge and understanding of the biological mechanisms and processes that underlie illness and health. Its practical applications are often unanticipated, although studies such as those to identify the genes that cause disease and the ways in which they do so are generally undertaken with the hope that success will provide the foundation for further research to develop means of preventing, diagnosing, or treating the disease.

Translational research has been variously defined (see, e.g., Woolf, 2008). This report generally follows the description developed by the IOM Clinical Research Roundtable, which distinguished two arenas of translational research (Sung et al., 2003). The first, which is the focus of this report, involves "the transfer of new understandings of disease mechanisms gained in the laboratory into the development of new methods for diagnosis, therapy, and prevention and their first testing in humans" (p. 1279). Such research aims to traverse what is sometimes called the "valley of death," an

---

[8] The United States saw approximately 12,900 new cases of tuberculosis reported in 2008 (CDC, 2009b), but more than 9.25 million new active cases were estimated worldwide in 2007 (WHO, 2009a). Approximately 1,500 new cases of malaria were reported in the United States in 2002 with a worldwide estimate of 350 million to 500 million new and previously diagnosed cases (CDC, 2007b). Tuberculosis and malaria are the subjects of substantial international research and development investments to improve treatments, and related initiatives seek to make treatments affordable for poor countries and individuals.

allusion to the shortfall in the applied research and support activities (e.g., establishing collaborations with industry, attending to intellectual property issues, and planning for FDA requirements) that is necessary to achieve this movement. The second area of translational research involves "the translation of results from clinical studies into everyday clinical practice and health decision making" (p. 1279), which is essential if patients, families, and society are to benefit.

Clinical research involves studies with humans. Chapter 5 discusses the stages of clinical research from the earliest human studies of safety and drug dosing through the usually complex investigations of safety and efficacy that are used to support FDA approval of a product.

Four stages or phases of *clinical research* are typically distinguished (Box 1-6). The focus initially is on establishing safety and then extends to include effectiveness (see, e.g., CDER, 1998). As discussed in Chapters 3 and 5, studies involving products to treat rare diseases often differ from

---

BOX 1-6
Types of Clinical Trials

Phase I trials initiate the study of candidate drugs in humans. Such trials typically assess the safety and tolerability of a drug, routes of administration and safe dose ranges, and the way the body processes the drug (e.g., how it is absorbed, distributed, metabolized, and excreted). They usually involve less than 100 individuals, often healthy volunteers.

Phase II trials continue the assessment of a drug's safety and dosing but also begin to test efficacy in people with the target disease. These studies may include a range of controls on potential bias, including use of a control group that receives standard treatment or a placebo, the random assignment of research participants to the experimental and control groups, and the concealment (blinding) from participants and researchers of a participant's assignment.

Phase III trials are expanded investigations of safety and efficacy that are intended to allow a fuller assessment of a drug's benefits and harms and to provide information sufficient to prepare labeling or instructions for the use of the drug. These studies may involve thousands of research participants and multiple sites.

Phase IV studies occur after a product is approved for marketing and are highly variable in their design. They are sometimes required by FDA but may be voluntarily undertaken by manufacturers. They are typically intended to provide further information about outcomes in clinical practice, e.g., in broader populations or over longer periods than studied in the trials used to support FDA approval.

studies that are typical for common diseases (e.g., by involving many fewer research participants).

The biomedical research enterprise overlaps with many aspects of medical *product development*. However, the latter typically is viewed as building on the discoveries of basic research and focusing on the preclinical and clinical studies necessary to demonstrate safety and efficacy as required for FDA to authorize the marketing of drugs and certain medical devices. The phrase *research and development* is commonly used for this spectrum of activity, which is usually undertaken by commercial firms.

Efficacy and Effectiveness

The achievement of desired results in controlled clinical studies (*efficacy*) is not the same as the achievement of desired results in actual clinical practice (*effectiveness*). After a product enters clinical use, problems may emerge that were not evident in clinical testing. Although FDA statutes and regulations use the term effectiveness to describe positive results reported in clinical trials, FDA review documents often employ the term efficacy rather than effectiveness in discussing clinical data used in approving a new drug.

When it approves a drug or medical device for marketing, FDA may require the sponsor to undertake postmarketing studies to provide additional evidence of safety or effectiveness or both. This report focuses on research to demonstrate safety and efficacy through the stage of clinical testing prior to FDA approval of a product.

2

Profile of Rare Diseases

After going from doctor to doctor, I tried to think of how the doctors must have felt. . . . This is what I think: "This woman is presenting this odd disease [lymphangioleiomyomatosis] that no one knows how to treat, obviously no cure for, and she and her husband are sitting here looking at me all moon-eyed desperate for help with this dilemma they have been blind-sided with. What am I to do? . . . There simply are no set standards for this, I'm as helpless as she is, yet she has come to me asking for my help."

Nutt, 2007

To have a rare disease is often to have a condition that goes undiagnosed for years while concerned physicians who have never seen the condition before may offer one diagnosis and then search for another when new or advancing symptoms belie the original diagnosis. Once accurately diagnosed, patients with rare conditions may be treated by physicians who have little evidence or guidance to help them—physicians who may experience the frustration imagined by the patient quoted above. Particularly when a condition is extremely rare, patients and families frequently have to travel long distances to consult with the few experts who have experience in treating and studying their rare diseases; patients and their families may even relocate to make access easier. Although the features of specific rare diseases can differ in myriad ways, the effects on life and functioning are often similar and are emotionally and financially devastating for the affected individuals and their families. Patients and family members may feel isolated and alone as they face the challenges of finding helpful information, learning a new medical language, and generally charting their way in a daunting new world.

As described in Chapter 1, some rare conditions are extremely rare, found in only a few or a few dozen people. Others occur in hundreds, thousands, or as many as 200,000 people in the United States. Many are genetic in origin or have a genetic component. Others arise from exposure to infections or toxins, from faulty immune responses, or occasionally from adverse responses to therapeutic interventions for other conditions. For many rare conditions, the causes are frustratingly elusive.

Although people may think of a rare disease as something that happens to someone else, rare diseases can afflict anyone, at any age. They can be acute or chronic. Many are debilitating and present an ongoing risk of death. Some are inevitably fatal given current medical options. Approved therapies are available to treat several hundred of these conditions, but most currently have no therapy that cures or modifies the disease itself.

For the rarest conditions, the literature may consist of a single published report describing a few individuals with a previously unidentified genetic syndrome. For other conditions, including a number of the relatively more common conditions such as cystic fibrosis, sickle cell disease, and some cancers, publicly and privately sponsored research has generated a knowledge base that may encompass epidemiology (including natural history studies), genetics, disease mechanisms, diagnostic tests and standards, biomarkers and outcome measures, effective treatments, and evidence-based guidelines for clinical services.

Faced with these realities, many patients and families turn to advocacy groups concerned with specific diseases or to umbrella organizations such as the National Organization for Rare Disorders (NORD) and the Genetic Alliance for support and for information about their condition and available resources. As discussed at the end of this chapter, they may also join together to create new organizations.

This chapter begins with a general overview of what is known about the epidemiology of rare diseases based on data and analyses from the United States and Europe. Epidemiologic studies can provide clues and directions for basic and clinical research to determine the causes and mechanisms of rare diseases and develop methods to prevent, diagnose, and treat these conditions. Subsequent sections of this chapter discuss the varied causes of rare diseases and examine in broad terms the range of available preventive, diagnostic, and treatment strategies for diverse rare diseases. The last section considers the impact of a rare condition on patients, families, and the broader community and recognizes the efforts by patients, families, and advocacy groups to try, in turn, to have an impact on the disease and those affected by it. Reflecting the large number of rare diseases, their great variability, and the scarcity of systematic information about the spectrum of rare diseases collectively, the chapter makes frequent use of examples.

EPIDEMIOLOGY OF RARE DISEASES

Defining and counting rare diseases is not straightforward. Difficulties in obtaining definitive diagnoses contribute, as do limitations in systems for reporting and tracking such diagnoses. In addition, as described in Chapter 1, countries have adopted different definitions of a rare disease, and researchers are continuously identifying new diseases or disease variants. Therefore, the epidemiology of rare diseases—including the determination of prevalence (the number of people affected at any one time), incidence (the number of new cases in a given year), and patterns of disease (e.g., age distribution) in the population—is inexact.

Moreover, some conditions that initially are classified as rare eventually outgrow that categorization. For example, when AIDS emerged in the United States, it fit the legislative definition of a rare disease—affecting fewer than 200,000 individuals. As the infection spread, as diagnostic capabilities and data collection systems improved, and as researchers developed effective treatments that reduced mortality without curing the disease, the total number of individuals with AIDS grew to nearly 470,000 by 2007 and the number of individuals with HIV infection exceeded 1.1 million (CDC, 2009c).[1]

If effective but not curative treatment can turn a rare disease into a common one, effective prevention can, conversely, turn a common condition into a rare disease. This is the case with many once common childhood infections such as mumps and measles. Public health officials are concerned, however, that factors such as the development of drug-resistant infectious agents and the opposition of some parents to childhood vaccinations could reverse the situation for some now rare diseases. The former concern—drug resistance—is partly a significant scientific challenge (i.e., developing new anti-infectives) and partly a public health and clinical practice challenge (i.e., discouraging overuse of antibiotics). Preventing negative health consequences from anti-vaccination sentiment involves public health expertise, social science research, clinician communication skills, and public policy responses.

---

[1] Under the Orphan Drug Act as described in Chapters 1 and 3, once a drug is designated as an orphan and undergoes further development, it then can be approved and qualify for 7 years of marketing protection even if the prevalence of the disease or condition at the time of approval exceeds the rare disease threshold.

Objectives, Types, and Uses of Epidemiologic Studies of Rare Diseases

The objectives of epidemiologic research in rare diseases include determining the extent, distribution, and burden of these diseases at the population level and helping identify factors that may cause or contribute to their development. Basic epidemiologic studies generate estimates of incidence and prevalence. For congenital disorders, the statistic often reported is the proportion of births (e.g., 1 in 5,000) affected by the condition. Estimates may include breakdowns by age, gender, race or ethnicity, place of residence, and other factors that may offer clues to causation for further investigation.

Epidemiologic data have a variety of policy uses, including providing the prevalence data to support an "orphan" designation for an investigational or already approved drug. Companies seeking this designation must provide the Food and Drug Administration (FDA) with documentation that the proposed indication or use for the drug involves fewer than 200,000 people in the United States.[2] For manufacturers seeking a Humanitarian Device Exemption, the FDA must document that the device is intended to treat or diagnose a disease or condition that affects fewer than 4,000 people in the United States per year.

Policy makers may also consider epidemiologic information on prevalence and disease burden—in combination with scientific, political, economic, ethical, and other factors—in making decisions about the allocation of resources for biomedical research. Decisions about research spending, for example, sometimes favor the relatively more common rare conditions such as ovarian cancer, neurofibromatosis, and sickle cell disease, but decision makers also have directed resources to extremely rare diseases, consistent with the value judgments underlying the adoption of special policies to encourage research on rare diseases. (See the analysis of National Institutes of Health [NIH] funding in Chapter 4.)

Natural history studies are another pillar of epidemiologic research on rare conditions. These studies track the course of a disease over time, identifying demographic, genetic, environmental, and other variables that correlate with its development and outcomes in the absence of treatment. Natural history studies have also generated important information about clinical (phenotypic) variation and have helped to identify subtypes of rare disorders that may be produced by different genes or by epigenetic factors that influence the effects of a gene. Such longitudinal studies are often a high priority for a rare disease organization or others interested in a poorly

---

[2] Rarely, as discussed in Chapter 3, a sponsor will ask for designation based on another option provided by the Orphan Drug Act: that a condition affects more than 200,000 in the United States but there is no reasonable expectation that the cost of developing a drug for that condition will be recovered from sales in the United States.

understood condition. Longitudinal studies of various sorts may also illuminate treatment effects.

Although natural history studies are not the primary focus of government- or industry-funded research, NIH and pharmaceutical companies as well as other entities do sponsor natural history studies of varying scope and complexity.[3] For example, members of the NIH Rare Diseases Clinical Research Network (see Chapter 5 and Appendix E) are undertaking such studies for a number of rare conditions, including several neurological disorders and several forms of vasculitis. Understanding the natural history of a disease is an important step in the development of therapies. As discussed in Chapter 3, FDA staff have identified the lack of such studies as a problem with some applications for approval of orphan drugs.

In 2008, participants in a workshop sponsored by the National Heart, Lung, and Blood Institute and the Office of Rare Diseases Research at the NIH discussed models for analyzing genotype-phenotype associations in rare diseases and made recommendations for more longitudinal studies and also for refinements in study protocols and better tools to evaluate the resulting data (NHLBI, 2008a). It is too early to judge whether these recommendations will yield more high-quality proposals, an improved infrastructure, and more funding for such studies, which are challenging even for common conditions. Recommendations in Chapters 4 and 5 address problems with tissue banking practices and arrangements that limit or complicate their use for natural history and other studies.

Many epidemiologic data for rare diseases come from studies of single diseases. These studies are sponsored by a multitude of different sources and employ a range of methods and data. Data for prevalence or incidence calculations may come from birth certificates or death certificates; hospital discharge, insurance claims, and other administrative databases; patient registries; special surveillance studies; and newborn and other screening programs.

National data collection programs tend to focus on more common conditions, but information about the prevalence and incidence of some

---

[3] For example, a search of the database ClinicalTrials.gov yielded 50 studies using the search term "natural history study" and 1,613 studies using the term "natural history." Among the NIH-supported natural history studies that involved rare conditions were studies of sickle cell disease (NCT00081523), neurofibromatosis type I (NCT00924196), hereditary hemorrhagic telangiectasia (NCT00004649), Rett syndrome (NCT00299312), stiff person syndrome (NCT00030940), Smith-Magenis syndrome (NCT00013559), and acromegaly (NCT00001981). The last cited study began in 1985 and continues. Examples of pharmaceutical company-funded studies include metachromatic leukodystrophy (NCT00639132, Shire); mucopolysaccharidosis I (NCT00144794, Genzyme); and infantile globoid cell leukodystrophy (NCT00983879, Zymenex A/S). (The numbers in parentheses are identifiers used for the ClinicalTrials.gov database, which was developed by NIH and FDA.)

rare conditions is generated through systematic disease tracking systems.[4] The Surveillance, Epidemiology and End Results (SEER) program of the National Cancer Institute (NCI) collects data on a number of cancers, including some that are relatively uncommon. At the Centers for Disease Control and Prevention (CDC), programs on infectious diseases and birth defects track and report data on several rare conditions. The Agency for Toxic Substances and Disease Registry (ATSDR) tracks data on exposures to toxic substances with a focus on hazardous waste sites. The American Association of Poison Control Centers aggregates surveillance data from regional poison control centers, which report information on a broad range of poisonings, including those resulting from prescription and over-the-counter drugs, household products, and insect bites.

As newborn screening programs become more consistent in the United States, they may provide firmer data on the birth incidence of a number of genetic conditions. Work is continuing to develop a standard framework for reporting the results of newborn screening tests as part of electronic health records and also for analysis of trends by public health agencies (see description at http://newbornscreeningcodes.nlm.nih.gov).

For many rare conditions, one difficulty confronting epidemiologic studies involves the lack of condition-specific codes in the World Health Organization's (WHO) International Classification of Diseases (ICD). The ICD provides the international standard diagnostic classification that is used for epidemiologic studies as well as for key health system management functions. To cite an example of the problem with lack of specific codes, a single ICD code (E75.2) covers Fabry disease, Gaucher disease, Krabbe disease, Niemann-Pick disease, Farber's syndrome, metachromatic leuko-dystrophy, and sulfatase deficiency. (Codes for endocrine, nutritional, and metabolic diseases can be viewed at http://thcc.or.th/ICD-10TM/ge70.htm.) At the urging of a European rare diseases task force, WHO has created an advisory group to make recommendations about coding improvements for rare diseases. That group has been circulating draft materials for comment, which will be followed by field testing; implementation of coding changes is not expected until after 2015 (Aymé, 2009; Tejada, 2009). This project is complex, but its recommendations, if implemented, should strengthen the foundation for epidemiologic and other research on rare diseases. Much of the preparatory work on rare disease coding has been conducted by Orphanet, a European information consortium (originally established by the French Ministry of Health) (Aymé, 2009). Orphanet is also the source of the prevalence data discussed below.

---

[4] International efforts are also important. For example, the International Network of Paediatric Surveillance Units, which does not include the United States, has supported studies that have described the molecular epidemiology and genotype-phenotype correlations for Rett syndrome, Prader-Willi syndrome, and Smith-Lemli-Opitz syndrome (Grenier et al., 2007).

Prevalence Data on Rare Diseases

It is estimated that FOP [Fibrodysplasia Ossificans Progressiva] affects about 3,300 people worldwide, or approximately one in two million people. Such statistics may be better grasped by the following example: if a large football stadium holds 100,000 fans, one would need to fill nearly 20 football stadiums to find one person who has FOP. At the present time, researchers are aware of approximately 700 people throughout the world who have FOP.

IFOPA, 2009, p. 3

"Who else has this rare disease? How many of us are there? What can I expect now? What is known or not known about this disease?" These are among the questions that patients and family members ask as they become, out of necessity, advocates for themselves or others. One step in learning about a rare disease is to determine its prevalence.

The prevalence of a disease in an area or jurisdiction may be expressed as the number, percentage, or proportion of people alive on a certain day who have been diagnosed with the disease. As described in Chapter 1, the European Union defines a rare disease as one with a prevalence of no more than 50 people per 100,000 population, whereas the United States sets a numerical maximum of fewer than 200,000 people in this country.

Prevalence is a function of both the incidence of disease (number of new cases reported in a given period) and the survival (duration of illness for self-limiting or curable diseases such as many infections). Table 2-1 displays NCI data that highlight how differences in survival affect the prevalence of three types of cancers with similar incidence rates but very different survival rates: poor for pancreatic cancer, intermediate for leuke-

TABLE 2-1 Differences in Prevalence for Three Cancers with Similar Numbers of New Cases per Year but Different Survival Rates, 2006

	Estimated New Cases (2009 estimate in parentheses)	Prevalence (complete)[a]
Thyroid	30,180 (37,200)	410,404
Leukemia (all types)	35,070 (44,790)	231,857
Pancreas	33,730 (42,470)	31,180 (invasive)

[a]As defined by SEER, complete prevalence represents the number or proportion of people alive on a certain day who have been diagnosed with a disease, regardless of when the condition was diagnosed.

SOURCES: Incidence: http://seer.cancer.gov/csr/1975_2003/results_single/sect_01_table.01.pdf; http://seer.cancer.gov/csr/1975_2006/results_single/sect_01_table.01.pdf. Prevalence: http://seer.cancer.gov/csr/1975_2006/results_merged/topic_prevalence.pdf.

mia (all types considered together), and good for thyroid cancer.[5] Survival for pancreatic cancer is so poor that the estimated number of new cases per year can be higher than the estimated number of people surviving at a given time during the year.[6]

The committee found no broad compilation of data on the prevalence or incidence of rare diseases in the United States. It did, however, locate a recent report from Orphanet that lists estimated European prevalence for almost 2,000 rare diseases (out of an estimated 5,000 to 8,000 such conditions) (Orphanet, 2009). The list has much in common with the NIH list of rare conditions cited in Chapter 1. The demography, living conditions, and other characteristics of Europe and the United States likewise have much in common. Thus, despite the limitations discussed below, the committee believes that the overall portrait of rare diseases prevalence in the Orphanet report is likely to approximate that in this country.

Figures 2-1A-D show the distribution of rare conditions according to prevalence as presented in the Orphanet report. They reveal an overall distribution that is highly skewed to very rare conditions. In fact, data for approximately 1,400 of the approximately 2,000 conditions (about 70 percent) consist only of case reports for individuals or families. For the conditions not included in the study, the distribution may be even more skewed given that the project began with what were thought to be the more common rare conditions (Eurodis, 2005).

In general, the limitations of the data in the Orphanet report include the use of single numbers for conditions with widely varying estimates of prevalence in the literature[7] and the lack of bibliographic citations and explanatory details.[8] The committee did not systematically check the data presented in the report, but it did note that a few of the listed conditions

---

[5] SEER identifies four primary types of leukemia: acute lymphocytic leukemia (ALL), acute myeloid leukemia (AML), chronic lymphocytic leukemia (CLL), and chronic myeloid leukemia (CML) but also reports data on several other types (Horner and Ries, 2007).

[6] An NCI working group has defined rare cancers as having an incidence of 40,000 or fewer cases rather than in terms of prevalence (Mikhail, 2005). This specification apparently relates to the specific challenges of clinical research involving populations that include many individuals who have undergone therapies, sometimes multiple therapies.

[7] For example, the prevalence report lists malignant hyperthermia (a rare, life-threatening reaction to certain anesthetics and other agents) with an estimated prevalence of 33 per 100,000 population, but a 2007 study published in the Orphanet journal cites a highly variable incidence from 1/5,000 to 1/50,000–100,000 anesthesia episodes (Rosenberg et al., 2007). For Prader-Willi syndrome, the prevalence report cites a figure of 10.7/100,000, whereas an article in an Orphanet-associated journal cited a range of 1/15,000 to 1/30,000 (Cassidy and Driscoll, 2009).

[8] The report does not include citations of source data but generally cites EMEA (European Medicines Agency), new scientific publications, gray literature, and expert opinion (Orphanet, 2009). Short overview discussions of individual conditions in the Orphanet database vary in the specificity of their citations of sources.

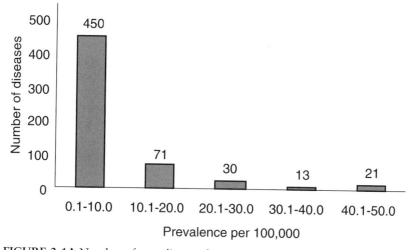

FIGURE 2-1A Number of rare diseases by prevalence up to 50/100,000.

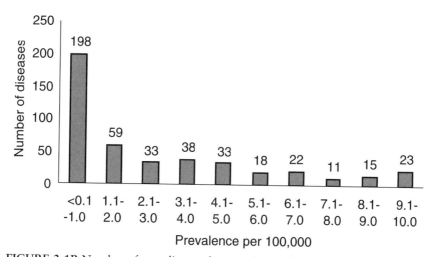

FIGURE 2-1B Number of rare diseases by prevalence of 10/100,000 or less.

(e.g., autism, pulmonary fibrosis) are not rare in the United States. The introduction to the report explicity notes (Orphanet, 2009, p. 2)

> a low level of consistency between studies, a poor documentation of methods used, confusion between incidence and prevalence, and/or confusion between incidence at birth and life-long incidence. The validity of the published studies is taken for granted and not assessed. It is likely that there

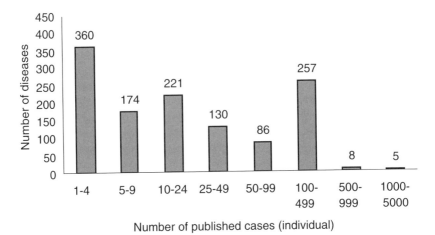

FIGURE 2-1C Number of rare diseases by number of individual cases in literature.

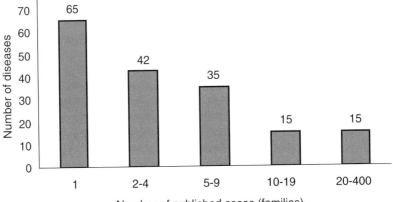

FIGURE 2-1D Number of rare diseases by number of family cases in literature.
SOURCE: Orphanet, 2009.

is an overestimation for most diseases as the few published prevalence surveys are usually done in regions of higher prevalence and are usually based on hospital data. Therefore, these estimates are an indication of the assumed prevalence but may not be accurate.

The factors cited illustrate problems inherent in trying to develop reliable prevalence estimates for rare conditions—individually and collectively. Again, notwithstanding these limitations, the committee expects that the data provide a rough approximation of the overall distribution of rare conditions, at least for the conditions included.

In part because data on many conditions are limited to case reports or special population studies, no well-supported estimate exists for the number of people collectively affected by rare diseases. A 1989 government report stated that 10 million to 20 million Americans had a rare condition (NCOD, 1989); the corresponding estimates in 2009 range from 25 million to 30 million (see, e.g., ORDR, 2009). The estimates were not accompanied by analyses or substantive citation of sources.

CAUSES OF RARE DISEASES

"How did this happen? Why did this happen to me? What can I do?" Individuals and families struggle with these questions as they try their best to grasp the meaning and impact of a rare disease diagnosis. In the past two decades, epidemiologic, molecular, and other research that takes advantage of scientific and technological advances in the biological sciences has greatly increased the number of rare diseases that have an identified cause—usually, although not invariably, genetic. The Orphan Drug Act, the Rare Diseases Act, and other policy initiatives discussed in this report have contributed to this knowledge by focusing attention, resources, and incentives on the study of rare conditions and products to treat them.

Knowing the genetic, infectious, or other cause of a disease does not necessarily mean that researchers understand the mechanism of the disease. For example, much remains to be learned about Von Hippel-Lindau syndrome, even though mutations in the *VHL* gene have been identified as the cause and another gene has been implicated in phenotypic variations (Woodward and Maher, 2006). Moreover, a number of more common rare diseases such as cystic fibrosis and sickle cell disease have known causes and reasonably well understood mechanisms but lack cures, satisfactory treatments, or preventive strategies. Nonetheless, identifying the cause of a condition is usually an important step in building the knowledge base for prevention or effective treatment.

Some rare conditions have multiple possible types of causes. For example, some forms of aplastic anemia, which is caused by damage to stem cells in the bone marrow and is diagnosed in about 500 to 1,000 people each year in the United States, are inherited (e.g., Fanconi anemia). More often, though, the condition is acquired as a result of a toxic exposure (e.g., benzene, chloramphenicol), an infection (e.g., hepatitis, herpes virus), radiation or chemotherapy, or another disease (e.g., rheumatoid arthritis) (NHLBI, 2009). Doctors sometimes cannot determine the cause for a specific patient.

For certain rare diseases that have been named and characterized for decades, investigators still have not determined the cause. For example, although the disease was identified decades ago, no cause is known for Gorham's disease, an extremely rare bone disorder that has been described under more than a dozen different names (LGDA, 2009). To cite other examples, the Vasculitis Research Consortium, which is part of the NIH-funded Rare Diseases Clinical Research Network, is investigating six forms of vasculitis (a group of rare conditions affecting blood vessels) for which the causes are not known (VCRC, 2010).

Genetic Causes

Notwithstanding the imprecision in the count of rare diseases and the difficulty of characterizing thousands of conditions, experts on rare diseases generally agree that the great majority of rare diseases—perhaps 80 percent or more—are genetic in origin (see, e.g., NORD, 2007; NIH, 2008). Many if not most are caused by defects in a single gene, for example, alpha$_1$-antitrypsin deficiency (which may cause serious lung or liver disease) and Friedreich's ataxia (a neurological disorder that may also be accompanied by cardiac and other problems). Multiple different mutations in that single gene may result in disease of varying features or severity. Other diseases, such as Fanconi anemia, have several named variants, each caused by a defect in a different gene (D'Andrea, 2010). Muscular dystrophy, which was once viewed as a single disease, now is described as having nine major forms, of which Duchenne muscular dystrophy may be the best known.

In some rare conditions, multiple genes may contribute collectively to manifestations of the disorder (Dale and Link, 2009). For example, a recent examination of Williams-Beuren syndrome describes one gene clearly identified as producing the condition's cardiovascular problems and seven others with suspected roles in producing other common features of the disease (Pober, 2010).[9] Continuing research on a number of "single-gene" conditions may suggest or identify additional (modifier) genes that influence the course of the disease, for example, the age at onset, severity, or organ system affected.

Rare genetic conditions are often inherited but may also arise as a result of sporadic or chance mutations. For example, about one-quarter of cases

---

[9] Multiple genes are also implicated in many common diseases such as diabetes, heart disease, and bipolar disorder, often in interaction with behavioral and environmental factors (such as smoking or air pollution) that complicate prediction, prevention, and treatment. Each generally contributes a small portion of the attributable risk. Early hopes that genetic studies would quickly lead to breakthrough therapeutic advances for these complex common conditions have generally not been fulfilled (see, e.g., Sing et al., 2003; Moore and Ritchie, 2004; Hyman, 2008).

of Marfan syndrome (a disorder of the body's connective tissues) may be caused by sporadic mutations that occur by chance in a sperm or egg cell of an unaffected parent (Dietz, 2009).

In addition, some diseases such as sarcoidosis are known or suspected to be heritable, but the specific genetic mutation or mutations have not yet been identified. For other diseases, known genetic causes do not explain all cases and other genes are suspected to play a role. Organizations supporting research on inherited conditions typically make gene identification a top priority as illustrated by the example of the Progeria Research Foundation in Chapter 1 and the examples in Appendix F. Fortunately, the scientific and technical advances cited in Chapter 4 are making gene identification easier, faster, and less expensive.

Infectious Agents

A number of rare diseases have infectious causes. Despite their rarity, some infections such as rabies, botulism, and Rocky Mountain spotted fever are relatively well publicized and feared. Others are truly obscure, for example, *Naegleria fowleri*. Newspapers and medical journals occasionally highlight cases of extremely rare infections such as Lemierre's syndrome, an often lethal disease (caused by *Fusobacterium necrophorum*) that was so nearly eliminated by the advent of antibiotics that it has been termed the "forgotten disease" (Boodman, 2009; Lu et al., 2009).

Some infections (e.g., those caused by *Balamuthia mandrillaris* and *Chromobacterium violaceum*) are thought to be rare worldwide (de Siqueira et al., 2005; Glaser et al., 2008). Others, however, are rare in wealthy countries but common in less economically developed countries. Some of these, for example, tuberculosis, were common in wealthy countries such as the United States before effective preventive measures or treatments were discovered and widely applied. One anxiety is that the development and spread of extremely drug resistant strains of tuberculosis and certain other diseases could—absent effective countermeasures—lead to their resurgence in areas where they are now rare. For example, the late 1980s and early 1990s saw a resurgence of tuberculosis in the United States when the number of cases reported rose by 20 percent and several outbreaks in hospitals affected both patients and staff (IOM, 2001).

As discussed in Chapter 1, public health experts and global nonprofit funders have highlighted several infectious diseases as neglected and have promoted international efforts to increase knowledge of these conditions, undertake intensive prevention campaigns, and develop affordable treatments. They also seek to make existing treatments affordable for poor patients and nations.

Research suggests that genetic factors may affect susceptibility to infectious agents, either increasing susceptibility or having a protective effect.

For example, research indicates that sickle cell trait contributes to resistance against malaria. Other genes are likely to affect susceptibility to malaria (Faik et al., 2009) and leprosy (Zhang et al., 2009).

Toxic Agents

Some rare diseases or conditions result from exposure to natural or manufactured toxic substances, including substances that appear as product contaminants. In the United States, examples include arsenic and mercury poisoning, mesothelioma (a cancer caused by exposure to asbestos), and eosinophilia-myalgia syndrome, which is associated with contaminated (or overused) tryptophan, a dietary supplement.[10]

It is likely that far more types of poisoning could be listed as rare conditions than are included in the list maintained by the Office of Rare Diseases Research (ORDR) at NIH. For example, the committee found newspaper reports of rare cadmium, chromium, phosphine, and other poisonings in the United States, but none is listed as a rare disease. These toxic substances are a concern of ATSDR.

Also not listed are rare poisonings caused by a variety of marine toxins that may contaminate seafood and that are tracked by the CDC (CDC, 2005). Likewise, Amatoxin poisoning, a rare and often fatal illness caused by *Amanita phalloides*—the "death cap" mushroom—is also not listed. Approximately 50 cases are diagnosed each year in the United States. Doctors who treat patients with this poisoning sometimes obtain FDA approval for emergency use of a milk thistle extract that is manufactured in Europe but that has not clinically evaluated or approved for marketing as a drug in the United States (Coombs, 2009).[11]

Some drugs have received orphan designation and approval for treatment of rare poisonings. For example, FDA has approved an orphan drug for the treatment of acute cyanide poisoning (hydroxocobalamin [Cyanokit]). Several agents have received orphan designations for treatment of snakebites, but only one has been approved (Crotalidae polyvalent immune fab [ovine] [CroFab] for certain rattlesnake and other snake bites).

---

[10] Dietary supplements are regulated by FDA, but under 1994 legislation (P.L. 103-417), manufacturers are usually not required to register their products with FDA, get marketing approval based on evidence of safety and effectiveness, or report adverse events possibly related to the use of the product. FDA may take action against an unsafe supplement once it has reached the market.

[11] The extract is, however, marketed as an herbal supplement, and a variety of unproved benefits have been asserted (NCCAM, 2008). Congress has directed that such supplements not be subjected to the same regulatory standards and review as medications.

Other Causes

Rare conditions may have a variety of other causes. Examples include conditions caused by nutritional deficiencies (e.g., beriberi, which results from thiamine deficiency and is rare in the United States [Medline Plus, 2008]) and injuries (e.g., commotio cordis, in which ventricular fibrillation and sudden death is associated with a nonpenetrating blow to the chest [Maron and Estes, 2010]).

Certain rare conditions are caused by the persistent adverse or toxic effects of treatment for another disease. For example, the ORDR list of rare diseases includes radiation-induced meningioma, which is a rare central nervous system tumor. Secondary cancers are a well-understood risk of radiation therapy and also chemotherapy. FDA has approved a few orphan drugs for the treatment of adverse effects of certain therapies for cancer and other conditions (e.g., dexrazoxane [Totect] for leakage of intravenous anthracycline into surrounding tissue and deferasirox [Exjade] for treatment of chronic iron overload from frequent blood transfusions).[12]

As is the case with illness caused by poisons, treatment-related illness is not a primary focus of rare diseases policy as such. Drug toxicity and safety in general are, however, major concerns of FDA and an array of other government efforts to protect patient safety. For example, progressive multifocal leukoencephalopathy (a rare brain infection that has been diagnosed in multiple sclerosis patients who have taken the drug Tysabri) has been the subject of several FDA safety notices (see, e.g., FDA, 2010a).

PREVENTION, DIAGNOSIS, AND TREATMENT

For rare diseases collectively, possible preventive, diagnostic, and treatment options and outcomes span a huge range. Some rare diseases are now preventable, many are not. Diagnosis is sometimes straightforward but often frustratingly slow. Cures exist for a few conditions but are a distant hope for most. For some conditions, disease-modifying therapies may allow a nearly normal life, whereas for others, the impact on morbidity and mortality may be very modest. Treatment of symptoms is the mainstay in many cases.

---

[12] Many adverse as well as positive reactions to medications may be explained by genetic variability. For example, malignant hyperthermia, which is included in the ORDR list, has been described as "a rare, life-threatening, autosomal-dominant, pharmacogenetic, anesthetic-related disorder that occurs in susceptible patients following the administration of a triggering agent" (Stratman et al., 2009). Another such condition listed by ORDR is 5-fluorouracil toxicity, which can occur in carriers of a mutation in the dihydropyrimidine dehydrogenase gene (Öfverholm, 2010).

This section and the next offer a broad, descriptive perspective on the range of preventive, diagnostic, and treatment measures; these topics could form the subject for a report in themselves. The discussion is intended to illustrate public health and clinical practices, rather than to evaluate them or provide recommendations.

Prevention

The prevention of rare diseases may take different approaches. Some preventive strategies are relatively simple but striking in effect, while others are complex and demanding. Some raise ethical questions. The discussion below considers primary and secondary prevention. Tertiary prevention, which involves treatment of evident disease to avoid further progression or suffering or to restore health or function, is considered here as treatment. (Other frameworks for prevention policies and research have been developed, particularly for mental disorders [see, e.g., IOM, 2004, 2009a].)

Primary Prevention

Primary prevention seeks to eliminate or reduce risk factors that cause disease. Prevention is a mainstay of the infection control programs of public health agencies. Common primary prevention measures include immunizations (which are usually aimed at conditions that are or have been relatively common) and hand washing and other basic sanitation measures that are employed to control both common and rare infections. These measures, particularly immunization, have made a number of once-common infections, such as chicken pox and measles, rare. Other public and private programs seek to reduce population exposure to toxic agents such as asbestos and mercury. Measures include bans or strict controls on the use of toxic agents and programs to clean up contaminated locations, including buildings in which asbestos is present and abandoned industrial or military sites that are multiply contaminated.

A different type of primary prevention is exemplified in the promotion of folic acid supplementation for women of childbearing age to prevent neural tube defects in their children. Neural tube defects that are listed as rare by ORDR include spina bifida and anencephaly. To prevent fetal exposure to harmful agents, many medications come with prominent warnings advising against use of the drug for pregnant women. Other drugs are approved with special precautions to limit the chance of fetal exposure. For example, thalidomide, a drug best known from the late 1950s for causing birth defects in children of mothers who were prescribed the drug for morning sickness, is now FDA-approved for treatment of two rare conditions (multiple myeloma and erythema nodosum leprosum). FDA required a restricted distribution program that is limited to registered physicians and pharmacists and to patients who agree to actions to minimize the risk of fetal exposure (Celgene, 2010).

Preventive measures for certain rare diseases sometimes involve very personal and intimate decisions about marriage and childbearing, and some measures may raise ethical questions. For a few serious genetic conditions, such as Tay-Sachs disease, thalassemia, cystic fibrosis, fragile X syndrome, and familial dysautonomia, screening and counseling programs have been developed to identify and advise individuals who carry the gene for the condition (Kaback et al., 1993; Gessen, 2008; Lerner, 2009; Zlotogora, 2009). High-risk couples may be advised about a range of options, including avoiding marriage to another person who is a carrier for the same disease, using contraceptive methods to avoid pregnancy, undergoing in vitro fertilization with embryonic screening, or obtaining prenatal screening with the possibility of pregnancy termination or planning for the birth of an affected child. After genetic testing and community-organized information counseling programs became available, the incidence of Tay-Sachs disease in the United States and Canada dropped by 90 percent from 1970 to 1992 for the Jewish population most at risk (Kaback et al., 1993). Individual or population genetic testing has also been linked to a significant decline in familial dysautonomia for which the incidence is the United States has reached as low as a single case in recent years compared to 10 to 12 cases in many of the years before testing became available in 2001 (Lerner, 2009). Some fear that the result will be less attention to treatment research and assistance for people who have an already rare disease of diminishing prevalence.

Secondary Prevention

Secondary prevention strategies involve screening or testing to identify a condition so that effective treatments can be provided to people before the onset of debilitating symptoms or complications. (Diagnosis when symptoms are evident is discussed below.) Newborn screening programs, which use biochemical or genetic blood tests, are prominent examples. In 2005, the American College of Medical Genetics (ACMG) recommended screening for 29 mostly inherited, serious, rare conditions (Watson et al., 2006). These recommendations were endorsed by a U.S. Department of Health and Human Services advisory panel on heritable disorders and genetic diseases in infants and children (Howell, 2005). As described by the ACMG, the conditions fall in five broad categories: organic acid metabolism disorders, fatty acid oxidation disorders, amino acid metabolism disorders, hemoglobinopathies, and other disorders.

According to a recent study, the "estimated number of cases of disorders that would have been identified in 2006 using the ACMG panel was

6,439, [which is] 32 percent more than the 4,370 that would have been identified otherwise" (Therrell et al., 2008, p. 1012). Four conditions (three hemoglobin disorders and congenital hypothyroidism) accounted for approximately 60 percent of this total, whereas nine of the screened conditions accounted for an estimated 15 or fewer cases.[13]

All states have newborn screening programs, although they vary in the conditions screened, particularly those outside the recommended core tests (NNSGRC, 2010). Technologies to expand the number of disorders screened are available. The CDC has created the Newborn Screening Translation Research Initiative (CDC, 2009d), and NIH has created the Newborn Screening Translational Research Network (NICHD, 2009). Aside from the availability of new screening technologies, the expansion of screening panels will be influenced by affordability (and possibly cost-effectiveness, taking into account the rate of false positive results), political considerations, and the continued emergence of new therapies that are beneficial when instituted early in life.[14]

Newborn screening may also trigger genetic testing and counseling of family members. It thereby offers a further opportunity for prevention when monitoring or early treatment can be effective in delaying or limiting the consequences of the condition for an affected sibling or other family member. Parents may first learn of their membership in a rare disease population after a child's screening.

In addition to allowing treatment at the outset to help prevent damage, the early identification of children with rare disorders can facilitate research by (1) providing a pool of potential research participants who have not developed advanced disease or serious disease-related complications and (2) allowing segmentation of potential participants by genotype (when genetic testing is available) to create more homogeneous study groups, which are important in complex conditions to differentiate the effects of treatment from the effects of other factors. Research use of retained samples from newborn screening programs has generated controversy about whether

---

[13] Ten of the disorders accounted for an estimated 100 or more cases, and four other disorders accounted for an estimated 50 or more cases.

[14] Despite the widespread and expanded adoption of newborn screening programs, some critics argue that such programs—or at least all elements of such programs—do not necessarily represent the best use of resources to promote child health compared, for example, to improved prenatal care for poor women (see, e.g., Atkins et al., 2005; Baily and Murray, 2008; Moyer et al., 2008). These critics call for more explicit comparisons with alternative policies of expected outcomes (benefits and harms) in relation to projected costs. Recent studies investigating the cost-effectiveness of newborn screening that include the costs of false positives have concluded that it generally compares favorably with other childhood interventions (see, e.g., Prosser et al., 2010).

such samples should be used in the absence of informed parental permission (Maschke, 2009).

Diagnosis

For many patients, diagnosis comes a frustratingly long time after symptoms first become evident. It follows countless tests and visits to different specialists and centers with multiple diagnoses considered and initially or eventually rejected. This kind of diagnostic odyssey for a rare condition is often described in television shows and newspaper stories about diagnostic mysteries.

A survey of 801 patients conducted in the late 1980s for the National Commission on Orphan Diseases found that approximately one in three reported that obtaining a diagnosis took from 1 to 5 years and one in seven reported that it took 6 years or more (NCOD, 1989). A European survey that focused on eight rare diseases (including cystic fibrosis, Duchenne muscular dystrophy, and Marfan syndrome) received nearly 6,000 completed surveys (Faurisson, 2004). Forty percent of respondents reported their first diagnosis was wrong, and 25 percent reported waiting between 5 and 30 years for a correct diagnosis. Accurate and timely diagnosis is especially important when early diagnosis can significantly affect the course of the disease.

For a few patients whose conditions have defied diagnosis, the NIH Undiagnosed Diseases Program, which was established in 2008, may help. From May 2008 to approximately December 2009, the program received more than 2,300 inquiries and more than 900 medical records, and it accepted 190 patients for evaluation (Garnett, 2010; see also Henig, 2009).

The diagnosis of many rare diseases has been limited historically by imprecise, cumbersome, or expensive testing and by limitations on physician and patient access to the most up-to-date information about rare diseases (including diagnostic criteria) and other diagnostic resources. Clinical specialization and subspecialization also contribute to the extent that specialists focus on their piece of a patient's complex of symptoms. For example, because of multiorgan involvement, patients with cystic fibrosis may be diagnosed by pulmonologists, gastroenterologists, allergists, or general pediatricians.

When patients or families seek medical help, the initial stages of diagnosis usually still depend on classic clinical practices—the physical examination and taking of a patient history, the use of blood and other laboratory tests, and the application of clinical knowledge and reasoning skills. One dilemma for clinicians and patients is that many rare diseases have neurological, digestive, or other symptoms that accompany a number of common and rare conditions, and depending on the disease and the individual patient, laboratory results may or may not be definitive. Physicians normally will consider common conditions that are consistent with the available information before considering rare conditions. The widely used clinical aphorism is, "When you hear hoofbeats behind you, don't expect to see a zebra."[15] Another diagnostic complexity is that a patient may have an atypical presentation of a common disease. Finally, a patient may have an atypical presentation of a rare disease, which may make it almost impossible to arrive at a diagnosis.

Although genetic tests are crucial to the diagnosis of many rare genetic conditions, the ordering of a specific test or set of tests typically depends on a clinician's evaluation and ability to recognize clues pointing to conditions for which genetic testing may be warranted. According to a unit of the publicly funded National Center for Biotechnology Information, approximately 1,500 tests are now available to assess whether a person carries a gene mutation associated with a specific disease (NCBI, 2009). That number, although growing, still falls considerably short of the number of rare diseases that are thought to be genetic. Examples of genetic conditions for which genetic tests are not commercially available include sitosterolemia (Steiner, 2009) and KBG syndrome (Brancati et al., 2006). NIH recently announced the creation of a registry of genetic tests (NCBI, 2010), and another database GeneTests, which is operated by the National Center for Biotechnology Information, has been available for several years (http://www.ncbi.nlm.nih.gov/sites/GeneTests/?db=GeneTests).

Physicians and patients may, however, be frustrated that some genetic tests are only available from a few laboratories based on decisions by patent holders (Cook-Deegan, 2008; Kesselheim and Mello, 2010). Moreover, testing may be very expensive and may not be covered by health plans. Some tests or genetic testing services are marketed not to physicians but to consumers, a development that has provoked considerable controversy (see, e.g., Schickedanz and Herdman, 2009; GAO, 2010a) as well as FDA and Congressional scrutiny (Carmichael, 2010). As discussed in Chapter 7, FDA regulates genetic tests that are packaged as test kits for laboratories that do genetic tests, but it generally does not regulate tests that are both produced and performed by laboratories. It is now reconsidering that approach.

Genetic counseling is recommended for individuals and families following the diagnosis of a rare genetic disorder to help them better understand the disorder, consider their options, and plan for the future. Family members may be advised about their options to be tested.

Many organizations that educate, assist, and advocate for patients with rare conditions seek to educate physicians about the disease. One goal is to increase the likelihood that physicians will recognize certain symptoms

---

[15] The expression was coined in a slightly modified form in the late 1940s by Dr. Theodore Woodward, a former professor at the University of Maryland School of Medicine in Baltimore (Sotos, 1989).

or constellations of symptoms as associated with a particular rare disease and will consider that disease among diagnostic possibilities that should be evaluated further. For example, the Cystic Fibrosis Foundation developed criteria to help standardize approaches to diagnosis (Rosenstein and Cutting, 1998).

Treatment

With the current state of medical science, most people here [with GIST] will never be "cured." . . . Thus, considering the alternative, I look forward to pills, surgeries and scans for decades to come (well, really, I am hoping for a cure or more effective treatments to arise sooner).

> Patient with GIST (gastrointestinal stromal tumor)
> Quoted at http://www.gistsupport.org/voices-of-gist/essays/brendas-war-on-gist.php

Discussions of treatment for rare diseases tend to focus on care for a single condition (e.g., Niemann-Pick disease) or a set of related conditions (e.g., lysosomal storage disorders). The *NORD Guide to Rare Diseases* (2003, with updated and expanded information available online) includes brief overviews of treatment for several hundred rare conditions, but the committee is not aware of reviews of treatment practices and options over the spectrum of rare diseases.[16] Various textbooks, online sites, and other resources advise on treatment for a broad range of infections, including some that are rare; other resources advise on treatments for a broad range of poisonings, again including some rare poisonings. Many rare diseases have been discovered relatively recently, so researchers have had limited time to work on identifying their causes and mechanisms of disease as the basis for investigating treatment targets or preventive strategies.

Some reviews have discussed treatment of genetic diseases with varying degrees of breadth. For example, a 1999 review of 372 genetic diseases reported that 34 percent had no effective treatment, 54 percent had treatments that produced partial responses, and 12 percent had treatments that produced complete responses (Scriver and Treacy, 1999). These numbers undoubtedly have changed in the past decade. For example, one of the authors of the 1999 study coauthored a 2008 review of treatment over a 25-year period for 65 conditions involving inborn errors of metabolism. This review reported that "the number of conditions for which there is no

---

[16] The Cochrane Collaboration has a cystic fibrosis and genetic disorders group that has developed 108 systematic reviews (or plans for reviews), including 61 reviews for various aspects of cystic fibrosis, 26 reviews for sickle cell disease, and 12 reviews for several conditions involving inborn errors of metabolism (see the list at http://www2.cochrane.org/reviews/en/subtopics/55.html).

response to treatment has progressively decreased; from 31 in 1983, to 20 in 1993, to 17 in 2008" (Campeau et al., 2008, p. 11). It also reported that the number of conditions that fully responded to treatment increased from 8 in 1983 and 1993 to 20 in 2008. As reasons for this progress, the authors cited "new small molecules, new enzyme replacement therapies, more conditions that can be treated by organ and cell transplantation, and new experimental approaches" (p. 11). These analyses involve small and highly selected subsets of all genetic diseases and are likely biased toward those that are well studied and for which there are treatments.

A 2004 textbook review of treatment for genetic diseases observed that treatments judged to be successful initially may later show their limitations (Nussbaum et al., 2004). This pattern may reflect the recognition over time of subtler manifestations of the disease, long-term adverse effects of treatment, and manifestations of the disease not recognized until treatments allowed longer survival. Because drugs are approved on the basis of relatively short-term clinical data involving unrepresentative patient populations, FDA often requires drug sponsors to undertake additional studies following the approval of a drug for marketing. The 2004 review linked the "unsatisfactory" state of treatment for genetic conditions to lack of identification of the causal gene; inadequate understanding of pathophysiology; and irreversible damage at the fetal stage before diagnosis.

Dietz (2010) recently reviewed therapeutic approaches to Mendelian disorders, focusing on approaches that use detailed knowledge of disease pathogenesis. This review, which is cited further in Chapter 4, explores how such understanding is contributing to investigations involving, for example, the replacement of deficient gene products (gene therapy, enzyme replacement therapy); the use of FDA-approved drugs in novel ways; the design of new small-molecule compounds; and the manipulation of gene expression. To repeat a theme of this report, research resources for rare diseases are limited, both collectively and individually. Nonetheless, basic and clinical research have yielded disease-modifying therapies for many conditions.

Table 2-2 illustrates the range of treatments—from surgery to diet and from stem cell therapy to environmental adaptation—that may be deployed for specific rare conditions. Some of these therapies have been used for decades, while others have emerged through technological advances. Many of the procedures cited are accompanied by complex pharmaceutical regimens—some short-term, others indefinite (e.g., use of immunosuppressive drugs following an organ transplant). As with any therapy, expected benefits are often accompanied by risks that may include significant harms. It is important for patients and families to understand and weigh both potential benefits and potential harms of treatment options.

Another way of looking at treatments for rare diseases is to consider

TABLE 2-2 Examples of Currently Available Treatments or Treatments in Development for Rare Diseases

Therapeutic Category	Treatment Example	Rare Condition
Small-molecule compounds	Imatinib	Chronic myelogenous leukemia
Protein therapies	Enzyme replacement therapy	Gaucher disease
Metabolic therapies	Sodium phenylbutyrate	Urea cycle disorders
Nutritional therapies	Phenylalanine-restricted diet	Phenylketonuria
Environmental modification or adaptation	Avoidance of sunlight	Xeroderma pigmentosa
Medical procedures	Phlebotomy	Hemochromatosis
Surgical procedures	Open heart surgery	Tetralogy of Fallot
Medical devices	Orthopedic implant	Thoracic insufficiency (e.g., Jeune syndrome)
Organ transplants	Combined liver-kidney transplant	Primary hyperoxaluria
Bone marrow or cord blood transplants	Bone marrow or cord blood transplant	Hurler syndrome
Stem cell transplants (investigational)	Neural stem cell transplant	Neuronal ceroid lipofuscinosis
Genetic therapies (investigational)	Exon skipping	Duchenne muscular dystrophy

SOURCE: This table draws from Nussbaum et al., 2004; Dietz, 2010; Maegawa and Steiner, in press.

the range of effectiveness of treatments or the variability in what is anticipated from the use of different therapies. Treatments may be

- curative,
- disease modifying, or
- symptom or function modifying.

Curative Treatments

Truly curative treatments for rare conditions are themselves rare. Immediate treatment may be completely successful for all or most cases of certain rare infections (e.g., *Tropheryma whipplei*) or certain rare poisonings (e.g., from snakebites or cyanide). Vitamin D supplementation generally cures rickets, although for one form (X-linked hypophosphatemic rickets), a combination of phosphate and a form of vitamin D will treat but not cure the condition (Imel et al., 2010).

Some rare anatomical defects can be corrected (essentially cured) with surgery, for example, coarctation of the aorta. Certain conditions that can be treated effectively with surgery, such as transposition of the great arteries or tetralogy of Fallot, have features beyond the intrinsic anatomical anomaly that require continued medical attention.

Organ transplantation is considered curative for a few rare conditions, for example, heart transplantation for hypoplastic left heart syndrome. For carefully selected subsets of patients, bone marrow transplantation or transplantation of stem cells from umbilical cord blood is, if successfully performed, considered a cure for Diamond-Blackfan anemia, Wiskott-Aldrich syndrome, and paroxysmal nocturnal hemoglobinuria as well as some cancers (Filopovich et al., 2007; Brodsky, 2009; Clinton and Gazda, 2009). Although they may be considered cures, such procedures come with significant short- and long-term health risks from the procedure itself and the necessary follow-up care (e.g., use of immunosuppressive drugs). Moreover, transplants are sometimes lifesaving but not curative. For example, umbilical stem cell transplant can save some children with infantile Krabbe disease from death, but they will still have major neurologic deficits (Duffner et al., 2009).

Disease-Modifying Treatment

Disease-modifying therapies are targeted to the underlying pathology of a disease in order to prevent its progression or otherwise limit the harm it creates. For example, with galactosemia, a potentially fatal disorder of galactose metabolism, the restriction of milk products immediately upon diagnosis through newborn screening will interfere with the pathology of the disease and prevent its severe manifestations. Children may still, however, experience various problems such as speech and language difficulties (Lai et al., 2008). Kidney transplantation is lifesaving but not curative for individuals who have nephropathic cystinosis; early initiation of disease-modifying treatment with cysteamine can significantly delay complications (Kleta and Gahl, 2004)

For many disease-modifying therapies, the treatment effect is short-lived and must be repeated indefinitely. Examples include enzyme replacement therapies for conditions such as Gaucher disease, which involves the ongoing use of a biologically created product to act in place of the enzyme that is missing or deficient as a result of a genetic defect. Depending on the condition, such therapy may be effective for some manifestations of the disease but not others (e.g., liver- and bone-related but not brain-related aspects of Gaucher disease) (Schmitz et al., 2007).

In some cases, the mechanism of action of a disease-modifying drug may not be clear. An example is riluzole, which is associated with a modest survival benefit for amyotrophic lateral sclerosis (Bellingham, 2010). Another example is hydroxyurea, which is the only disease-modifying therapy identified for sickle cell disease (Segal et al., 2008).

Rational drug design specifically aims to develop new drugs based on knowledge of disease biology. This strategy holds promise for many rare conditions for which no disease-modifying therapies are known. Current treatment for these conditions still emphasizes treatment of symptoms and prevention of complications.

Symptomatic and Functional Therapies

Symptomatic treatments are vital to patient well-being for many chronic rare conditions, especially when more definitive therapies are not available. Painful and distressing symptoms of many rare as well as common diseases include pain, nausea, bladder or bowel dysfunction, itching, dizziness, movement limitations, and speech dysfunction to name a few. Treatments also seek to treat or prevent other disease- or treatment-related complications, for example, infections (such as the bronchitis or pneumonia caused by cystic fibrosis or primary ciliary dyskinesia), anemia (such as that associated with hereditary spherocytosis), and delayed growth (such as that associated with X-linked hypophosphatemic rickets).

To temper symptoms and preserve or improve physical, intellectual, and emotional functioning, clinicians may use a wide variety of therapeutic methods. These include medications, nutritional agents, surgical procedures, psychotherapy, physical and occupational therapy, complex medical devices (e.g., sophisticated communication devices), and less complex devices (e.g., braces).

The above discussion emphasizes the physical dimensions of treatment. Care-giving extends well beyond the physical to include psychological, spiritual, and practical support. These dimensions of care may be especially significant for individuals and families facing serious illness. Genetic counseling is important for individuals and families facing the new diagnosis of a genetic disorder. Also, because many rare disorders are fatal, end-of-life care is important to help patients (to the extent they are able to participate) and families plan for an expected but not necessarily predictable death and to make difficult decisions about the site and nature of care. After a death, continued support can help families and others cope with grief and other consequences of loss.

Delivering Preventive, Diagnostic, and Treatment Services

A variety of factors—including lack of knowledge, lack of resources, or failure to follow recommendations—may interfere with a physician's or patient's use of effective diagnostic techniques, preventive measures, and treatments. Although this report focuses on research and development and not the movement of effective treatments or preventive or diagnostic measures into practice, that movement is crucial if the benefits of research are to be realized in the lives of patients and their families.

One common mission of advocacy organizations is to educate clinicians about rare conditions as a means of improving the provision of care, including the appropriate consideration of new diagnostic and therapeutic options. Depending on the condition and the organization, other strategies may include the development of clinical practice guidelines, quality improvement and assessment programs (including incentives for meeting quality standards), and continuing medical education and consumer education activities.

This section briefly discusses just a few issues in health care delivery that may affect the availability or quality of care provided to people with rare conditions. It does not examine the development and use of clinical practice guidelines, the challenges of emergency care, the role of electronic health records or information systems, or the cost or financing of services. Chapter 6, however, examines health plan coverage and reimbursement of orphan drugs, and Chapter 7 examines coverage and reimbursement of devices marketed for small populations under a Humanitarian Device Exemption.

Specialized Centers for Rare Diseases

For both common and rare diseases, the creation of medical centers or medical practices specializing in the diagnosis and treatment of a disease is a frequent strategy to improve the quality and consistency of care. For rare diseases, specialized centers can offer consultations to outside clinicians, develop care guidelines based on available evidence and experience, and serve as an established referral site in emergencies or other situations in which local resources are insufficient. These centers can also provide a base for research.

One of the early priorities of the Cystic Fibrosis Foundation (CFF) was the establishment of a network of accredited care centers. From two centers at the outset in 1961, CFF now accredits 115 care centers as well as 95 adult care programs (CFF, 2008, undatedb). The foundation has also designated 10 centers as basic research centers and more than 70 as sites for its Therapeutics Development Network (CFF, undatedb).

In 1972, Congress authorized the creation of comprehensive research and treatment centers for sickle cell disease. These centers were subsequently established by what is now the National Heart, Lung, and Blood Institute. In 2007, the American Society of Hematology recommended a number of revisions in the program "to ensure that clinical research is conducted in a milieu where federally funded comprehensive care programs include a much larger proportion of children and adults with sickle cell disease than is currently served by existing centers, networks, and other governmental support programs" (ASH, 2007). In addition, the organization has recommended changes in the program to promote multidisciplinary, multicenter, collaborative research and more resources for translational research.

Among other examples of specialized centers to improve care delivery, the Children's Tumor Foundation has created a Neurofibromatosis Clinic Network of affiliated clinics that meet operational principles established by an advisory board. The organization had recognized 38 such clinics in the United States by the end of 2008 (CTF, 2009). The CDC funds comprehensive treatment centers, including more than 130 for hemophilia, 8 for thrombosis and hemostasis, and 6 for thalassemia (CDC, 2009b).

In addition to bringing together comprehensive expertise and resources to address an array of patient needs, specialized care centers make it easier for sponsoring organizations and others to establish and monitor the quality of care and other standards. For rare diseases, however, the evidence base to establish standards may be limited, and the number of patients may be too small for some statistical tracking tools to be very useful.

For extremely rare diseases, networks of comprehensive care centers are the exception, although individual medical centers may still be recognized as loci of clinical expertise. Examples include many of the institutions participating in the NIH Rare Diseases Clinical Research Network (see Chapter 5).

In addition to a focus on systems of care, a priority for many advocacy organizations has been to help patients and families identify individual physicians with some experience and expertise with extremely rare conditions. Organizations may provide a list of physician contacts, as exemplified by the website of the International Fibrodysplasia Ossificans Progressiva (FOP) Association, which lists physician contacts, including clinical researchers at the FOP Research Laboratory at the University of Pennsylvania (who are also cited as emergency contacts). In addition, as noted earlier, NIH has created the Undiagnosed Diseases Program, which sees patients through the NIH Clinical Center.

Pediatric-Adult Care Transition

Children form a substantial part of the population with rare conditions. Although many rare diseases are fatal in infancy or childhood, early diagnosis and improved treatment for a number of conditions have increased the number of infants and children who survive to adulthood. For this group, the transition from pediatric or adolescent to adult care is often a matter of acute concern to the young people themselves, their families, and the professionals who care for them. One review of the importance of managing this transition noted that even in situations when the need was long anticipated, for example, for children with phenylketonuria (PKU), the response has still fallen short (Scriver and Lee, 2004).

Table 2-3 highlights characteristics of child and adolescent health that may affect the transition from pediatric to adult care for children with serious chronic conditions. To the extent that young people in transition lose health insurance through a parent's work-based coverage or under Medicaid, the shift from pediatric to adult care may create additional complications and risks. Medicaid covers a range of special services for children that are not usually covered for adults and that may be particularly important for children with severely debilitating rare conditions.

For many serious chronic conditions that begin at birth or in childhood, children's hospitals usually have a depth of expertise and multidisciplinary inpatient and outpatient care coordination that will not be matched by other medical centers that treat adults (IOM, 2007). Treatment of serious, chronic, rare conditions often involves multiple specialties such as medical genetics, neurology, gastroenterology, psychiatry, endocrinology, and physical therapy. Particularly for conditions that still often result in death in early adulthood, the adult center may have no specialists with experience treating those conditions.

Recognizing the complexities of and deficiencies in chronic care coordination generally, the American College of Physicians (ACP, 2004) has followed the American Academy of Pediatrics (AAP, 2002) in endorsing the concept of the medical home as a centerpiece for medical care and other coordination. In principle, the implementation of this concept would sup-

TABLE 2-3 Characteristics of Child and Adolescent Health That May Affect the Complexity of Health Care Transitions

Simpler Transition	More Complex Transition
Single health condition	Multiple health conditions
Low risk of future health problems	High risk of future health problems
No dependence on medical equipment	Reliance on life-sustaining medical equipment
Rare acute illness, medically stable	Frequent acute episodes, medically unstable
Few medications	Multiple medications, medication problems
No cognitive impairments	Profound mental retardation
No physical impairments	Serious physical impairments
Mentally healthy	Mentally ill
No behavioral concerns	Serious behavioral concerns

SOURCE: IOM, 2007 (adapted from Kelly et al., 2002).

port smooth transitions from pediatric to adult care for children with rare conditions.

IMPACT OF RARE DISEASES ON PATIENTS, FAMILIES, AND COMMUNITIES

I found that families don't have feelings. . . . Individuals do. My feelings about this were different from my wife's, and those are different from my daughter's. Everyone has their own, very individual experience. That has had an important impact on how our family has dealt with all of it. It's something that all families need to recognize when they are going through a shared experience like this. Just because you feel or react one way, doesn't mean your wife or children are experiencing the same thing in the same way. It was quite a thing to realize.

Hollaway, 2007

Rare diseases take their toll on all involved, from affected individuals and their families and friends, to the health professionals who care for them, to their communities, and the larger society. Many rare diseases result in premature death of infants and young children or are fatal in early adulthood. Such premature deaths can have lifelong effects on parents, siblings, grandparents, and others close to a family. Frequently, rare conditions produce devastating long-term functional, physical, and mental disabilities that strain families' emotional and economic resources. Even for rare conditions that are less severe, the isolation, the uncertainty about the course of the disease, and the frequent lack of effective treatments can have a significant impact.

Just as rare conditions vary, individual and family experiences with debilitating or life-threatening illness clearly vary—as do their responses. The effects of rare conditions on patients and families and their responses are often shaped by socioeconomic status, including differences in income and education. Better outcomes may be linked to medical and nonmedical actions that take such differences in financial and nonfinancial resources into account. Patient and family values also vary. Advocacy groups and educators encourage health care professionals to respect these values as they help patients and families understand what they are facing and make decisions about care and treatment.

High and burdensome costs are not unique to rare diseases, but a number of factors can push patient, family, and societal costs higher for rare conditions than for more common ones. The search for an accurate diagnosis can be not only time-consuming but also expensive. Medications developed specifically for rare conditions can be extraordinarily expensive, costing tens or even hundreds of thousands of dollars per year. Many rare conditions are diagnosed in childhood and then affect individuals for decades. Many individuals require extensive, long-term supportive care that is not covered by Medicare or private health plans, although Medicaid may cover such services for those who qualify. Even for relatively well-off individuals and families, the expenses associated with life with a rare disease can be a significant burden.

For both individuals and family members, the economic impact of rare diseases extends to lost productivity, lost wages, or the inability to find manageable work with flexible leave, health insurance, and other key benefits. Notwithstanding laws against discrimination based on disability or genetic information (notably the Genetic Information Nondiscrimination Act of 2008, P.L. 110-233), employers may fear the consequences of hiring a person with evident health problems and may take health (including the health of an employee's family members) into account when making hiring or layoff decisions. For small employers, a single health plan member with extraordinary medical costs can lead to unaffordable premiums for the entire group of employees. As described in Chapter 6, if it survives calls for its repeal, the Patient Protection and Affordable Care Act of 2010 (P.L. 111-148) should make access to insurance easier for many people with rare conditions and should limit certain restrictions on coverage, for example, a lifetime cap on benefits.

> *I did not choose this work as my career; the vocation was bestowed on me more than 14 years ago when my two children were diagnosed with a genetic disease called pseudoxanthoma elasticum.*
>
> Terry, 2009

The physical, emotional, and financial impact of a rare disease on individuals and families has motivated many of them to try, in turn, to have an impact on the disease and others affected by it. They have joined together to form support and advocacy organizations—some focused on individual conditions, others encompassing a number of related conditions, and yet others such as NORD and the Genetic Alliance acting as umbrella organizations and advocates. Although not focused solely on rare conditions, the Genetic Alliance convenes a range of activities to help rare disease and other groups develop, function effectively, and collaborate. NORD likewise provides assistance to rare disease groups, including newly organized groups.

Some groups (e.g., the Vasculitis Foundations, which was founded in 1986 as the Wegener's Granulomatosis Association) have moved from a concentration on a single condition to a focus on a group of related conditions, some of which previously had not had an organized voice. Such movement reflects both the biological reality that knowledge about one condition may be more generally relevant and the organizational reality that consolidation can bring operational efficiencies and greater public recognition (see, e.g., Hoffman, 2006).

Many advocacy organizations take on multiple roles, including providing information, supporting patients and families in obtaining needed clinical and other services, offering emotional support, educating clinicians, shaping public policy, and promoting research. Patients, families, and advocacy groups have been a driving force in public policy. Notably, they pressed for the passage of the Orphan Drug Act and the creation of the Office of Rare Diseases Research at NIH. They likewise were active in working for passage of the Genetic Information Nondiscrimination Act and creation of the compassionate allowances program that allows people with a number of rare conditions to qualify quickly for Social Security Disability Insurance (see Chapter 6). Some rare disease groups and their umbrella organizations argue that efforts to influence public policy should take this broad approach rather than focus on funding or other policies aimed at individual rare diseases (see, e.g., Farmer, 2009; Terry, 2010).

As is true for organizations associated with common diseases such as breast cancer or cancer generally, rare disease groups often aim to engage and have an impact on the broader community through public awareness and fundraising efforts. Walks, runs, bike races, telethons, celebrity appearances, and other events involve people in highly visible activities that draw attention to rare conditions and the toll they take. In addition, NORD and other groups promote awareness of rare diseases generally, including through activities associated with Rare Diseases Day.

Of particular relevance for this report, individuals, families, and advocacy groups have also mobilized to promote the study of rare diseases and the development of products to treat these diseases. In some cases, research is the primary focus of advocacy organizations. Although groups may focus mainly on raising money for research and advocating for more public funding for research, some take more active roles. For example, they may work with researchers by organizing group members to participate in clinical studies, provide personal data for natural history studies, contribute tissue samples, and volunteer in other ways (see, e.g., Farmer, 2009; Frohnmayer and Frohnmayer, 2009; Terry, 2009). They also can direct research to issues of most concern to patients and families (Nijsten and Bergstresser, 2010). The Office of Rare Diseases Research at NIH has made involvement of advocacy groups an important feature of the Rare Diseases Clinical Research Network.

Organizational strategies and agendas for supporting research vary depending on the state of knowledge, the organization's financial resources, the concerns of organizational founders, and other factors. As discussed further in Chapters 4 and 5 and Appendix F, some patient organizations have promoted partnerships with industry and public agencies and devised new models of "venture philanthropy" to bridge the gulf between basic research findings and approved therapies (see, e.g., IOM, 2008, 2009b; Kelley, 2009; Ashlock, 2010).

In sum, rare diseases have a profound impact on patients and families, but patients and families, in turn, have an impact on the world around them when they organize with others to inform their communities, influence public policy, and stimulate research. Sometimes separately but also in concert, rare disease organizations and their umbrella organizations have worked together on a broad agenda that includes funding for research and technological innovations that will identify the mechanisms of rare diseases and translate these findings into studies that ultimately lead to better ways to prevent, diagnose, and treat these diseases. As this report illustrates, the confluence of scientific advances and policy initiatives provides new opportunities to accelerate this progress.

3

Regulatory Framework for Drugs for Rare Diseases

Many people think of FDA as the judge—the agency that reviews the data and either gives a thumbs up or a thumbs down to each application. If it were only so easy. Before FDA can make any decision, we have to figure out what it means for a product to be safe and effective . . . we have to determine the right standards to apply.

Margaret Hamburg,
Commissioner of Food and Drugs, 2010

As highlighted by its commissioner, the work of the Food and Drug Administration (FDA) involves complex judgments about how the agency should fulfill its multiple, complex responsibilities. One area of complexity involves judgments about what evidence is sufficient to support the agency's approval of medicines intended for people with rare diseases. More broadly, both FDA and Congress face complicated assessments and, often, a shortage of definitive information when they weigh the potential for a policy to promote the public health by encouraging innovation and access to new therapies against the potential for that policy to expose the public to unsafe or ineffective products.

Certain regulatory requirements undoubtedly lead pharmaceutical companies to put aside some drug development efforts that they might otherwise initiate or continue. Generating the evidence to support approval of a drug is costly and time-consuming for companies, and the potential always exists that pivotal clinical studies will not support safety or efficacy. In addition, the way requirements are implemented may lead companies to put aside some potentially beneficial, innovative products, for example, if they expect or encounter difficulties in obtaining answers to questions or advice on trial design or if the review of their applications for approval of a product is slow or inconsistent across FDA review divisions. When companies consider regulatory costs and uncertainties in addition to the expected size of the market, candidate drugs that could meet the needs of small populations may be particularly vulnerable.

Recognizing that regulations to protect the public's health may also create barriers to market entry for new drugs and medical devices, Congress has created a variety of policies to encourage the development and speed the evaluation of innovative products to meet serious unmet health needs. A leading example is the Orphan Drug Act (P.L. 97-414), which provides protection from competition (i.e., exclusive marketing rights), tax credits for certain clinical development expenses, grant support, and other incentives for sponsors to develop drugs for people with rare diseases. Sponsors are usually for-profit pharmaceutical or biotechnology companies, but not-for-profit research organizations and even state agencies have occasionally sponsored applications for the designation and approval of an orphan drug. For example, the California Department of Health Services created the product, conducted the clinical trials, and received approval to market botulism immune globulin (BabyBIG) for treatment of infant botulism, a rare condition caused by *Clostridium botulinum* (Masiello and Epstein, 2003; Arnon, 2007). Development of the drug was supported by an FDA orphan products grant.

Policies on orphan drug development operate within the broader framework of FDA regulations. This chapter, therefore, begins by reviewing the basics of drug and biological product regulation before discussing policies to encourage the development of drugs for small populations, specifically the Orphan Drug Act of 1983. The latter discussion also compares patent protections with protections provided by market exclusivity as defined below and presents summary data on orphan drug designations and approvals. After a review of concerns about the adequacy of agency resources in relation to its responsibilities, the chapter concludes with recommendations that focus on the consistency and quality of FDA guidance and review of orphan drugs and the need to ensure that product development research funded by the National Institutes of Health (NIH) is designed and conducted to meet FDA requirements.

Because the regulation of medical devices differs significantly from that for drugs, Chapter 7 examines the regulation of medical devices and policies to encourage the development of devices for small populations. That discussion covers policies on diagnostic devices, including policies on the codevelopment of drugs and companion diagnostics and policies on combination products (e.g., those combining a drug and a device).

GENERAL FRAMEWORK FOR THE REGULATION
OF DRUGS AND BIOLOGICS

This report generally uses the term drug to encompass both pharmaceuticals and therapeutic biological products. Many policies to promote the development of products for people with rare diseases apply to both types of products. This section discusses the basic regulation of drugs defined as chemical compounds, the regulation of biological products, and other general regulatory provisions (e.g., those intended to speed the approval of drugs for serious and life-threatening conditions) that may have particular relevance for orphan drugs.

Basics of Drug Approval

When Congress passed the Federal Food, Drug, and Cosmetic Act in 1938, it prohibited the misbranding of drugs (i.e., the making of false therapeutic claims) and required their labeling with directions for safe use (Swann, 2003). It also required sponsors of new drugs to notify FDA prior to their being placed on the market and to submit certain safety data to support their approval by the agency for marketing in interstate commerce. In 1962, Congress added a requirement that FDA assess the effectiveness of new drugs before approving them, gave FDA increased authority over clinical studies used to support applications for approval, and established policies to promote good manufacturing practices.[1] In 1984, Congress defined a route for the approval of generic copies of previously approved brand-name drugs by eliminating the requirement that sponsors of generic drugs conduct their own clinical trials of safety and effectiveness. This action made the development of generic drugs much more attractive to industry. The Center for Drug Evaluation and Research (CDER) is responsible for administering these policies.

For a sponsor that is ready to initiate clinical studies of a promising drug, whether for a common or a rare condition, the first formal step is to file an Investigational New Drug (IND) application. An IND application describes available information about the drug, for example, data from already conducted animal and other studies indicating that it is reasonable to initiate studies with human participants. The application also provides detailed information about the proposed initial clinical trial strategy. As described below, FDA has various mechanisms that allow consultation

---

[1] This report defines efficacy as the achievement of desired results in controlled trials and effectiveness as the achievement of desired results in usual clinical settings. FDA statutes and regulations use the term effectiveness to describe positive results reported in clinical trials, although FDA review documents often employ the term efficacy rather than effectiveness to refer to clinical data used in approving a new drug.

to assist sponsors in designing and conducting trials that will meet FDA standards. In many cases, a sponsor will seek assistance from FDA on the preparation of an IND application. Sponsors are required to keep the FDA informed of changes in trial strategy.

If the sponsor concludes that the results of its clinical trials will support FDA approval of a drug, then the sponsor files a New Drug Application (NDA), which FDA must review and approve before a drug can legally be marketed. For generic drugs, the requirement is for approval of an Abbreviated New Drug Application (ANDA). Sponsors may file supplemental applications for approval of new indications for a drug, new formulations, and other purposes.

To secure FDA approval to market a drug, sponsors must provide substantial evidence of the drug's safety and effectiveness for its intended use. As described in statute (21 USC 355(d)), substantial evidence

> means evidence consisting of adequate and well-controlled investigations, including clinical investigations, by experts qualified by scientific training and experience to evaluate the effectiveness of the drug involved, on the basis of which it could fairly and responsibly be concluded by such experts that the drug will have the effect it purports or is represented to have under the conditions of use prescribed, recommended, or suggested in the labeling or proposed labeling thereof. If the Secretary determines, based on relevant science, that data from one adequate and well-controlled clinical investigation and confirmatory evidence (obtained prior to or after such investigation) are sufficient to establish effectiveness, the Secretary may consider such data and evidence to constitute substantial evidence for purposes of the preceding sentence.

For many years, FDA interpreted the plural term "investigations" in the statute as requiring at least two phase III clinical studies to support new drug approval, with some rare case-by-case exceptions (e.g., drugs for a life-threatening or severely debilitating disease when one large, well-designed, multicenter study showed robust results) (53 Fed. Reg. 41516, 41521). In the FDA Modernization Act of 1997 (P.L. 105-115), Congress added a sentence clarifying that data from one adequate and well-controlled study, together with confirmatory evidence obtained before or after that study, can constitute "substantial evidence" of effectiveness for any new drug.

FDA regulations specify further details about characteristics of adequate and well-controlled studies (21 CFR 314.126; see also CDER-CBER, 1998). Summarized, they state that studies and study reports should

- provide a clear statement of purpose;
- permit a valid comparison of the experimental group with a control group;

- employ suitable methods to assign study and control groups and otherwise to minimize bias;
- use clear, reliable methods to define and assess responses of research participants; and
- employ appropriate methods to analyze study results.

Generally, FDA has recognized the following types of controls in clinical trials: placebo concurrent control; dose-comparison concurrent control; no-treatment concurrent control; active treatment concurrent control; and historical control. FDA may also accept results from uncontrolled trials as corroborating evidence. In principle, the agency may waive certain of the requirements. As discussed below, it has sometimes done so in approving orphan drugs.

In addition to regulations, FDA has developed a number of documents that provide additional guidance to industry on the design and conduct of trials to support approval. For example, the agency recently issued one draft guidance document on the use of adaptive designs for clinical trials and another on noninferiority clinical trials.[2]

Some drugs currently on the market have never been approved by the FDA because they were on the market before enactment in 1938 of the Federal Food, Drug, and Cosmetic Act. In recent years, FDA has moved to require companies that sell such drugs to seek approval (Derbis et al., 2008). Colchicine (which is discussed in Box 3-3 and in Chapter 6) is an example of a previously unapproved drug that was approved for a common use and for an orphan indication in 2009.

---

[2] The draft guidance defines an *adaptive design clinical study* "as a study that includes a prospectively planned opportunity for modification of one or more specified aspects of the study design and hypotheses based on analysis of data (usually interim data) from subjects in the study. Analyses of the accumulating study data are performed at prospectively planned timepoints" (CDER-CBER, 2010a, lines 66-69). The guidance notes that changes based on such analysis "may make the studies more efficient (e.g., shorter duration, fewer patients), more likely to demonstrate an effect of the drug if one exists, or more informative (e.g., by providing broader dose-response information)" (lines 38-40). A working group of the Pharmaceutical Research and Manufacturers of America has also developed materials on adaptive design, including training courses and white papers (see http://www.biopharmnet.com/doc/doc12004-01.html).

The other CDER-CBER guidance document explains that *noninferiority trials* involve comparison of an investigational drug with an active treatment (an active control). They seek to demonstrate "that any difference between the two treatments is small enough to allow a conclusion that the new drug has at least some effect or, in many cases, an effect that is not too much smaller than the active control" (CDER-CBER, 2010b, p. 2). Such trials are more difficult to interpret because they depend on a result that is not directly measured (i.e., whether the active treatment had the effect expected). They may be used because investigators consider a placebo- or no-treatment controlled trial to be unethical or because they want to compare the efficacy of active treatments.

Regulation of Biologics

Biological products are made from living organisms and may be composed of cells or tissues or of sugars, proteins, or nucleic acids or complex combinations of these substances. Examples of such products include vaccines, blood-based clotting factors, antitoxins, therapeutic proteins, and monoclonal antibodies. The regulatory status of this diverse set of products is not easily summarized, and the following discussion simplifies or ignores some details.

For purposes of this report, the main points about the regulation of biologics are that most biologics are also drugs and as such are generally held to the same standards of safety and efficacy as apply to nonbiologic drugs. In addition, the incentives of the Orphan Drug Act (360bb(a)(1)) are available to sponsors of biologics. Most biologics are approved on the basis of a Biologics License Application (BLA) as provided for in the Public Health Service (PHS) Act, although "by historical quirk" certain biologics have been approved as drugs under the Food, Drug, and Cosmetic Act (Schact and Thomas, 2009). (The location of regulatory authority in the PHS act reflects the early regulatory history of biologics, particularly that related to rules to ensure the safety of vaccines.) Title VII of the Patient Protection and Affordable Care Act of 2010 (P.L. 111-148) revised the definition of biological product under the PHS act to include all proteins (except for chemically synthesized polypeptides). As described later in this chapter, the law also created a pathway to FDA approval for "biosimilar" biologics that is analogous to that created for generic drugs.

In 2003, FDA transferred responsibility for review and approval of most therapeutic biologics from the Center for Biologics Evaluation and Research (CBER) to CDER. The types of products transferred to CDER include most proteins intended for therapeutic use (e.g., interferons, enzymes); agents that modify immune system response (other than vaccines and allergenic products); monoclonal antibodies; and certain other products intended to alter production of blood cells (FDA, 2009b). CBER continues to oversee vaccines, antitoxins, antivenins, venoms, allergenic products (e.g., allergy tests and shots), blood, and blood products. Thus, depending on the category, some orphan biologics are regulated by CDER and others by CBER.

Treatment Use of Investigational and Certain Other Drugs

Since the 1980s, Congress and FDA have created procedures to allow treatment use (i.e., other than research use) of investigational drugs. Because many patients with rare diseases have debilitating and life-threatening conditions for which no approved drugs are available and because the clinical trial process and drug approval process are lengthy, these patients and their families may be particularly anxious for access to a drug that has enough promise to be under investigation in a clinical trial. A major concern is that "treatment use" policies and their application should not jeopardize patient safety or impede the conduct of research to assess a drug's safety and efficacy.

In 2009, FDA issued revised regulations on treatment use of investigational drugs. In general, the agency allows expanded access in three categories of patient populations: individual patients, intermediate-sized groups, and large groups.[3] Box 3-1 summarizes the general determinations necessary to approve such use and also includes those that apply specifically to individual patient use. The conditions that must be satisfied in order to justify expanded use become more extensive as the size of the population to be treated increases. Although the rules provide that treatment use of an investigational drug should not compromise clinical study of the drug, this criterion may be hard to meet for a drug aimed at a very small population with few potential research participants.

Speeding and Facilitating Review and Approval of New Drugs

In the decades after Congress required FDA review of efficacy as well as safety and as the volume and complexity of applications for the approval of new drugs grew, pharmaceutical companies, patient and consumer advocacy groups, and others complained that the length of time for reviews and decisions was excessive and costly. To provide additional resources for FDA and to speed reviews, the Prescription Drug User Fee Act of 1992 (P.L. 102-571) and subsequent renewals and revisions have authorized FDA to collect user fees from companies seeking approval of new drugs. FDA in consultation with industry, consumer groups, and others established specific performance goals related to review times, sponsor requests for meetings, responses to sponsor appeals of decisions, and other processes. FDA strongly encourages sponsors of drugs for rare diseases to seek pre-IND meetings to discuss development strategy.

Sponsors of orphan drugs are exempt from user fees, but they benefit generally from the additional resources the fees provide to FDA. The fees collected by the agency have allowed it to hire hundreds of additional

---

[3] In addition, the regulations provide for the use of the expanded access mechanism to allow a physician to provide an approved drug that is subject to a Risk Evaluation and Mitigation Strategy (REMS) to a patient who is not otherwise eligible. The expanded access provision might be invoked, for example, when a REMS restricts an approved drug to patients who have certain lab test results and a particular patient does not meet that criterion. In commentary on the rules, FDA stated that it would monitor the impact of the rule on expanded access to drugs that are covered by a REMS.

BOX 3-1
Options for Patients to Obtain Access to Investigational
Drugs When the Primary Purpose Is to Diagnose,
Monitor, or Treat a Patient's Disease or Condition

To permit treatment of a patient with an investigational drug under an expanded access program, FDA "must determine that:

(1) The patient or patients to be treated have a serious or immediately life-threatening disease or condition, and there is no comparable or satisfactory alternative therapy to diagnose, monitor, or treat the disease or condition;

(2) The potential patient benefit justifies the potential risks of the treatment use and those potential risks are not unreasonable in the context of the disease or condition to be treated; and

(3) Providing the investigational drug for the requested use will not interfere with the initiation, conduct, or completion of clinical investigations that could support marketing approval of the expanded access use or otherwise compromise the potential development of the expanded access use."

Individual patient use, including in emergencies

FDA may permit an investigational drug to be used for the treatment of an individual patient by a licensed physician. . . . (1) The physician must determine that the probable risk to the person from the investigational drug is not greater than the probable risk from the disease or condition; and (2) FDA must determine that the patient cannot obtain the drug under another IND or protocol. . . . *Safeguards* (1) Treatment is generally limited to a single course of therapy for a specified duration unless FDA expressly authorizes multiple courses or chronic therapy. (2) At the conclusion of treatment, the licensed physician or sponsor must provide FDA with a written summary of the results of the expanded access use, including adverse effects. (3) FDA may require sponsors to monitor an individual patient expanded access use if the use is for an extended duration. (4) When a significant number of similar individual patient expanded access requests have been submitted, FDA may ask the sponsor to submit an IND or protocol. . . .

SOURCE: 74 Fed. Reg. 40900. (Note: this excerpt excludes sections on options involving use by intermediate-sized and large groups.)

---

employees, but the adequacy of FDA resources to fulfill its responsibilities continues to be a major concern as discussed below (see, e.g., FDA Science Board, 2007; IOM, 2007; GAO, 2009a). For drugs that are intended for use with serious or life-threatening conditions for which unmet needs for treatment exist, FDA has instituted additional options—fast track status, accelerated approval, and priority review—to speed reviews and provide more extensive and timely guidance to sponsors about the nature of the evidence that is needed to support approval (FDA, 2009a; Schact and Thomas, 2009). Sponsors of orphan drugs frequently qualify for these mechanisms, and one analysis indicated that applications for orphan drugs were more likely than other applications to have done so (Seoane-Vazquez et al., 2008).

For applications that qualify for *fast track status*, companies submit modules of an NDA on an ongoing basis for a "rolling review" by FDA as the modules are submitted. This allows more frequent consultation with FDA on various issues related to the entire application for approval, including sections on preclinical studies; early phase I and phase II clinical trial results; and phase III studies. Most important, as the final clinical trials are completed and the results are reviewed, all of the other modules of the NDA are essentially completed.

In some cases, another option is *accelerated approval,* which allows the use of surrogate endpoints that are not considered well established but that are determined to be "reasonably likely to predict clinical benefit." FDA rules define surrogate endpoint as "a laboratory or physical sign that is used in therapeutic trials as a substitute for a clinically meaningful endpoint that is a direct measure of how a patient feels, functions, or survives and that is expected to predict the effect of the therapy" (57 Fed. Reg. 13234 at 13235; see also Fleming, 2005). FDA then requires postapproval studies to develop further evidence about benefits and risks based on clinical outcomes.

According to a recent study by the Government Accountability Office (GAO), FDA used the accelerated approval process to approve 90 drugs based on surrogate endpoints between 1992 and November 20, 2008 (GAO, 2009a). Of these 90 drugs, 79 were for cancer, HIV/AIDS, or inhalation anthrax.

The successful and timely completion of the required postapproval studies has proved challenging. Products can remain on the market for an extended period without conclusive evidence of safety and clinical benefit (Fleming, 2005).

The GAO report expressed concern that several required postmarketing studies remained open and that FDA did not have a satisfactory system for monitoring study progress. At the time of the GAO study, no drugs that had gone through accelerated approval had been withdrawn from the market based on the results of follow-up studies. Since then, one company has announced the withdrawal of such a drug (gemtuzumab ozogamicin for injection [Mylotarg]) after a postapproval study failed to demonstrate benefit (Pfizer, 2010). FDA announced that it would seek the withdrawal of one drug based on failure to complete required studies (Karst, 2010), and it could seek withdrawal for another drug after postmarket study findings did not confirm the preapproval studies (Stein, 2010).

For *priority reviews,* FDA sets a goal of completing application reviews within 6 months compared to a standard review goal of 10 months. For orphan drug applications involving new molecular entities, a recent analysis reported that the proportion with priority review status increased from 35 percent for the period 2000 to 2002 to 50 percent in the period 2006-2008; for orphan products identified as "significant biologics," the corresponding increase was from 17 to 67 percent (Tufts Center, 2010). In addition to granting priority review status directly, FDA may also award priority review vouchers when approving a drug for a neglected tropical disease; such vouchers can be used to obtain priority review for a subsequent drug application and can also be sold or otherwise transferred to another sponsor (21 USC 360n).

Another mechanism to facilitate review and, equally important, reduce regulatory uncertainty is the *Special Protocol Assessment*. It allows FDA to provide expedited assessment of the adequacy of certain clinical trial protocols and to reach agreements with sponsors on the design and size of trials to support efficacy claims in marketing applications (CDER-CBER, 2002b). Once an agreement is reached, it generally cannot be changed by FDA or the sponsor. Normally, Special Protocol Assessments are available only after the end of phase II trials. However, for sponsors of drugs for rare conditions, they can be arranged after the end of phase I trials (Anne Pariser, Associate Director for Rare Diseases, FDA, May 14, 2010, personal communication).

Requirements That May Apply After Marketing Approval

When FDA grants approval to a sponsor to market a drug, it may specify certain postmarketing requirements. As noted above, postmarketing studies to develop additional evidence about benefits and risks are required for products approved under accelerated approval procedures. In addition, under the Pediatric Research Equity Act of 2003, FDA may require that companies conduct pediatric studies of drugs, but orphan drugs are explicitly exempt from these requirements. As discussed later in this chapter, sponsors may also voluntarily commit to undertake specified postmarketing studies, including pediatric studies requested by FDA under the Best Pharmaceuticals for Children Act.

As provided under the Food and Drug Administration Amendments Act of 2007, FDA may also require a postmarketing Risk Evaluation and Mitigation Strategy (REMS) if it determines that such a mechanism is necessary to ensure that the benefits of a drug outweigh its risks. A REMS might include (1) a medication guide to be distributed to patients with each prescription; (2) a communication plan for educating health care providers; or (3) one or more elements to ensure safe use (CDER-CBER, 2009). The latter might include special physician training or certification, certification of dispensing pharmacies, provision of additional information for physicians, limitation of availability to patients in specified settings, patient monitoring and agreement to certain terms of use, and inclusion of patients in a registry. Such registries are not considered research, but postmarketing studies may be conducted using the information collected (e.g., clinical and laboratory data or outcomes data).

The committee has no comprehensive information on the extent to which orphan drugs are approved with postmarketing study requirements or commitments or with REMS requirements. Later in this chapter, Box 3-3 includes examples of orphan drugs approved with postmarketing study provisions.

Access to Information on Clinical Data to Support FDA Approvals

In response to 1996 and subsequent legislation, CDER has begun to post information on the basis for its judgments about new drugs, including those approved as orphan drugs. These descriptions include assessments by agency reviewers of the quality and results of the clinical trials submitted to support approval. Information from these reviews is presented in the next section of this chapter to illustrate the range of evidence that FDA may accept in particular cases. FDA now also makes available online the staff reviews and company presentations provided to its expert advisory committees when those groups have been asked for advice on a product application. Transcripts of the meetings may provide further information, for example, in responses to questions about the materials submitted. Staff analyses (and associated discussion) may also be available for drugs that are considered during an advisory committee meeting. Reviews for generic drugs are generally not publicly available.[4]

Notwithstanding FDA actions to provide more details about the basis for its approval of a new drug, many details about drug trials are treated as confidential and not made public by FDA. As discussed in Chapter 5,

---

[4] For example, in 2009, FDA approved generic chenodeoxycholic acid as an orphan drug for the treatment of gallstones. The drug was approved for this indication in 1983 as one of the first orphan drugs but was subsequently withdrawn from the market. A summary of the 2009 FDA review, including any data on the safety and effectiveness generated since 1983, is not public, although it might be obtained eventually through an inquiry under the Freedom of Information Act. In 2004 and 2007, different companies received orphan drug designations for the drug's use to treat cerebrotendinous xanthomatosis (CTX). (Orphan drugs designations and approvals are found at http://www.accessdata.fda.gov/scripts/opdlisting/oopd/index.cfm.) Advocates for patients with CTX noted the effort invested in obtaining the 2009 FDA approval (but did not note that the approval was for gallstones) and emphasized that the company distributing the drug "has committed to ensuring that all CTX patients will have access" to the drug through a specialty pharmacy (CTXinfo.org, 2010). That company received a new orphan designation in 2010 for the CTX indication.

FDA does not make public its negative decisions or the clinical assessments on which they are based, except when staff presentations to advisory committees detail negative assessments of the information presented by sponsors. Securities and Exchange Commission regulations for publicly traded companies may require that they publicly report failed trials and similar information that is relevant to investors or potential investors. These reports typically do not have the specificity found in an FDA review or a top-tier peer-reviewed medical journal (Fisher, 2002).

Some information about studies undertaken to support FDA approval may also be found elsewhere. In the 1997 FDA Modernization Act, Congress required sponsors of drugs intended for serious or life-threatening conditions to submit basic information about certain clinical trials to a publicly accessible database—what is now ClinicalTrials.gov (CDER-CBER, 2002a).[5] The database became available online in 2000; as of April 2010, it included information on more than 89,000 trials (see http://clinicaltrials. gov/ct2/info/about). The Food and Drug Administration Amendments Act of 2007 required sponsors or principal investigators to submit to Clinical-Trials.gov "basic results" of certain studies performed in support of drugs and devices that FDA has approved (Section 801 of P.L. 110-85; see also Tse et al., 2009).

In 2010, as part of a "transparency" initiative at FDA, the agency published several draft proposals for comment (FDA, 2010b). Among the proposals are that the agency would disclose "when a drug or device is being studied and for what indication, when an application for a new drug or device has been submitted or withdrawn by the sponsor, whether there was a significant safety concern associated with the drug or device that caused the sponsor to withdraw an application, and why the agency did not approve an application" (Asamoah and Sharfstein, 2010, p. 3; see also Chapter 5). Another would allow the agency to explain that an orphan drug may represent an important therapeutic advance even if the application for the drug has been abandoned or withdrawn by the sponsor for business or other reasons. In general, the provision of more information about the reasons that drugs that are not approved or are withdrawn before approval would be particularly valuable to guide possible further investigation of drugs proposed for the treatment of rare diseases.

---

[5] The act required the Secretary of Health and Human Services (through the Director of the National Institutes of Health) "to establish, maintain, and operate a data bank of information on clinical trials of drugs for serious or life threatening diseases and conditions." If a sponsor identifies "a specific instance when disclosure of information would interfere with enrollment of subjects in a clinical investigation," FDA will consider a request to exclude that information (CDER-CBER, 2002a).

REGULATORY POLICY TO PROMOTE INNOVATION AND DEVELOPMENT OF ORPHAN DRUGS AND BIOLOGICS

SECTION 1. (a) This Act may be cited as the "Orphan Drug Act". (b) The Congress finds that

(1) there are many diseases and conditions, such as Huntington's disease, myoclonus, ALS (Lou Gehrig's disease), Tourette syndrome, and muscular dystrophy which affect such small numbers of individuals residing in the United States that the diseases and conditions are considered rare in the United States;

(2) adequate drugs for many of such diseases and conditions have not been developed;

(3) drugs for these diseases and conditions are commonly referred to as "orphan drugs";

(4) because so few individuals are affected by any one rare disease or condition, a pharmaceutical company which develops an orphan drug may reasonably expect the drug to generate relatively small sales in comparison to the cost of developing the drug and consequently to incur a financial loss;

(5) there is reason to believe that some promising orphan drugs will not be developed unless changes are made in the applicable Federal laws to reduce the costs of developing such drugs and to provide financial incentives to develop such drugs; and

(6) it is in the public interest to provide such changes and incentives for the development of orphan drugs.

Preamble to the Orphan Drug Act (P.L. 97-414)

As discussed in Chapter 1, enactment of the Orphan Drug Act in 1983 followed several years of effort by policy makers and advocates for people with rare diseases to understand and devise appropriate responses to industry reluctance to incur the costs of discovering and developing drugs for small or otherwise economically unattractive markets. Early analyses of the problem tended to refer to drugs of limited commercial value with later descriptions referring to orphan drugs for rare diseases (see, e.g., Interagency Task Force, 1979). Except in its title, the 1983 law does not use the term orphan drug.

The initial statutory definition of rare disease or condition referred to "any disease or condition which occurs so infrequently in the United States that there is no reasonable expectation that the cost of developing and making available in the United States a drug for such disease or condition will be recovered from sales in the United States of such drug" (see Sec. 526(a)(2) of the original act). After FDA and companies found it difficult to apply this definition, Congress in 1984 changed to the definition to specify that a rare disease or condition is one that affects "less than 200,000 persons" in the United States or affects "more than 200,000 in the United States and for which there is no reasonable expectation that the cost of developing and making available in the United States a drug for such disease or condition will be recovered from sales in the United States" (21 USC 360bb). A drug may also qualify for orphan status when it is intended for a subset of individuals with a particular disease or condition as long as the subset is medically plausible and affects fewer than 200,000 people in the United States. A number of orphan designations and approvals involve such subsets, for example, patients with a recurrent cancer or with a condition that is not responsive to standard treatments.[6]

Because rare is defined in terms of the U.S. population or market, the incentives of the Orphan Drug Act also apply to drugs for conditions that are uncommon in this country but may be very common worldwide. For example, in 2009, FDA approved artemether-lumefantrine (Coartem, NDA 22-268) as an orphan drug for treatment of acute, uncomplicated malaria, which is rare in the United States but not in many developing countries.[7]

Incentives for Orphan Drug Development

The Orphan Drug Act covers drugs and biologics. Except for the orphan products grants program, the incentives do not extend to medical devices (see Chapter 7). Box 3-2 summarizes the primary incentives for drug development provided by the Orphan Drug Act and other laws.

In economic terms, the Orphan Drug Act in combination with other FDA policies offers both "push" and "pull" incentives (see, e.g., Reich, 2000; Grabowski, 2005). Push incentives, which are intended to subsidize or lower research and other development-related costs, include research tax credits, orphan products grants, consultation with staff on acceptable research designs, and exemption from user fees. Pull incentives include the market exclusivity provision as well as the mechanisms to speed and facilitate review of drugs that were described earlier. The provision for

---

[6] In the case of antibacterial agents, FDA has noted in discussions with the Infectious Diseases Society of America that a disease or condition should not be confused with an etiologic agent and that a drug to treat a subset should not also be an appropriate treatment for all those with the condition (Tollefson, 2008). For example, if antibiotic was used to treat people with multidrug-resistant disease and was also used to treat people with disease that was not resistant, then the former group would not be a medically plausible subset. If the disease in question affects fewer than 200,000 people in the United States, then the subset issue is irrelevant.

[7] FDA also awarded the sponsor a transferable priority review voucher for a future product application as authorized by Congress in 2007 to promote the development of drugs for certain tropical diseases. This award drew criticism because the drug, although not previously approved in the United States, had been authorized for marketing in 85 countries, beginning in 1999 (Anderson, 2009).

BOX 3-2
Primary Incentives Provided by the Orphan Drug Act

• Seven years' marketing exclusivity from the date of marketing approval of a drug with an orphan designation. During this period, no other sponsor may obtain approval of the same drug for the same use except under limited circumstances, but FDA may approve a different drug for the same indication. Exclusivity is available to patented as well as unpatentable drugs. (See discussion of patents and exclusivity in a later section.)

• Tax credit of up to 50 percent for qualified expenses for clinical research to support approval of an orphan drug.

• Grants to support clinical development of products for use in rare diseases.

• Exemption (through the FDA Modernization Act of 1997) from several kinds of user fees that are normally charged sponsors. For fiscal year 2010, the fee for an application requiring clinical data was $1,405,500 (or $702,750 if for a supplemental application requiring such data) with different amounts for other fees (74 Fed. Reg. 5524).

• Recommendations from FDA staff to sponsors about nonclinical and clinical studies that would support approval of a drug for a rare disease. Other special assistance, such as accelerated approval or fast track or priority review, may also be available for sponsors of orphan drugs.

---

marketing exclusivity is generally regarded as the most significant incentive under the Orphan Drug Act.

Before sponsors can apply to have a drug approved under the Orphan Drug Act and before sponsors are eligible for incentives such as orphan products grants, they must apply for and receive an orphan designation for the drug from the FDA's Office of Orphan Products Development (OOPD). To obtain a designation, sponsors are expected to describe the drug's proposed use, provide evidence that the prevalence of the target condition or a medically plausible subset of a condition is below 200,000, and justify the drug's promise for the proposed use. If sponsors are relying on the cost recovery rationale, they must submit supporting data related to the cost of their development activities (including the allocation of costs if the research involves more than one indication); costs for past and future production and marketing activities; projections of sales associated with the orphan indication; data on any overseas approvals and sales; and other information.

More than one sponsor can receive an orphan drug designation for the same drug for the same indication. However, except under limited circumstances, only the sponsor that receives the first FDA approval can receive orphan drug marketing exclusivity. A manufacturer may obtain multiple orphan designations and approvals for different indications for the same product.

FDA can revoke an orphan designation if it finds significant inaccuracies or omissions in the data submitted in support of a designation (as authorized at 21 CFR 316.29). In 2007, FDA revoked the designation for a pancreatic enzyme product on the grounds that more accurate data indicated that the target population (people with exocrine pancreatic insufficiency) exceeded 200,000 at the time of designation (Wasserstein and Karst, 2007). (Designation is not affected if the target population grows to exceed 200,000 after designation but before approval.) In addition, if a sponsor fails to produce sufficient quantities of an approved orphan drug, the director of OOPD has authority—never invoked—to withdraw the product's exclusive marketing rights (21 CFR 316.36).

Exclusivity and Patents

The incentives provided by market exclusivity for orphan drugs need to be understood in the context of both patent law and other policies granting exclusivity for drug sponsors. Patent law provides an important means for innovators to protect their inventions or intellectual property from competitors. It gives patent holders the exclusive right to produce, use, or sell the patented invention for a specified period (35 USC 271(a)). Patents are issued by the U.S. Patent and Trademark Office and, under current law, extend for 20 years from the date of submission of the patent application.

By the early 1980s, the research and development process for new drugs combined with the time required for FDA review had reduced the effective patent life for the average new drug to well below the 17 years then available under patent law (Flannery and Hutt, 1985). In the Drug Price Competition and Patent Term Restoration Act of 1984 (P.L. 98-417, widely known as the Hatch-Waxman Act), Congress provided for the restoration of a portion of the patent term consumed by clinical studies and FDA review. In general, patent term restoration is limited to 5 years and an effective period of (postapproval) patent protection of 14 years.

The provisions on patent term restoration were part of a larger bill that established a pathway for FDA to approve generic versions of brand-name drugs. The goals were to make less expensive versions of brand-name drugs more widely available to consumers while still providing incentives for pharmaceutical companies to develop novel drugs (Mossinghoff, 1999;

Glover, 2007). To accomplish the latter objective, the legislation created two new "data exclusivity" rules.

The first exclusivity rule provides that truly innovative drugs—new chemical entities (also called new molecular entities)—receive a 5-year period of data exclusivity, during which the sponsor of a generic drug must submit a full New Drug Application that relies on its own preclinical and clinical data. At the end of 5 years (4, if the generic drug applicant chooses to challenge the innovator's patents), the applicant can submit an ANDA that need only show that its product is the same as, and bioequivalent to, the innovator's product.[8]

The second exclusivity rule provides that other applications for approval that are supported by clinical data (e.g., those involving new formulations of the drug) receive 3 years of exclusivity. Again, during the period of exclusivity, generic versions can be approved only if sponsors provide their own clinical data on safety and efficacy.[9]

In 1997, Congress enacted the Best Pharmaceuticals for Children Act (as part of the FDA Modernization Act) to encourage the testing of pharmaceuticals for children. If a company conducts pediatric studies in response to a written request from FDA and complies with various requirements relating to these studies, the law provides for an extension of 6 months to the exclusivity periods described above. Thus, for example, the 5-year prohibition on the submission of an abbreviated application becomes 5 years and 6 months.

The market exclusivity incentive for orphan drugs is broader than the various types of exclusivity discussed above. During the period of exclusivity, FDA *cannot* approve an application from a different manufacturer

---

[8] A generic product is the same as the innovator product if it has the same active ingredient, route of administration, dosage form, and strength (CDER, 2003). The law permits differences in these characteristics, with prior agency approval, if no clinical data are needed to establish the safety or effectiveness of the generic product. Generally, a generic drug is bioequivalent to the innovator product if there is not a significant difference in the rate and extent of absorption of the drug when administered at the same molar dose of the therapeutic ingredient under similar experimental conditions.

[9] Congress also tied the timing of generic drug approval to certain patents covering the innovator drug. For any unexpired patent that claims the brand drug or a method of using the brand drug, a generic applicant is required to choose between waiting for the patent to expire or challenging the patent (as invalid or not infringed). If the generic applicant chooses to wait, FDA may not approve the generic application until the patent expires. If the generic applicant challenges the patent, then complex patent litigation provisions are triggered. As a practical matter, under these provisions, if the drug is a new chemical entity and the innovator enforces its patent by bringing a lawsuit, the generic application cannot be approved until 7.5 years after approval of the brand drug. In some situations, litigation is still going on at the end of this time. In these cases, FDA may approve the generic drug, and the generic company may market the product, although it markets "at risk" of substantial damages if it loses the patent case.

for the same orphan drug and the same indication—even if that sponsor provides independent clinical data of safety and efficacy. An exception is available if the sponsor who has the orphan drug approval agrees to the additional approval or is found to be unable to supply sufficient quantities of the product.

Another exception is that under rather convoluted regulations, if a competitor demonstrates clinical superiority for its version of the same orphan drug for the same indication, then its version is not considered to be the "same drug." Therefore, it may also be approved with orphan drug exclusivity.[10] At least three products have been approved on the basis of this exception—oral fludarabine phosphate, octreotide acetate (Sandostatin LAR), and histrelin acetate (Supprelin LA) (Karst, 2009b) FDA's regulations describing when one drug is the "same" as another for purposes of orphan drug exclusivity were drafted broadly to provide strong incentives for orphan drug development.

One analysis estimated that orphan drug exclusivity adds approximately 0.8 year of protection from competition beyond that typically provided by patents (Seoane-Vesquez et al., 2008). (The analysis was based on 99 relevant orphan new molecular entities [NMEs] out of a total of 115 compared to 421 relevant nonorphan NMEs out of a total of 520.) The authors of the analysis found that a relatively low percentage of orphan drugs classified as NMEs had a generic competitor enter the market immediately after the expiration of orphan exclusivity. They concluded that generic entry for many drugs was limited not only by orphan exclusivity but also by continuing patent protection as well as the small patient populations and low expected profits.

Program Administration

At FDA, the OOPD is generally responsible for promoting the development of products for rare diseases. Its specific tasks include designating orphan drugs (including reviewing claims about the prevalence of a rare

---

[10] The regulatory language, which was added in the early 1990s, reads as follows: "Same drug means: (i) If it is a drug composed of small molecules, a drug that contains the same active moiety as a previously approved drug and is intended for the same use as the previously approved drug, even if the particular ester or salt (including a salt with hydrogen or coordination bonds) or other noncovalent derivative such as a complex, chelate or clathrate has not been previously approved, except that if the subsequent drug can be shown to be clinically superior to the first drug, it will not be considered to be the same drug. (ii) If it is a drug composed of large molecules (macromolecules), a drug that contains the same principal molecular structural features (but not necessarily all of the same structural features) and is intended for the same use as a previously approved drug, except that, if the subsequent drug can be shown to be clinically superior, it will not be considered to be the same drug" (21 CFR 316.3(b)(13)(i), (ii)).

disease and the promise of a product), administering the orphan products grants program, and disseminating information to the public. Other responsibilities include reviewing and approving applications for the designation of a Humanitarian Use Device and administering the new grants program for pediatric medical device consortia (see Chapter 7). A 2001 study by the Office of the Inspector General of the Department of Health and Human Services concluded that the "Office of Orphan Products Development provides a valuable service to both companies and patients" (OIG, 2001b, p. 2).

As part of its information dissemination activities, the OOPD maintains a website with relevant information, including a database on designated and approved orphan drugs. Other initiatives include

- offering workshops for companies, academics, and others on applying for orphan drug designation;
- analyzing characteristics of orphan drugs, including the nature of rare conditions targeted and the reasons designated drugs do not progress to approval as a basis for identifying possible drugs worth further attention;
- identifying promising candidates for orphan tropical diseases;
- working with other governments, entities, or agencies to harmonize or coordinate policies and procedures internationally; and
- cooperating with the National Institutes of Health to offer a course on the science of small clinical trials.

The OOPD recently posted a database of products that have received orphan status designation (which means that they have been found promising for treating a rare disease) and that also have already been approved by FDA for the treatment of some *other* disease (Goodman, 2010). These products have thus advanced a considerable way through the process of drug development and therefore may be less risky for companies than developing a new drug.

Roles of CDER in Orphan Drug Approval

As is the case for other drugs, CDER is responsible for reviewing and approving NDA applications for orphan drugs. In general, the review divisions of CDER are organized around therapeutic areas such as neurology and gastroenterology.

Recently, FDA announced the creation of a new position within CDER, the Associate Director for Rare Diseases, who will serve as the center's lead person on issues involving orphan drugs and rare diseases. Responsibilities will include

- serving as the primary contact for the rare diseases community;
- assisting developers of drug and biologic products in understanding and following relevant regulatory requirements;
- coordinating the development of policies within CDER for the review an approval of drugs for rare conditions; and
- encouraging collaboration among CDER scientists and clinicians.

The creation of this position is an important development. Realizing its promise will require adequate resources and staff support.

Overview of Orphan Drug Designations and Approvals

Since the beginning of the program, the OOPD has granted more than 2,100 orphan drug designations, and CDER has approved more than 350 for marketing. Only three drugs have been approved based on the cost recovery rationale (Timothy Coté, M.D., Director, Office of Orphan Products, May 2, 2010, personal communication; see also Karst, 2009b). Two of the three drugs were previously approved for use with common conditions.[11]

Appendix B presents summary data on approved orphan drugs. Highlights from this paper and other sources include the following:

- The number of orphan drugs designated each year has grown substantially in recent years, increasing from 69 in 2000 to 165 in 2008 (Coté, 2010). The number of designated drugs gaining marketing approval in 2000 was 13 and in 2008, 15.
- Of the orphan drugs approved from 1983 through 2007, 22 percent were biologics (Seoane-Vezquez et al., 2008).
- Between 1983 and 2007, orphan-designated drugs had a shorter FDA review time on average (1.6 years) than nonorphans that were approved as new molecular entities (2.2 years) (Seoane-Vezquez et al., 2008).
- Orphan drugs accounted for more than 30 percent of all drug approvals in 2008 (Coté, 2009).
- From 2000 to 2008, orphan drugs accounted for 22 percent of the

---

[11] Buprenorphine hydrochloride (Subutex, approved as the analgesic Buprenex in 1981) and buprenorphine with naloxone (Suboxone) received orphan designations in 1994 and marketing approval in 2002 (both for treatment of opioid dependency). Company sales projections to support cost recovery claims are not public (Schulte and Donovan, 2007). FDA approved an orphan designation for raloxifene (Evista) in 2005 and approved the drug in 2007 for use to reduce the risk of invasive breast cancer in postmenopausal women with osteoporosis and the risk of invasive breast cancer in postmenopausal women at high risk for invasive breast cancer. It was originally approved in 1997 for treatment of osteoporosis in postmenopausal women.

innovative drugs (NMEs) approved by FDA and 31 percent of the innovative biologics (Tufts Center, 2010).

• Oncology drugs dominate orphan drug approvals, accounting for 36 percent of approvals from 2000 to 2006 (Coté, 2010). The other categories accounting for more than 5 percent of approvals include drugs for metabolic disorders (11 percent), hematologic-immunologic disorders and neurologic disorders (7 percent each), infectious or parasitic disorders (6 percent), and cardiovascular conditions (5 percent).

• Most drug approvals are for a single indication. A notable exception involves human growth hormone, versions of which account for 14 approvals involving 6 unique products (i.e., products that have the same manufacturer and the same ingredients). Among the 346 orphan drugs approved through 2009, there were 279 distinct products (Appendix B).

• Among 108 qualifying orphan drugs that were approved under an NDA from 1984 to 1999 and were still available in 2010, 55 percent had generic equivalents on the market that were manufactured by a competing company (Appendix B).

• As of early 2009, 33 previously approved orphan drugs were no longer on the market, of which 12 had no chemically identical approved alternative drugs (Wellman-Labadie and Zhou, 2009). In October 2009, a generic drug that was chemically identical to one of the 12 discontinued drugs (chenodeoxycholic acid [Chenix], approved in 1983) received a new orphan drug approval for the same indication (Chenodal, ANDA #091019).

Although the committee heard criticisms that the incentives and processes for promoting orphan drug development have been more effective in stimulating drug development for the more common rare conditions than for very rare conditions, data on orphan designations suggest that approvals are concentrated neither in the higher reaches of the rare diseases prevalence range (100,000 to <200,000) nor at the lowest end of the range (diseases with affected individuals numbering in single or double digits). The median population prevalence for drugs with orphan designations is 39,000 (Coté, 2009). Of 326 products approved before 2009, 83 (25 percent) were for conditions with U.S. prevalence of less than 10,000 patients.[12]

---

[12] As discussed in Chapter 1, very low prevalence rare diseases account for a substantial proportion of the conditions for which prevalence information was reported in the 2009 Orphanet prevalence report. Not surprisingly then, data reported by Heemstra et al. (2009) using an earlier Orphanet report (but excluding diseases with prevalence of less than 0.1/100,000) showed that the more common conditions (10/100,000 to 50/100,000) were more likely to have a U.S. or European orphan drug designation than the less common rare diseases.

Orphan Product Grants Program

Orphan product grants support the clinical development of products for use in rare diseases or conditions for which no current therapy exists or for which the proposed product will be superior to the existing therapy. The program extends beyond drugs and biologics to include medical devices and medical foods. Grant funding typically extends for up to 3 years for phase I trials and up to 4 years for phase II and III trials.[13] In FY 2010, the amount available for orphan product grants (new and continuing projects) was approximately $15.2 million (Goodman, 2010).

As of May 2010, the online listing of grants showed that a total of 517 product research grants had been awarded over the life of the program; 70 grants were active at that time. Many of the grants involved early-stage clinical trials to develop initial information on safety and efficacy. Approximately a dozen grants were for studies of medical devices. The majority (approximately 90 percent) of the awards have gone to universities or other nonprofit organizations (Tufts Center, 2010).

By early 2010, FDA had approved or cleared for marketing 43 of the grant-supported products (Katherine Needleman, M.S., Director, Orphan Grants Program, FDA, March 10, 2010, personal communication). Of these approvals or clearances, 36 involved drugs (one of these was for a combination drug-device product) and 7 involved devices. According to a recent review, sponsors with orphan product grants reported that 22 percent of their clinical development programs led to approvals, whereas the approval success rate was 16 percent for major pharmaceutical or biotechnology companies (Tufts Center, 2010). Sometimes a grant will lead to useful knowledge about the use of a drug in the form of peer-reviewed publications (FDA, 2010c), but the sponsor may not pursue the additional work needed for approval of a product.

An orphan products grant may offer the only funding available to academic researchers to develop proof-of-concept results indicating that their product works on a targeted disease. Such results may then attract industry funding to pursue further testing to support FDA approval. As discussed later in this chapter, funding for the program has lagged far behind in inflation and has thus limited the reach of this focused grant program.

---

[13] Grants may be awarded up to $200,000 (or up to $400,000 in total direct plus indirect costs) per year for up to 4 years. A fourth year of funding is available for phase II or III clinical studies (75 Fed. Reg. 47602-47603).

Issues in the Orphan Drug Approval Process: Applying
Standards and Identifying Problem Areas

Rare diseases present significant challenges to the system for approving drugs for entry to the market. The life-threatening and progressive nature of many rare diseases, combined with the small number of patients available to participate in clinical studies, often makes it impractical or impossible to conduct research using the same models used for more common conditions. A primary goal for FDA should be to facilitate development of therapeutics for rare disorders by promoting predictability, consistency, and reasoned flexibility in the regulatory process within and across its review units.

The committee was not able to find systematic information on the nature or consistency of FDA advice or judgments about adequate toxicology, carcinogenicity, or other preclinical studies for orphan drugs or about acceptable surrogate endpoints for studies involving such drugs. It is aware of concerns about the consistency of judgments across review divisions of CDER and the reasonable application of review criteria to studies of drugs to treat serious rare conditions that have no approved treatment. One of the recommendations at the end of this chapter calls a more detailed analysis of FDA approval (and disapproval) decisions than is possible with public data. Chapter 5 includes recommendations for NIH and the FDA Critical Path Initiative related to surrogate endpoints for rare diseases.

Evidence of Efficacy Accepted by FDA

Following the standards described earlier, FDA approves orphan drugs on the basis of clinical studies that are considered adequately controlled and sufficient to establish efficacy when the nature of the population and condition for which the drug is intended are taken into account. The committee found no comprehensive information on the characteristics of studies used to support orphan drug approvals.

From a variety of sources, it determined that the approvals of orphan drugs do not necessarily follow the pattern for approvals of drugs for common conditions, for which FDA often asks for evidence from two phase III trials. For example, Appendix B presents an analysis of medical officer reviews for drugs approved from 2007 to 2009. (Before 2007, these reviews were not consistently public.) For the 44 drugs approved during this period, the author located full medical officer reviews for 30. (The remaining 14 drugs included 9 clotting factors or immune globulins, 4 previously approved drugs, and 1 other product.) For the 30 drugs collectively, the medical reviews reported a total of 71 trials evaluating efficacy. The trials enrolled a median of 179 participants, and treatment lasted a median of 8.5 weeks. Of the 71 trials, 55 were considered pivotal trials that provided key evidence of efficacy. They included 30 phase III studies, 17 phase II studies, 1 phase I study, and 4 phase IV studies (which were conducted following FDA approval of the drug for a different indication).

In this sample, 13 of the 30 orphan drugs were approved based on a single efficacy trial, including 8 based on a single phase III trial; 4 based on a single phase II trial; and 1 based on a single phase I trial. Among the 55 pivotal trials, 27 had a double-blind design, 5 were single-blind, and the remaining 23 did not have blinding. Twenty-six trials used placebo controls, and 11 used active comparators. Thirty-eight studies were randomized. Thirteen were single-arm studies.

Box 3-3 presents examples of the different kinds of efficacy studies that FDA has accepted in approving orphan drugs. The examples suggest considerable variability and flexibility in the evidence that FDA has

---

BOX 3-3
Examples of Variations in Types of Efficacy Studies
Accepted by FDA in Orphan Drug Approvals

In 2010, FDA approved carglumic acid (Carbaglu) for the treatment of acute hyperammonemia resulting from a deficiency of the enzyme N-acetylglutamate synthase (NAGS). NAGS deficiency is an extremely rare condition that can be fatal without treatment. The sponsor submitted data from a retrospective, unblinded, controlled case series for 23 patients who were treated for a median of 7.9 years (range 0.6 to 20.8 years). Complete data were available for 13 patients. The summary review stated that "although the retrospective case series data . . . are not derived from traditionally defined adequate and well controlled investigations, the plasma ammonia level data submitted for review do stand as evidence 'on the basis of which it could fairly and responsibly be concluded by experts that the drug will have the effect it purports or is represented to have'" (Greibel, 2010, p. 1 quoting Section 505(d) of the Food, Drug, and Cosmetic Act). The approval letter from FDA specified a number of postmarket study requirements, including a registry to obtain long-term safety information over a 15-year period (Beitz, 2010).

Alglucosidase alfa (Myozyme) was approved in April 2006 as enzyme replacement therapy for Pompe disease, a rare autosomal recessive lysosomal storage disease. Without treatment, infants with the disease usually die by 18 months of age from respiratory and heart failure. Myozyme was approved based primarily on the results of a randomized, open-label, historically controlled study in 18 infantile-onset patients. The ventilator-free survival rate for the treated infants was 83 percent at 18 months of age compared to 2 percent survival in the age-matched historical comparison groups of 61 patients. Among other postmarket studies, the sponsor agreed to two long-term studies to collect additional clinical data, including growth and development information (Beitz, 2006).

Before colchicine (Colcrys) received orphan drug approval in 2009 for familial

considered sufficient to support approval. The first two examples, which have the least traditional evidence supporting approval, involve extremely rare conditions. The third example involves a drug that had never been approved by FDA but had a long history of use for gout (see note earlier in this chapter).

Some data point to differences in the evidence supporting approvals of orphan compared to nonorphan drugs. An analysis of accelerated approvals for NMEs in oncology found that 73 percent of those approved from 1995 through 2008 for nonorphan indications were supported by phase III studies compared to 45 percent of NMEs approved for orphan indications (Richey et al., 2009). The authors also found that the orphan NMEs were more likely than the regular NMEs to have difficulty completing the follow-up confirmatory studies. Another study by Mitsumoto and col-

Mediterranean fever (FMF), FDA had indicated to the sponsor that "in principle, the application for FMF could potentially rely solely on . . . published articles in the scientific and medical literature" since the drug had a long history of use (Roca, 2009, p. 10). (FDA required a dosing study to support approval of the drug for gout flares, an indication that is not rare.) In approving the application for FMF, FDA relied on three randomized, double-blind, placebo-controlled clinical trials (out of 74 studies cited by the sponsor) that involved a total of 48 participants. The sponsor incurred expenses for the literature review; the clinical trials had been funded by others. (See also discussion in Chapter 6.)

Sorafenib (Nexavar) has orphan drug approvals for treatment of advanced renal cell carcinoma and unresectable hepatocellular carcinoma. It was approved for the latter indication based on a randomized, double-blind, placebo-controlled, multicenter, international trial involving 299 study participants randomized to the investigational drug and 303 to a placebo. The primary endpoints were overall survival and time to progression. Overall survival for the test drug was 10.7 months versus 7.9 months for the placebo. The study was stopped early based on prespecified efficacy criteria (Llovet et al., 2008). The approval letter included reminders of postmarketing study commitments related to the earlier approval of the drug for renal carcinoma; it also specified additional postmarketing commitments (Justice, 2007).

Collagenase (Xiaflex) has orphan drug approval for treatment of Dupuytren contracture, a debilitating hand deformity. It was approved on the basis of results from two randomized, double-blind, placebo-controlled studies, one with 302 individuals with the condition, the other with 66 participants. The primary endpoint was proportion of patients who achieved a specified reduction in the contracture within 30 days after the final injection. For the larger study, 64 percent of the participants receiving the test drug achieved the specified response compared to 7 percent of those receiving the placebo. For the smaller study, the comparable figures were 44 percent and 5 percent (Rappaport, 2010).

leagues (2009) compared approvals for neurological drugs and found that of 20 recently approved nonorphan drugs, all had at least two randomized, placebo-controlled, double-blind clinical studies compared to 32 percent of the 19 approved orphan drugs. The mean number of trial participants in the former was 506 compared to 164 for the latter.

These analyses underscore the importance of sound alternative trial designs for use in studies involving small populations. They likewise support the importance of efforts undertaken by FDA and NIH to educate their personnel as well as investigators and sponsors about the most appropriate study designs.

Moreover, the analyses point to the need for more detailed examinations of CDER approvals, both to identify the extent and dimensions of variability in reviews and to assess the extent to which variability represents a reasoned approach to differences in the conditions and drugs being reviewed. These differences might relate to differences in the prevalence and nature of the disease, differences in mode of action of the drug, or other such factors. A recommendation at the end of this chapter calls for this kind of assessment as a basis for developing guidelines for CDER reviewers and providing guidance to sponsors.

Problems with Submitted Studies

FDA does not release medical reviews or other details when it rejects a sponsor's application for approval of a drug. As a result, information about the problems with these applications—including problems with study designs as well as problems with the interpretation of study results—is often limited.

CDER staff have, however, identified a number of problem areas that may be encountered with sponsors of studies of drugs for common conditions but that may more often be encountered with sponsors of studies of orphan drugs, including academic investigators funded by NIH (Pariser, 2010). Box 3-4 summarizes some of the problems with applications and supporting studies. Certain of the cited problems involve primarily procedural or administrative issues (e.g., incomplete applications). Some of these problems may reflect sponsor inexperience with FDA policies and practices as well as situations in which guidance from FDA may not be sufficiently clear or specific, as discussed further below. Other problems, in particular, the lack of natural history studies, reflect the challenges and expense of rare diseases research and orphan product development as mentioned in Chapter 2.

BOX 3-4
Examples of Problem Areas for Sponsors Developing Evidence for Orphan Drug Approval

• Incomplete NDA applications

• Toxicology studies not completed on a timely basis

• Inadequate characterization of the chemical compound

• Lack of advance communication with FDA about adequacy of plans for clinical trials

• Lack of natural history studies to characterize the disease process, including variability in disease severity, symptom stability, and outcomes

• Poor use of early-phase safety and dosing studies to inform phase III or pivotal studies

• Inadequate trial design, including lack of formal protocols, poorly defined questions, inadequate control groups, and lack of validated biomarkers and appropriate surrogate measures

---

SOURCE: Pariser, 2010.

Concerns About FDA Reviews and Guidance

In addition to problems that FDA finds with submitted applications and research designs, some sponsors and investigators have raised questions about the quality and consistency of FDA reviews of orphan drugs, the appropriateness of its standards for approval, and the adequacy of current agency guidance (see, e.g., Radcliffe, 2009; Kakkis, 2010). Criticisms include

• lack of adequate resources at CDER, including resources for advance meetings or other discussions with sponsors about trial design and outcomes measures and for development of written guidance;

• inadequate reviewer understanding of the rare disease (including what constitutes an acceptable surrogate endpoint) that is the subject of a particular approval application;

• variability in reviewer understanding of trial designs and analytic methods that have been designed for studies involving small numbers of participants;

• inconsistency in the application of review standards across the review divisions of CDER; and

• insufficient or delayed guidance for sponsors on various issues, including the use of "small *n*" study designs and methods and the specification of acceptable subsets of rare conditions to meet prevalence requirements for orphan drug designation (the second of which is an issue for the OOPD rather than CDER).

More fundamental is the argument that different standards of evidence should be applied to approval for orphan drugs given the difficulties of doing conventional trials for many extremely rare conditions, including those conditions that progress over very long periods. The rationale is that even if a drug works, research may not be able to demonstrate safety and efficacy (especially if the effect is subtle) when only a few dozen patients are known to have the condition. As described above, FDA has, in fact, approved drugs for a number of extremely rare diseases on the basis of evidence that it judged met the standards for approval.

Responses to Problems

In response to some of the criticisms of the substance and the implementation of the Orphan Drug Act, Congress in 2009 required FDA to appoint a review group to make recommendations about "appropriate preclinical, trial design, and regulatory paradigms and optimal solutions for the prevention, diagnosis, and treatment of rare diseases" (P.L. 111-80). A second group is to focus on neglected diseases of the developing world. Within a year of establishing the review groups, FDA must report to Congress on its findings and recommendations, and approximately 6 months later it must issue guidance and internal review standards based on the recommendations. (These provisions have been informally termed the Brownback-Brown amendments to the Agriculture, Rural Development, Food and Drug Administration, and Related Agencies Appropriations Act of 2010 [P.L. 111-80].)

After considering the criticisms related to the adequacy of researcher and reviewer understanding of acceptable trial designs and analytic methods for small populations, FDA and NIH collaborated on a multisession course on the science of small clinical trials. The course was first offered in 2009 to FDA and NIH staff and then revised and offered in 2010 to all interested parties. In 2010, registration closed after 1,300 participants enrolled. (This information was provided at the registration site for the program, http://small-trials.keenminds.org/.)

In addition, as discussed above, FDA recently created the position of Associate Director for Rare Diseases to provide a central resource within CDER and to assist developers of orphan drugs and biologics in understanding and meeting regulatory requirements. The Associate Director will also coordinate work to develop CDER policies and procedures specific to the review and approval of orphan products and to promote training of CDER staff in relevant methodologies.[14]

FDA RESOURCES AND ORGANIZATION

From a resource perspective, the strength of FDA support for the development of safe and effective products for people with rare diseases rests on at least two major elements. One involves resources for FDA generally but particularly the Center for Drug Evaluation and Research, which reviews most orphan drug applications. The second involves resources for the Office of Orphan Products Development, which is the focal point for efforts to promote orphan product development and directly funds grants for that purpose.

Agency-wide Concerns

Although concerns about the adequacy of FDA funding and capacities are hardly new, they have been particularly intense in recent years. A 2007 Institute of Medicine report on drug safety found that the FDA system was impaired by "serious resource constraints that weaken the quality and quantity of the science that is brought to bear on drug safety; an organizational culture in CDER that is not optimally functional; and unclear and insufficient regulatory authorities particularly with respect to enforcement" (IOM, 2007, p. 4). The report noted the dependence of the agency on user fees and expressed concern that reporting requirements "associated with the user-fee program are excessively oriented toward supporting speed of approval and insufficiently attentive to safety" (p. 6). The report included many recommendations for strengthening the drug safety system, including the creation of a public-private partnership to "prioritize, plan, and organize funding for confirmatory drug safety and efficacy studies of public health importance" (p. 8) and increased funding to support drug safety and efficacy activities.

Also in 2007, the FDA Science Board released a subcommittee report asserting that the "nation is at risk if FDA science is at risk" and that FDA science is indeed at risk (p. 2). The "demands on the FDA have soared due to the extraordinary advance of scientific discoveries, the complexity of

---

[14] CDER has developed a number of policy and procedure manuals that are intended to promote consistency in staff advice and reviews on a range of topics, for example, statistical analysis and templates for reviews of NDAs. The Medical Policy Coordinating Committee "serves as a forum for CDER scientists and policy development staff to identify and discuss medical and medical-related regulatory issues that may call for the development and implementation of medical and regulatory policies and guidances" (CDER, 2009).

the new products and claims submitted to FDA for pre-market review and approval, the emergence of challenging safety problems, and the globalization of the industries that FDA regulates," whereas "resources have not increased in proportion to the demands . . . [so] that the scientific demands on the Agency far exceed its capacity to respond" (p. 3). In brief, the numbers of personnel are insufficient, the agency is reactive rather than leading in the development of regulatory science, and its surveillance mission suffers from lack of staff and inadequate information technology.

A group that lobbies for increased resources for FDA has compared FDA funding trends to those for the CDC and reported that the CDC and FDA had roughly equivalent funding in FY 1985 but that the budget for the former has grown at a compounded average rate of 11.4 percent compared to 7.1 percent for FDA. The CDC's FY 2010 budget was $6.37 billion compared to $2.35 billion for FDA (Alliance for a Stronger FDA, 2009).

The FDA Science Board report identified eight areas of scientific and technological advances that are particular challenging for the agency: "systems biology (including genomics and other "omics"), wireless healthcare devices, nanotechnology, medical imaging, robotics, cell- and tissue-based products, regenerative medicine, and combination products" (p. 4). Although the report did not specify a particular level of increased funding, it suggested that another group's recommended increase of 15 percent per year for 5 years "would still be insufficient . . . to initiate and support all the changes necessary" for the agency to fulfill its mission (p. 8).

FDA has recognized the need to take advantage of scientific developments to improve the way medical products are developed and evaluated. For example, the Critical Path Initiative, which was created in 2004 and emphasizes public-private collaborations, has focused on certain areas of particular relevance to products for rare diseases, including improving the development of biomarkers and modernizing the science of clinical trials (FDA, 2009d). In addition, the Advancing Regulatory Science Initiative is intended to strengthen the science base for product evaluation by providing better evaluation tools, standards, and pathways. It includes as one focus the setting of standards for products with people with unmet health needs (Hamburg, 2010b). Of note is that a research grants program to support the initiative is being funded primarily under the auspices of NIH with the NIH Common Fund providing $6 million and the FDA providing $750,000 for FY 2010 to FY 2012. Box 3-5 summarizes the research objectives. The announcement of the initiative included several examples of projects that might be funded and would reinforce elements of the Critical Path Initiative, for example, the development of new or improved biomarkers and the development of clinical trial strategies for more rapidly and efficiently evaluating the safety and efficacy of FDA-regulated products.

BOX 3-5
NIH Request for Applications on Advancing Regulatory Science Through Novel Research and Science-Based Technologies (February 24, 2010)

Purpose. This regulatory science initiative encourages grant applications that propose to study the applicability of novel technologies and approaches to the development and regulatory review of medical products (including drugs, biologics, and devices).

Research Scope. Applications should fall within five broad categories:

(1) New tools and methodologies for assessing medical product safety and efficacy (including drugs, biologics, and devices and point of care diagnostics);
(2) Novel information technologies and statistical models that can improve product evaluation and inform regulatory decisions;
(3) Strategic design of research in "omics" and systems biology to better inform regulatory decision-making and support product development;
(4) Research on rare diseases/small sample size populations; and
(5) Novel approaches addressing optimal study designs for clinical trials.

This initiative will contribute to the overall goals of improving regulatory science by supporting research in at least one area of medical product development ranging from in vitro and in vivo product characterization and evaluation through clinical studies and to a manufactured, approved product.

SOURCE: NIH, 2010b.

Center for Drug Evaluation and Research

According to the 2007 Science Board report, in 2006 CDER regulated drugs accounting for $275 billion in pharmaceutical sales, and it also regulated some 5,000 domestic and foreign manufacturers of these pharmaceuticals. For FY 2006, the report showed total funding of just under $508 million of which about $298 million (58 percent) came from congressional appropriations with the rest provided by user fees. For FY 2009, total funding for the CDER was just over $656 million, of which about $300 million (45 percent) came from appropriations. In addition to resources, CDER and other FDA centers faced significant personnel challenges in recruitment, retention, performance, and professional development. The Science Board report noted the absence of good measures of performance in areas such as review of new product applications for safety and efficacy and the fact that neither CDER nor other parts of the agency could obtain all the expertise they needed without the involvement of external scientists.

The initiation of user fees allowed a considerable increase in staff conducting reviews of new drugs, from 600 in 1996 to 1,320 in 2004—a 125 percent increase that was associated with a substantial decrease in review times (IOM, 2007). FDA performance reports suggest that the agency has done better at meeting its goals for review times than its procedural goals such as timely response to requests for meetings. For example, the FY 2008 goal for scheduling what it terms type B meetings (which include pre-IND meetings, end of phase I meetings, end of phase II meetings, and pre-NDA-BLA meetings) was to have 90 percent scheduled within 60 days, but the actual performance was 58 percent as of September 2008 (FDA, undated). The goal for Special Protocol Assessments was to respond to a sponsor's request for evaluation of a protocol design with 45 days; performance was near the goal at 86 percent.

The importance of resources for meetings with sponsors is suggested by a 2006 consultant report that examined the review of NDAs. Sponsors that had met with agency staff were more likely to gain approval of their NDA at the first review than were sponsors that did not meet with FDA (Booz Allen Hamilton, 2008).

A 2007 IOM report on drug safety argued that more staff resources were needed to take on a variety of tasks, many of them relevant to drugs for rare diseases. These tasks include the development of more consistent approaches to risk-benefit assessment, the release of more information on safety and effectiveness, and the creation of a public-private partnership for planning confirmatory drug safety and efficacy studies.

Office of Orphan Products Development

Within FDA, the FY 2010 budget for the Office of Orphan Products Development is $22.1 million, including $15.2 million for the orphan products grants, $3 million for the pediatric device consortia grants, and $3.8 million for program administration including salaries and program operations. The figure for the orphan products grants program includes an additional $1.2 million that was internally provided to the grants program in FY 2010 to support certain continuing and noncompeting awards (FDA, 2010c; Katherine Needleman, M.S., Director, Orphan Grants Program, FDA, September 3, 2010, personal communication).

Although funding for the grants program rose in absolute and inflation-adjusted amounts for most of the program's first dozen years, absolute funding has declined in some years since then. Funding in constant dollars has, in any case, been dropping since FY 1995. The Food and Drug Administration Amendments Act of 2007 increased the authorization for the grants program to $30 million through FY 2012, but appropriations remain at only about half that amount. Because funding has not kept pace with inflation, the grants program cannot operate at the same level as it did in the 1990s much less at an enhanced level to accelerate the orphan product development.

RECOMMENDATIONS

Most assessments credit the Orphan Drug Act with encouraging more investment by drug companies in the development of products for people with rare conditions. In general, the Office of Orphan Products Development is viewed positively as a helpful resource and successful advocate, especially given its modest resources. The primary criticism is that its budget for orphan products grants is seriously inadequate. More generally, Congress is widely viewed as having provided inadequate resources for FDA to conduct or support a wide range of research and consultation to support its mission (see, e.g., FDA Science Board, 2007; IOM, 2007). This research includes, for example, work on biomarker identification and validation and research on the codevelopment of drugs and companion diagnostics that would benefit the development of products (including, in some cases, medical devices) for rare conditions.

Although the committee focused on FDA activities related to products for rare diseases rather than the agency overall, it concluded that an underfunded and understaffed agency provides an uncertain and in some respects weak and unstable environment for the maintenance of strong agency-wide efforts to (1) promote the development of orphan drugs; (2) offer high-quality, scientific and regulatory guidance to those engaged in orphan drug development; (3) provide sophisticated reviews of applications for drugs and biologics that appropriately apply statutory criteria to challenging data; and (4) establish and monitor reasonable requirements for continued collection of safety and efficacy data once an orphan drug is approved. Thus, the committee supports generally the recommendations of other IOM committees and other groups for building a stronger FDA.

With respect to orphan drug development specifically, the creation by FDA of the new position of Associate Director for Rare Diseases within CDER is a positive and important step. The Associate Director should be able to provide an important resource to CDER review staff. The creation of the position in itself should serve as a signal that the review of drugs and biologics intended for small populations needs special consideration and expertise related to appropriate research and analytic methods. Fulfilling the responsibilities assigned to the new position of Associate Director for Rare Diseases will take resources, including additional staff and support from senior FDA officials. As this report was being completed, legislation had been introduced to provide $1 million in funding that would support the hiring of staff (NORD, 2010).

In general, the new emphasis on rare diseases expertise in CDER should find further support in the agency's increasing recognition of the need for advances in regulatory science, as shown by the new joint NIH-FDA Leadership Council and the grants program described above. One area for further attention is continued work on innovation in clinical trial and analytic strategies for small populations.

A broad goal for the new rare disease initiative at CDER should be to promote reasonable consistency and at the same time reasoned flexibility in the review of similarly situated products (e.g., products for diseases with reasonably similar prevalence, targets, time frames of effect, and other characteristics). Evaluations of specific evidence, even when informed by solid understandings of trial design and clinical and scientific issues, may still have a subjective element; experts do disagree. The realm of subjectivity can, however, be constrained by an appreciation of the factors that contribute to variability and the development of criteria to guide reviews.

RECOMMENDATION 3-1: The Center for Drug Evaluation and Research (CDER) should undertake an assessment of staff reviews of applications for the approval of orphan drugs to identify problems and areas for further attention, including inconsistencies across CDER divisions in the evaluations of applications that appear to present similar issues for review. Based on this assessment, CDER should

• **develop guidelines for CDER reviewers to promote appropriate consistency and reasoned flexibility in the review of orphan drugs, taking into account such considerations as the prevalence of the disease, its course and severity, and the characteristics of the drug; and**
• **use the analysis and the review guidelines to inform the advice and formal guidance provided to sponsors on the evidence needed to support orphan drug approvals.**

CDER should make public the primary results of its assessment and consult with outside experts in developing the guidelines called for in this recommendation. The guidelines would be applied across CDER review divisions and would be adjusted to reflect advances in the biomedical and regulatory sciences. They might include supplemental materials, for example, a series of illustrations of successful applications, possibly involving templates for certain elements.

The assessment might suggest the need for additional disorder-specific expertise to be recruited for sponsor consultations and some product reviews. Depending on the results of its analysis of reviewer decisions and on consultations with experts in rare disorders and others, FDA could propose to define one or more classes of rare conditions for which it would create tailored criteria for the approval of products and for the specification of requirements of longer-term assessments of safety and efficacy following approval. It could, for example, propose a special review class for rare disorders that are characterized by rapid progression and early death or severe and irrevocable loss of critical function. The criteria for this class would then cover major issues for trial design and application review (e.g., toxicology studies, carcinogenicity studies, surrogate endpoints, number and type of efficacy studies).

The process for devising new guidelines and guidance would be developed to be consistent with statutory requirements and FDA's broad responsibilities for protecting the public from unsafe and ineffective products. The recommendation above focuses on CDER because it is the locus of the majority of orphan drug reviews, but the agency should consider a similar analysis of CBER reviews and, in the meantime, apply the guidelines to CBER reviews when relevant.

In conducting the analyses proposed above, FDA can be expected to develop a clearer understanding of the current adequacy of the evidence submitted with applications for orphan drug approvals, including the appropriateness of clinical trial designs. This understanding may, in turn, suggest how pre-IND and other meetings might help sponsors of drugs for rare diseases develop adequate preclinical and clinical evidence. It may also suggest the need for modifications in written guidance for sponsors.

In addition to evaluating reviews of orphan drugs, CDER should specifically examine the use of small clinical trials. This analysis should build on the educational work already undertaken by FDA and NIH.

RECOMMENDATION 3-2: The Center for Drug Evaluation and Research should evaluate the extent to which studies submitted in support of orphan drugs are consistent with advances in the science of small clinical trials and associated analytic methods. Based on its findings, CDER should work with others at FDA, NIH, and outside organizations and experts, as appropriate, to

- adjust and expand existing educational programs on the design and conduct of small clinical trials;
- specify which CDER and NIH personnel should complete these educational programs;
- revise guidance for sponsors on trial design and analysis and on safety and efficacy reviews of products for rare diseases; and
- support further work to develop and test clinical research and data analysis strategies for small populations.

The identification of possible problem areas in clinical trial designs and drug approval reviews may also help guide efforts for CDER, the OOPD, and NIH to work collaboratively on mechanisms to ensure that NIH-funded product development studies are planned and conducted to be consistent with the requirements for FDA approval. These mechanisms would need to cover NIH grant reviews and other activities related not only to awards for phase III studies but also to awards for certain kinds of preclinical and early-phase clinical studies. One step could be for NIH to require investigators for preclinical studies of therapies for rare diseases to demonstrate their understanding of FDA procedures and requirements. In addition, NIH and FDA might also develop an education module specifically for NIH grant applicants. More generally, timely meetings and other communications between FDA staff and sponsors should reduce the likelihood that the investment of sponsors and research participants with rare diseases will be used unproductively or even wasted.

> **RECOMMENDATION 3-3: To ensure that NIH-funded product development studies involving rare diseases are designed to fulfill requirements for FDA approval, NIH and FDA should develop a procedure for NIH grantees undertaking such studies to receive assistance from appropriate CDER drug review divisions that is similar to the assistance provided to investigators who receive orphan products grants. NIH study section review of rare disease clinical trial applications should involve reviewers who are knowledgeable about clinical trials methods for small-populations. For all sponsors of drugs for rare diseases, CDER should have resources to support sufficient and adequate meetings and discussions with sponsors from the earliest stages of the development process.**

With respect to the Office of Orphan Products Development, the committee was concerned about the low level of funding for the orphan grants program, which as described above, has for several years had a declining budget as calculated in constant dollars. Clearly, however, the funding history for the program does not reflect the scientific and technological advances described in Chapter 4.

Notwithstanding increased interest by companies in orphan products and some initiatives by NIH that should assist orphan product development, the committee concluded that funding for the orphan products grants program is seriously inadequate and has undermined an important resource for nonprofit and commercial entities seeking to translate promising discoveries into approved products for people with rare diseases. It would be reasonable to argue, at the minimum, for an increase to the $30 million authorized in the Food and Drug Administration Amendments Act of 2007. That would allow more qualified researchers to benefit from this focused product development program and take advantage of the expertise and experience of the Office of Orphan Products Development. In addition, the committee encourages FDA to work with NIH on a systematic process for referring to NIH worthy orphan product grant applications that FDA lacks funding to approve. FDA has, from time to time, done this, and the expectation of new resources at NIH as described in Chapter 5 provides a rationale for a more formal referral process.

The next chapter reviews some of the scientific and technological advances that are making it faster, easier, and less expensive to undertake basic discovery research to understand the biology of rare diseases and identify targets for therapeutic development. Chapter 5 examines the preclinical and clinical stages of drug development. Although the recommendations in the next two chapters focus on NIH and private-sector activities, Chapter 5 includes a recommendation for FDA's Critical Path Initiative to define criteria for the evaluation of surrogate endpoints for use in trials of products for rare conditions. Overall, the recommendations in the next two chapters should not only help accelerate rare diseases research and orphan product development but also increase the likelihood that marketing applications based on NIH-funded research meet the standards for FDA approval.

4

Discovery Research for Rare Diseases and Orphan Product Development

I could see there was a transformation of cancer treatment on the horizon thanks to breakthroughs in biochemistry and genomics. I wanted to be part of that, which is why I was a physician-researcher. . . . By the late 1980s, C.M.L. [chronic myeloid leukemia], though rare, was a cancer that scientists knew a lot about. We knew, for instance that a chromosomal abnormality existed in every C.M.L. patient. We knew that this abnormality created an enzyme that caused the uncontrolled growth of cancer cells. . . . If you want to develop targeted chemotherapies, C.M.L. is the disease to study. We know the most about it—and, if we can figure out a way to block this enzyme, we can turn off the cancer switch.

Interview with Brian Druker (Dreifus, 2009)

The research undertaken by Brian Druker and his colleagues and predecessors offers a classic example of the foundation that basic research builds for the subsequent development of therapies for rare diseases. Breakthroughs in biochemistry and genomics, as well as advances in computational tools, have transformed the process of research and drug development. The process begins with basic laboratory studies that reveal the molecular mechanisms of disease, which related to a chromosomal abnormality in the case of chronic myelogenous leukemia (CML). This foundation leads to the discovery of biomarkers for rare conditions and the discovery of potential biological targets on which drugs can act. The target in CML is a rogue enzyme created by the mutated chromosomes, which triggers uncontrolled cell growth. Once a target is defined, the process shifts from basic research to the discovery of a therapeutic approach. Imatinib mesylate (Gleevec), the drug discovered by Druker, specifically deactivates the enzyme target in CML. It was approved by the Food and Drug Administration (FDA) in 2001 and is now used not only for CML but also for other rare cancers. Increased knowledge of kinase inhibitors (of which imatinib was the first) is supporting the development of more potent, second-generation drugs for CML that may also be less susceptible to resistance (Sawyers, 2010).

Today, as a result of scientific and technological innovations, much of the basic research initially undertaken with CML could be done more quickly, inexpensively, and easily. For example, identification of the genetic cause of conditions that are clearly inherited used to involve speculative approaches and laborious analytical tools. The sequencing of the human genome has spawned an array of rapid and relatively inexpensive DNA analysis tools that have the potential to foster more targeted and efficient therapeutics development for rare diseases. Advances in the scientific understanding of disease mechanisms likewise are helping researchers focus more efficiently and effectively on potential therapeutic targets. As a result, the future holds the promise of continued innovation that will further accelerate biomedical research to the benefit of patients with rare as well as common diseases.

As discussed in Chapter 1, research on rare diseases can illuminate disease mechanisms and therapeutic opportunities for more common diseases. Box 4-1 briefly summarizes several additional examples of rare diseases research that have yielded broader knowledge.

Many of the same approaches and techniques are used to study both rare and common diseases, but research on rare diseases faces some special barriers and constraints. One is the sheer number of rare diseases, an estimated 5,000 to 8,000. Many of the challenges stem from the low prevalence that is the defining characteristic of rare diseases. Particularly for extremely rare conditions, the small numbers of affected individuals means a dearth of biological specimens, which severely limits studies of disease mechanism and etiology. Small numbers also constrain epidemiologic research and clinical trials as highlighted in Chapters 3 and 5. Other challenges include the limited funding for research and a limited number of investigators committed to the study of rare conditions.

The basic research tools available to investigators have advanced dramatically over the past 20 years, with new approaches continuing to evolve, both in the laboratory and from the use of computational biology. Along with new and better tools, models for supporting discovery research have also undergone a transformation in recent years. This chapter briefly examines the implications for rare diseases research of a number of current research strategies for both target discovery and therapeutic discovery. The next chapter focuses on product development, particularly from the perspective of companies and their academic and government collaborators

BOX 4-1
Examples of Research on Rare Diseases with
Implications for Treatment of Common Conditions

Some of the most effective treatments for coronary artery disease (a very common condition) were first established during the study of a rare condition called *familial hypercholesterolemia*. The disease was ultimately linked to mutations in the gene for the low-density lipoprotein receptor that coordinates the uptake of cholesterol from the blood. This work laid the foundation for the development and use of drugs (specifically, statins) that inhibit the rate-limiting enzyme in cholesterol synthesis, hydroxymethylglutaryl (HMG)-CoA (coenzyme A) reductase, in the lowering of circulating cholesterol and the prevention of coronary artery disease and myocardial infarction (Stossel, 2008).

Patients with a rare condition called *osteoporosis-pseudoglioma syndrome* have loss-of-function mutations in the low-density lipoprotein receptor-related protein-5 (LRP5), while mutations causing rare conditions associated with high bone mass and density produce increased LRP5 function. Subsequent work showed that LRP5 normally inhibits serotonin production in the gut. Inhibition of gut serotonin production has emerged as a promising treatment for common causes of osteoporosis including the loss of bone mineral density associated with aging and menopause (Haigh, 2008; Long, 2008).

Aortic aneurysm is the cause of death in about 1 to 2 percent of individuals in industrialized countries, but its cause is largely unknown and medical treatments are lacking. During the study of *Marfan syndrome*, a rare connective tissue disorder associated with a high risk of ascending aortic aneurysm and tear, researchers showed that aneurysm development and progression is associated with increased activity of transforming growth factor β (TGF-β), a molecule that instructs cellular behavior. It was subsequently shown that interventions that inhibit TGF-β, including administration of a neutralizing antibody or the angiotensin II type 1 receptor blocker losartan, could attenuate or prevent many manifestations of Marfan syndrome in mouse models. Responsive Marfan phenotypes included aortic aneurysm, skeletal muscle myopathy, pulmonary emphysema, and degeneration of the mitral valve. This work prompted the launch of the first clinical trial for Marfan syndrome based upon a refined understanding of disease pathogenesis, specifically assessing the efficacy of losartan in attenuating aortic root growth. Alteration of TGF-β activity was subsequently linked to other rare (e.g., Loeys-Dietz syndrome) and common (e.g., bicuspid aortic valve with aneurysm) presentations of aortic aneurysm (Jones et al., 2009). Losartan has also proved effective in the treatment of TGF-β-induced myopathy in a mouse model of Duchenne muscular dystrophy (Cohn et al., 2007).

who are evaluating and undertaking the complex work needed to transform promising research discoveries into products that are safe and effective for patients in need. All along this continuum from basic research through clinical trials, infrastructure and innovation are needed to accelerate the development of therapies for people with rare diseases. The discussion here focuses on the role of government, industry, academic investigators and institutions, and advocacy groups. Other groups also contribute, for example, organizations such as the American College of Medical Genetics.

Both this and the next chapter discuss the infrastructure for rare diseases research and orphan product development and "innovation platforms" to encourage and support collaborative work. Such collaboration is needed to bridge the gulf—sometimes referred to as the "valley of death"—between basic research findings and beneficial products, especially in the stages that precede clinical studies of efficacy. Early initiatives to bridge the gulf included public policies such as the Amendments to the Patent and Trademark Act of 1980 (P.L. 96-517, commonly known as the Bayh-Dole Act). That legislation encouraged cooperation among academic institutions, other nonprofit organizations, and small businesses to commercialize research discoveries funded by the federal government (Schact, 2007). Efforts continue to successfully engage government, academic, nonprofit, and commercial entities as collaborators in translating research discoveries into safe and effective drugs and medical devices. First, however, must come the discoveries.

TARGET DISCOVERY

Most rare diseases have a genetic etiology, but the molecular pathogenesis has been defined for a relatively small number of rare diseases. For most of this small group, a specific gene alteration is recognized as responsible for the disorder, and for a subset, understanding of the pathogenesis extends to identification of the function of the affected gene product. For an even smaller subset, investigators have described targets such as specific molecules or physiologic pathways that are amenable to therapeutic modification. The next sections discuss some particular areas of research advances and their prospects for increasing understanding of the molecular pathogenesis of rare diseases. Such understanding provides the basis for modern drug discovery.

Traditional Genetic Studies

Because most rare diseases are caused by defects in a single gene, identification of a mutated gene is the logical starting point for research in most cases. Although the standard approach to mapping the chromosomal location of the gene of interest has used candidate gene analysis or linkage analysis, these methods are inherently slow and often cumbersome.

Many factors can limit the utility of genetic mapping studies for rare disorders, notably the lack of large families with multiple affected, surviving individuals. Early death and other disease-related causes of reduced reproduction contribute to this lack as does the general decline in family size associated with economic and social development. Recent technological advances have enabled researchers to employ genome-wide association studies to identify genetic variation that contributes to the pathogenesis of common disorders, as well as some of the most prevalent rare diseases such as juvenile idiopathic arthritis (see, e.g., Thomson et al., 2010). These studies depend on large patient populations and on an inherent assumption that the predisposing alleles or haplotypes are both ancient and shared among unrelated affected patients, effectively precluding this approach for small patient populations with high locus or allelic heterogeneity. Impaired reproductive fitness, a feature of many rare disorders, imposes allelic heterogeneity and would therefore implicitly disqualify this approach as a strategy for research on these disorders. Although some critics of genome-wide association studies argue that they have not been terribly informative with regard to individual risk of disease, the studies have highlighted pathways whose relevance to a particular disease had been unsuspected (Hirschhorn, 2009). Fortunately, additional tools for genetic research are now available.

Study of Modifier Genes and Epigenetics

Variation in secondary genes can alter primary gene effects and related pathways and can attenuate or mask underlying disease predisposition. Studies of these secondary genes are likely to inform the development of novel therapeutic strategies. For many rare and common disorders, there is considerable phenotypic variation among individuals with the same underlying primary disease gene mutation. This can be particularly striking when wide phenotypic variation is seen within individual families. For example, in X-linked adrenoleukodystrophy (a metabolic disorder that causes neurological damage), some affected family members have onset of neurodegeneration and death in childhood, whereas others show mild manifestations of disease such as isolated adrenal insufficiency that first manifests in adulthood. Yet other family members may be entirely asymptomatic (Maestri and Beaty, 1992; Moser et al., 2009).

The study of modifier genes can be facilitated through the use of inbred mouse strains that often show wide variation in disease severity based upon the genetic background on which a primary disease-causing mutation occurs. Animal models also offer the ability to use targeted genetic or pharmacologic perturbations to test focused hypotheses regarding modifier genes and pathways. The identification of modifier genes is of particular value in rare diseases, where diagnosis is already difficult due to the small number of cases.

Beyond germline genetic variation, modification of DNA (e.g., DNA methylation, histone acetylation) contributes to rare disorders such as the Prader-Willi syndrome and Angelman syndrome (Adams, 2008), but it may be even more important as a contributory factor in modulating gene expression and, therefore, disease predisposition and severity. These epigenetic modifications are likely acquired as the result of an array of exposures (e.g., prenatal exposure to tobacco smoke) and experiences (e.g., stress). Investigators are now using microarray and sequencing to analyze methylation patterns as biomarkers that can have clinical value.

Whole Genome Sequencing, Gene Expression Analysis, and Exome Sequencing

Whole genome sequencing provides a complete analysis of the entire complement of an individual's DNA. It can now be used to identify genetic variants associated with rare diseases in individual patients or families (Lupski et al., 2010; Roach et al., 2010). The cost for sequencing has fallen dramatically, but it remains resource intensive and challenging because each exome contains a large number of polymorphisms (variants), only one of which is typically the primary gene alteration (Lifton, 2010; Wade, 2010).

Microarray methods, which are used to comprehensively assess which genes are transcribed and which are not active in making proteins, are not diagnostic for genetic diseases. They can, however, be helpful in working out pathways that are dysfunctional in both genetic and acquired rare disorders (Wong and Wang, 2008). Experimental methods to interrupt gene expression in cell culture systems and animal models include the introduction of target-specific microRNAs, a tool that has been used to confirm the role of genes and pathways in the pathogenesis and modulation of disease.

Exome sequencing is a promising new approach to the search for disorder-causing genes for rare diseases (Kuehn, 2010; Tabor and Bamshad, 2010). The method focuses on the less than 5 percent of the genome that actually codes for protein. With this method, identification of genes associated with disorders of previously unknown etiology is possible using DNA from as few as two to four patients (Ng et al., 2009; Johnston et al., 2010). This approach provides a particular advantage to rare diseases, given that biological specimens are often scarce. It is expected to accelerate the rate of identification of gene defects for rare diseases.

Proteomics and Metabolomics

Researchers have made significant progress in the cataloging of genetic variation and its correlation with disease predisposition, initiation, and progression. Parallel initiatives for protein variation are also important.

Proteomics is the science of detecting, identifying, and quantifying the products of gene translation and represents another approach to uncovering variation that underlies the pathogenesis of rare diseases. A single gene can generate an array of protein species based upon alternative translational start and stop sites and splicing. The derived proteins can be further diversified in relative abundance, structure, and function by posttranslational modifications including phosphorylation, glycosylation, acetylation, and tagging for degradation. Proteomics analyses can detect primary perturbations that cause disease (e.g., congenital disorders of glycosylation), pathogenetic or compensatory pathway activation (e.g., the activation of kinases through quantitative analysis of substrates for phosphorylation), and candidate proteins for validation as biomarkers to aid in diagnosis, prognostication, or therapeutic trials (e.g., newborn screening by tandem mass spectrometry or detection of increased circulating levels of cardiac muscle-specific enzymes after myocardial infarction) (see, e.g., Duncan and Hunsucker, 2005; Haffner and Maher, 2006; Suzuki et al., 2009; Van Eyk, 2010). One challenge is that proteomic analysis requires expensive equipment (e.g., mass spectrometry) and data analysis tools, which means that this technique is usually centralized in special laboratories.

Metabolomics involves the study of the small-molecule metabolites found in an organism. As in proteomics, mass spectrometry can be used to detect abnormal metabolic products, to diagnose rare diseases, and to understand alterations in relevant biological pathways. An example is the elucidation of a series of synthetic enzyme deficiencies that result in the production of abnormal bile acids leading to serious liver, neurologic, connective tissue, and nutritional disorders (Heubi et al., 2007).

Systems Biology and Bioinformatics

With the aid of translational bioinformatics (Schadt et al., 2005a; Vodovotz et al., 2008), the construction of molecular networks and pathways relevant to specific rare disorders is increasingly possible. Bioinformatic analyses of data from gene expression arrays, proteomics studies, and clinical observations on patients with rare diseases can define signatures of fundamental disease mechanisms (Dudley et al., 2009; Patel et al., 2010; Suthram et al., 2010). Integration of this information with signatures of drug activities or therapeutic responses could intuitively promote discovery regarding the etiology, pathogenesis, and treatment of unclassified or poorly understood disorders (Schadt et al., 2005b). For example, if two diseases show overlapping or identical signatures, established treatments for one might benefit the other. Drugs that show signatures that oppose those seen for certain diseases emerge as candidate therapies. Bioinformatic methods can screen known chemical compounds for structural characteristics that predict desired drug activities that are potentially beneficial for patients with rare diseases. Identification of drugs with overlapping signatures will promote the informed testing and substitution of agents that might show greater efficacy or other desirable characteristics such as reduced toxicity. Through these approaches, it should be possible to identify multiple intervention target sites for some disorders.

Conversely, studies of biological networks can also identify common pathways for multiple rare diseases that are biologically related. For example, a more comprehensive understanding of the molecular basis for lysosomal function may provide an opportunity for interventions that are beneficial for an array of lysosomal disorders (Sardiello et al., 2009). More broadly, this capability may open the door for the discovery of single therapies that can benefit multiple rare disorders and, potentially, also more common diseases.

The promise of systems biology is built on the availability of molecular and genetic data, combined with the development of valid computational methods for integrating these data into predictive models of disease (Schadt, 2005a). Although most genomic sequences are available in publicly accessible databases, many experimental biological data as well as clinical trials data are not collected or stored in a way that ensures broad access to the information. Thus, as discussed later in this chapter, the infrastructure for rare diseases research and product development should include structures and processes for sharing research resources, including data and biological specimens.

THERAPEUTICS DISCOVERY

Once basic research is performed and findings implicate a specific biological target, which could be an enzyme, a product of a biochemical pathway, an altered gene, an epigenetic mechanism, or a combination of the above, then the search begins for an appropriate therapeutic agent. Sometimes recognition of a molecular defect can point directly to potential therapies.

Effective therapies can either inhibit deleterious or excessive functions or restore missing functions, both of which can result from gene mutations. In the former category, for example, the finding that transforming growth factor β (TGF-β) plays a role in the development of aortic root aneurysms in Marfan syndrome led to studies of an inhibitor of TGF-β (angiotensin II type I receptor inhibitor losartan) that are currently in phase III trials (Dietz, 2010). A large number of monoclonal antibodies are available to modulate exuberant immunologic, inflammatory reactions in rare as well as more common diseases. Imatinib successfully treats CML and other cancers by inhibiting tyrosine kinases. Increasingly, small interfering RNAs (siRNAs) are being tested as inhibitory drugs, systemically and by direct instillation into the central nervous system and other tissues (Dykxhoorn and Lieberman, 2006).

A few disorders can be treated with "curative" therapies that restore missing functions. Examples of such conditions and treatments include congenital hypothyroidism (replacement of thyroid hormone), bile acid synthetic enzyme deficiencies (oral bile acid therapy), biotinidase deficiency (biotin vitamin therapy), and celiac disease (dietary avoidance therapy). Still, for most rare diseases an obvious and easy therapeutic remedy is elusive or beyond current scientific capabilities. As discussed in Chapter 2, for most rare conditions, treatment is limited to symptomatic therapies (see, e.g., Campeau et al., 2008; Dietz, 2010).

High-Throughput Screening of Compound Libraries

When a potentially relevant target for an identified disease is validated, chemists then mount an intensive search for chemicals that might modify the target or targets. They screen vast compound libraries that are primarily assembled and secured within pharmaceutical companies to develop a list of potential "hits" that might some day become a "lead compound" and eventually new medicine, almost always after extensive "medicinal" chemistry to improve various properties of the parent compound and turn it into a drug suitable for testing in humans. This sophisticated process can be divided into three distinct steps: (1) development and maintenance of large compound libraries, (2) specific assay development, and (3) high-throughput screening.

Assays are analyses that quantify the interaction of the biological target and the compound that the researchers are investigating. They also might measure how the presence of the compound changes the way in which the biological target behaves. The chemical compounds tested in these assays are maintained in large compound libraries, which may contain more than 5 million chemicals. Products from natural sources such as plants, fungi, bacteria, and sea organisms can be integrated within compound libraries. Most compounds, though, are derived through the use of chemical synthesis techniques, in which researchers create chemical compounds by manipulating "parent" chemicals. They might also use combinatorial chemistry, in which researchers create new but related chemical compounds and test them rapidly for desirable properties. Sometimes companies will provide compounds to laboratories for low-volume screening, or alternatively the assay for the molecular target can be provided to a company where it will be optimized for high-throughput screening.

Testing the expanding number of available biological targets against thousands or millions of chemical entities requires highly sophisticated screening methods. Researchers use robotics, for example, to simultaneously test thousands of distinct chemical compounds in functional and binding assays. Academic researchers with expert knowledge of specific pathways may guide the development of assays in collaboration with industry. The chemical compounds identified through this kind of screening can provide powerful research tools that contribute to a better understanding of biological processes. This, in turn, may lead to new targets for potential drug discoveries.

The purpose of this chemistry stage is to refine the compound. Hundreds and possibly thousands of related compounds may be tested to determine if they have greater effectiveness, reduced toxicity, or improved pharmacological behavior, such as better absorption after a patient takes the drug orally.

To optimize the molecules being investigated, scientists use computers to model the structure of the lead compounds and how they link to the target protein—an approach to structure-based design known as in silico modeling (silico referring to the silicon technology that powers computers). This kind of structural information gives chemists a chance to modify lead molecules or compounds in a more rational way. This refinement process is called lead optimization, which may produce a drug candidate that has promising biological and chemical properties for the treatment of a disease.

Once a candidate drug (or group of candidates) is developed and its effectiveness in altering the molecular target is verified, then animal studies begin to determine whether the drug can be absorbed through the gastrointestinal tract for oral delivery, whether adequate levels of the drug are achieved in the blood, how the drug is metabolized in the body and excreted, and whether it actually reaches the molecular target defined by the basic research. In addition, if an animal model of the rare disease exists (through genetic alterations), this provides researchers with an opportunity to gather a preclinical proof of therapeutic concept, which can be very important before the compound enters development. This process of drug discovery for rare diseases is no different than that for common diseases—the costs and infrastructure required for both are significant.

Methodological Approaches to Biologics Discovery

For a biologic product (e.g., a specific protein, enzyme, peptide, antibody, or vaccine), the discovery phase varies considerably from the process for a small-molecule drug described above. It requires different areas of expertise, some of which can be found at academic institutions and others of which are available at biotechnology and pharmaceutical companies.

If the defect in a specific rare disease is due to deficiency of a specific protein, then human protein replacement therapy may be a feasible approach. To accomplish this, the replacement protein can either be isolated from other animals or, more commonly, be expressed in microorganisms or plant, nonhuman mammalian, or human cells after introduction of a gene encoding the desired human protein (so-called recombinant expression). This process can be extremely complicated. Some proteins require specific modifications (called posttranslational modifications) that are only accomplished by specific organisms or cell types. Other proteins require artificial modifications to target them to a specific tissue or cell type or to facilitate their uptake into cells, if that is where their critical function resides. For example, for some lysosomal enzyme deficiency diseases, it is critical to target the replacement protein for uptake in liver or muscle cells, whereas for other diseases, the replacement protein must have different modifications that promote uptake by reticuloendothelial cells (Grabowski and Hopkin. 2003). Not all obstacles have found solutions. Currently, a sizable number of rare diseases that affect the brain present a major challenge since many biologics lack the ability to cross from the circulation into the central nervous system (the so-called blood-brain barrier). Researchers continue to investigate strategies for overcoming this problem (see, e.g., LeBowitz, 2005; Valeo, 2010).

Given this complexity, there is no single path to success for biologic therapeutics. Rather, the opportunities and obstacles must be elucidated for each disease, and the approach must be tailored accordingly—a truly daunting task for thousands of rare disorders. Nevertheless, biologics have strong appeal because they have the potential to address the etiologic foundation of a disease process (e.g., through replacement of a deficient protein), to prevent diseases (e.g., with vaccines), or to harness the power of the immune system to achieve target specificity and to diversify the output of potential therapeutic agents (e.g., by production of an antibody that neutralizes a deleterious protein). Good examples include clotting factor proteins to treat hemophilia, vaccines to prevent smallpox or measles, and antibodies to treat multiple forms of cancer (Reichert et al., 2005).

Restoration of functional levels of missing molecules includes enzyme replacement therapy, available for several lysosomal storage diseases. Among these are Gaucher disease, Fabry disease, mucopolysaccharidosis I and VI, and Pompe disease (Lim-Melia and Kronn, 2009). Enzyme therapy is also employed for one form of severe combined immunodeficiency, adenosine deaminase deficiency (Aiuti et al., 2009). These approaches have required research efforts to express the protein yeast, bacteria, plant, or mammalian cell systems at small laboratory scale to provide sufficient enzyme for research studies. Enzyme therapy does not correct central nervous system dysfunction because an enzyme does not cross the blood-brain barrier. An approach, not yet successful, has been to make this barrier transiently permeable, and hematopoietic stem cell transplantation is being explored to restore the brain's capacity to make protein on its own (Hemsley and Hopwood, 2009).

Other Forms of Therapy Applicable to Rare Diseases

Cell Therapy

Cell therapies for rare disorders are largely confined to blood and marrow transplants to repopulate key cell subpopulations through differentiation of hematopoietic stem cells. Examples include a diverse range of rare disorders including degenerative neurologic disorders such as Krabbe disease (Escolar et al., 2006), Fanconi anemia (Kelly et al., 2007), and metabolic storage diseases such as the mucopolysaccharidoses (Sauer et al., 2004). Blood and marrow transplantation offers the opportunity for long-term correction but is attended by major risks (especially when using unrelated donors) such as failure of reconstitution, graft versus host disease, severe infections owing to immune suppression, and death. Current research efforts are aimed at reducing or eliminating these side effects. Undoubtedly, blood and marrow transplants will be studied for efficacy in additional rare diseases.

Cell therapies beyond blood and marrow transplantation have the potential through tissue engineering to reconstitute organ tissues that have been injured as a result of a rare disorder. New cell therapies will utilize embryonic or adult stem cells that can be programmed to differentiate into a mature cell of choice. It is likely that initially targeted disorders for cell therapies will be the more commonly occurring organ system injuries such as myocardial infarction. Nonetheless, cell therapies hold promise for rarer events and disorders, and human clinical trials of stem cells as potential therapy for rare diseases have begun (see, e.g., Steiner et al., 2009).

Gene Therapy

Gene therapy has been successful in limited circumstances. The overall goal of traditional gene therapy is to deliver a normal gene to compensate for one that is either dysfunctional or absent in a specific rare disease. Attempts to deliver genes with viral or other vectors directly to organs such as the lung for cystic fibrosis or the liver for metabolic disorders or hemophilia (High, 2009) have not yet been therapeutically successful. Attempts to introduce the factor IX gene into hemophilia patients using adeno-associated virus (AAV) have demonstrated factor production but have been attended by hepatoxic immunologic reactions (High, 2009).

More recently, correction of several rare disorders has been accomplished by inserting genes with retrovirus vectors into the patient's hematopoietic stem cells and returning these cells to the patient to restore lost function. This approach seemed to provide successful correction for severe combined immunodeficiency, but it also induced malignant transformation of lymphocytes in several of the treated patients, halting the further use of this approach pending the ability to overcome this serious adverse event (Aiuti et al., 2009; Hacein-Bey-Abina et al., 2010). Similarly, promising results for treatment of chronic granulomatous disease with gene-modified autologous stem cells have been accompanied by unanticipated serious adverse outcomes (Stein et al., 2010). The use of self-inactivating lentivirus vectors may circumvent some of the problems attributable to retrovirus vectors (Neschadim et al., 2007).

High (2009) recently reported the finding of improved vision after direct injection of an AAV vectored wild-type gene necessary for production of visual pigment into the subretinal space of patients with Leber congenital amaurosis. Other recent successful gene therapies have also been reported (see, e.g., Bainbridge et al., 2008; Cartier et al., 2009). These achievements provide renewed hope, but gene therapy is currently considered experimental and is tightly regulated. Extensive research will be needed to create gene therapies that provide efficient, stable, and safe correction across a range of rare disorders. Future research should overcome many of the current barriers to corrective gene therapy including avoidance of insertional mutagenesis and deleterious immunologic responses, maintenance of gene expression, and promotion of the targeting, engraftment, and viability of genetically altered cells. The research to achieve these goals may require decades.

Combined gene and cell therapy also demonstrates promise. Mesenchymal stem cells can repopulate injured tissues, but can also be genetically programmed to enhance their benefit. For example, mesenchymal stem cells that have been genetically programmed to produce interleukin-10 have been shown to protect against reperfusion injury in transplanted rat lungs (Manning et al., 2010). This strategy has also been studied in treating osteogenesis impefecta (Chamberlin et al., 2004). Continuing support of improved and novel approaches to gene therapy is important for rare diseases, which for the most part have genetic causes that will often be difficult to treat with simpler therapies.

Diagnostics

Rare disorders are identified in a variety of ways, including by physical examination for clinical phenotypes, by biochemical assays, by testing for chromosomal abnormalities, by testing for gene mutations, and by imaging to detect structural and functional abnormalities. There are many rare diseases for which no diagnostic tests are available. These diseases must be diagnosed on the basis of carefully defined clinical characteristics. Box 4-2 highlights some of the enabling technologies to support advances in diagnostics.

As noted earlier, detection of gene mutations is accelerating for rare diseases, and new methods such as whole exome sequencing promise even greater momentum. Once the primary genes are identified, the development of laboratory tests for rare disorders becomes feasible. (As described in Chapter 7, many diagnostic tests are regulated as medical devices. FDA has recently indicated that it will seek to regulate some genetic tests, although the specifics have yet to be determined.) In addition, genotyping now allows for identification of classical disease subtypes, an increasingly important step in designing and prescribing effective therapeutic agents. Finally, genetic testing for polymorphisms of genes coding for drug metabolizing enzymes (pharmacogenetics) will be increasingly useful for identifying drug responders and nonresponders with rare as well as common diseases.

In addition, research in the area of development of new technologies for newborn screening is advancing reasonably quickly; most targeted conditions are rare diseases (see Chapter 2). For example, tandem mass spectrometry for the direct assay of enzymes in dried blood spots has been applied to newborn screening for Krabbe disease (Li et al., 2004). As new biomarkers are described, cheaper and more facile diagnostic methods will

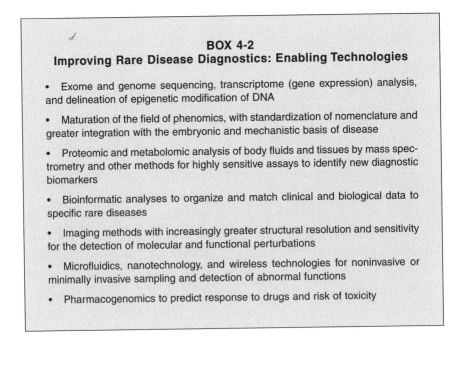

BOX 4-2
Improving Rare Disease Diagnostics: Enabling Technologies

• Exome and genome sequencing, transcriptome (gene expression) analysis, and delineation of epigenetic modification of DNA

• Maturation of the field of phenomics, with standardization of nomenclature and greater integration with the embryonic and mechanistic basis of disease

• Proteomic and metabolomic analysis of body fluids and tissues by mass spectrometry and other methods for highly sensitive assays to identify new diagnostic biomarkers

• Bioinformatic analyses to organize and match clinical and biological data to specific rare diseases

• Imaging methods with increasingly greater structural resolution and sensitivity for the detection of molecular and functional perturbations

• Microfluidics, nanotechnology, and wireless technologies for noninvasive or minimally invasive sampling and detection of abnormal functions

• Pharmacogenomics to predict response to drugs and risk of toxicity

undoubtedly be developed and used at an early age to identify presymptomatic rare conditions.

If DNA sequencing and interpretation of sequence data can in the future be carried out at low cost, it is conceivable that whole exome or whole genome sequencing will be productive for early diagnosis or even for newborn screening (Collins, 2009). The responsible application of such testing will require a comprehensive assessment of ethical, economic, practical, and social implications.

Genetic tests will, in all likelihood, include not only the identification of single nucleotide polymorphisms of the primary gene but also of DNA copy number variations, modifier gene polymorphisms, gene expression profiles, and the determination of epigenetic modification of DNA or histones that bear on gene expression and, therefore, the clinical manifestations. This extended genetic testing, when coupled with meticulous patient phenotyping, has the potential to explain clinical variation within defined rare disorders and offers opportunities to more accurately predict the clinical course of the disease. Such diagnostic information will be useful in guiding decisions about the timing of therapeutic interventions and their intensity. As is true of most diagnostic testing, genetic testing also may identify variants of uncertain significance that puzzle clinicians and do not yet assist decisions about patient care.

In addition to genetic markers, other biomarkers may be useful in predicting disease severity or progression. They may include specific patterns of peptides and metabolites identified by proteomic or metabolomic analysis. In selected disorders, longitudinal assessments of environmental exposures may predict variation in outcomes (e.g., for patients with cystic fibrosis who are exposed to tobacco smoke).

INFRASTRUCTURE FOR BASIC RESEARCH AND DRUG DISCOVERY FOR RARE DISEASES

As highlighted above, the basic research tools available to investigators have advanced dramatically over the past 20 years, with new approaches continuing to evolve. Along with them, models for providing the infrastructure necessary for discovery research have also undergone a transformation in recent years. This section describes some elements of the necessary infrastructure, including animal models, patient registries and biospecimen repositories, research funding, and training and also describes innovations in the area of sharing data and other resources, which can lower the considerable costs of basic and translational research.

Although collaboration and innovation in the sharing of data and other scarce resources are particularly useful for advancing research on rare diseases, commonly cited barriers include concerns about the protection of intellectual property. These concerns involve legal, technical, and financial issues related to the patent process itself, but they also derive from the significance of intellectual property, broadly construed, to the success of institutions and individuals. The committee was not asked to examine the protection of intellectual property, but it is importance to recognize that such protection through the issuing of patents and copyrights is a fundamental element of the infrastructure linking biomedical research to product development. The passage of the Orphan Drug Act was in part a response to the lack of incentives for companies to investigate rare diseases applications of off-patent or unpatentable drugs (Asbury, 1985). Although the patenting process is the same for products for common and rare diseases, questions about the status of patents on genes and proteins may present special challenges for rare genetic diseases research that relate to development of new drugs (discussed in Chapter 5).[1]

At the institutional level, developing feasible mechanisms for data and resource sharing in both academic and commercial research is not a straightforward process (see, e.g., Cohen and Walsh, 2008; So and Stewart, 2009). For example, university technology transfer offices have been criticized for being slow and cumbersome. Moreover, because the patenting process is costly, institutions with limited resources may be forced to choose which discoveries they will seek to protect and which they will not. In these circumstances, the limited commercial prospects for many products for rare diseases may influence institutions to bypass future commercialization opportunities, and the lack of patent protection may discourage the sharing of data and materials with potential collaborators.

At the individual level, investigators' desires for professional advancement and stature as well as their property interests in discoveries may sometimes impede and sometimes support sharing and collaboration. One study of access to genetic data and materials reported that nearly 50 percent of genetic researchers have encountered negative responses to their requests for data or materials related to published research (Campbell et al., 2002; see also Schofield et al., 2009). Reasons cited for denying access included not only desires to protect the commercial value of the intellectual property but also to maintain publication opportunities. Another factor cited was the cost of producing the data or materials requested.

Although barriers are significant, a range of infrastructure and information sharing innovations can be cited, including several that operate

---

[1] A 2006 National Research Council report *Reaping the Benefits of Genomic and Proteomic Research: Intellectual Property Rights, Innovation and Public Health* (NRC, 2006) examined these questions. Recently, in a case involving gene patents held by Myriad Genetics, the ruling of a federal district court would, if upheld on appeal, invalidate or restrict patents on individual genes (Pollack, 2010).

under the auspices of the National Center for Biotechnology. One example is GenBank, which is a National Institutes of Health (NIH) database of publicly available DNA sequences that have been submitted by individual laboratories or from large-scale sequencing projects (Benson et al., 2008). A significant incentive for such submissions is the requirement by scientific journals for deposition to GenBank or a similar database so that an accession number will be included in a published article.

Also, a significant response to institutional, individual, and other barriers to information access has been the requirement by NIH that applicants for grants that exceed $500,000 include a plan for "timely release and sharing of final research data from NIH-supported studies" (NIH, 2003, unpaged). In addition, some private organizations such as the Myelin Repair Foundation have grant provisions to speed information sharing (MRF, 2010; see also Schofield et al., 2009). More examples of initiatives to increase access to information and other infrastructure resources are described below and in Chapter 5.

Animal Models

Development of disease models in animals yields major opportunities for discovery of the genetic and biochemical basis for rare diseases, the identification of therapeutic targets, and the testing of new drugs and biologics for efficacy and safety. A number of genetic diseases occur naturally in animals (e.g., hemophilia B in dogs [Kay et al., 1994]), and various techniques exist for creating such models when they do not exist in nature. Mouse models are common, but simpler, more rapidly reproducing models such as the zebrafish are also valuable where genetic mouse models do not fully recreate human disease. Technological advances have allowed the development of long-sought alternative animal models for Huntington disease (monkey) and cystic fibrosis (pig) (Wolfe, 2009), but satisfactory animal models still await many rare diseases, for example, Smith Lemli Opitz syndrome (Merkens et al., 2009).

Mouse models, and occasionally other animal models, can be created using both forward and reverse genetic manipulation. Forward genetics involves the altering of specific genes to change their expression patterns and products. Although expensive and time-consuming, this approach is now a fundamental experimental strategy and has been an important contributor to research advances for an array of rare diseases. Reverse genetics is carried out by exposing animals to mutagenic agents and identifying genetic disorders by careful genotyping and phenotyping of the animals. Using this approach, a lethal skeletal dysplasia was created in mice that led to the identification of a deficiency of the GMAP-210 gene in these mice as well as in human achondrogenesis type 1A (Smits et al., 2010). The ability to carry out these studies requires animal (especially mouse) manipulation and maintenance facilities that are now available in most major academic research centers. Adequate funding for these studies is a challenge for fledgling research programs.

Expanded development and access to genetically modified mice that are relevant to rare diseases will promote research progress and accelerate work aimed at identifying potential therapeutic agents for rare diseases. Other research approaches have used cultured cells from mouse models of rare disease. Mice with humanized livers can be a boon for drug toxicity testing. Interestingly, it was research on tyrosinemia, a rare disease that led to this model (Azuma et al., 2007). Progress at the preclinical stage will undoubtedly be aided by the creative use of human cells, both normal and those derived from patients with genetic defects. An emerging option may be the in vitro generation of normal or disorder-specific differentiated cells from human pluripotent cells.

Mice with genetic disorders are collected, studied, and made available to researchers by various organizations, including the National Cancer Institute (http://mouse.ncifcrf.gov/) and the Jackson Laboratories, which also offers cells, tissues, and other products and services (http://jaxmice.jax.org/). One initiative of the Friedreich's Ataxia Research Alliance was to arrange with Jackson Laboratories to make mice available so that researchers no longer had to maintain their own research animals (Farmer, 2009).

Patient Registries and Sample Repositories

Patient registries can address many obstacles faced in the study of rare disorders including provision of a centralized source of information regarding disease incidence, prevalence, regional or temporal clustering of cases, and natural history or response to treatment. They can also serve as a recruitment tool for the launch of studies focused on disease etiology, pathogenesis, diagnosis, or therapy. (Chapter 5 discusses the role of patient registries in clinical studies.) In addition, patient registries can form the basis for the development of support networks and national or regional patient advocacy groups.

When combined with genetic information, patient registries can inform the correlation of patient genotype with the distribution, onset, severity, or progression of clinical manifestations or response to treatment (phenotype-genotype correlations). In essence, for rare disorders it is necessary to collect as much information as possible on as many patients as possible to discriminate predictive patterns from chance correlations, to validate these patterns using statistical methods, and to apply them productively in individual patient diagnosis, prognostication, counseling, and management (i.e., individualized medicine). Patient registries can be organized for a specific diagnosis (e.g., the Cystic Fibrosis Foundation [CFF] Patient Registry), a class of phenotypically related diagnoses (e.g., the National Registry of Genetically Triggered Thoracic Aortic Aneurysms and Cardiovascular Conditions [GenTAC]), or even a particularly important clinical event or outcome that is common to many conditions (e.g., the International Registry of Acute Aortic Dissections). Decisions about whether a registry should attempt to capture a comprehensive or representative sample are often influenced by disease prevalence. For example, the GenTAC cohort derives from five centers with a high surgical volume of patients with aortic aneurysm, whereas for the CFF registry, centers accredited by the CFF make a concerted effort to enter prescribed data elements for all patients. The CFF approach, in which designation as an accredited center and funding are linked to participation in the registry effort, has proven remarkably effective; more than 25,000 individuals are included in the registry (CFF, 2009). CFF-accredited centers also provide rich genotypic information and use standardized and evidence-based diagnostic and management guidelines based in part on national registry data analyses. This approach can serve as a model for certain other rare disorders, although it will be limited to patient advocacy groups or other coordinating entities that have substantial sophistication, organization, and resources to exert as leverage.

In addition to patient registries, a number of advocacy groups have promoted the development of repositories of biospecimens. In recognition of the challenges this undertaking presents for many groups, the Genetic Alliance Biobank provides infrastructure coordination for multiple rare diseases, and it includes clinical records and questionnaires as well as biological materials (Genetic Alliance, 2010). This type of federated approach also lowers the barriers for access to patient samples by individual researchers.

The National Disease Research Interchange, a federally funded private organization, takes a different approach to biospecimens (http://www.ndriresource.org/). It provides academic and industry researchers with a national human tissue and organ retrieval system. The organization recently created an alliance with a number of rare diseases organizations to increase awareness of its resources and develop new resources, including the National Rare Disease Biospecimen Resource.

Given the scope of the challenge to strengthen patient registries and other aspects of the research infrastructure for many or all rare disorders, it seems highly practical and desirable for NIH to be positioned as a central partner if not the leader in this effort. Later in this chapter, Recommendation 4-1 proposes that NIH collaborate on a comprehensive system of shared resources for discovery research on rare diseases. In Chapter 5, Recommendation 5-3 calls for NIH to support a collaborative public-private partnership to develop and manage a freely available platform for creating or restructuring patient registries and biorepositories for rare diseases and sharing de-identified data. Many complex details will need to be considered to implement these recommendations.

Funding of Basic Research and Drug Discovery for Rare Diseases

The discussion below focuses on government and nonprofit organizations as funders of basic research on rare diseases, but it also includes some data and some concerns related to the financing of clinical studies. In general across many sectors of the economy, industry funds relatively little basic research, both as a percentage of total industry funding of research and development and in comparison to federal government funding (AAAS, 2009). In health care, publicly funded basic research is a foundation for pharmaceutical development.

NIH and Other Federal Agencies

As with other basic biomedical research in the United States, the major funding source for basic research on rare diseases is undoubtedly NIH. The committee was not, however, able to determine the amount of NIH funding directed to all conditions that are identified as rare. It understands that the Office of Rare Diseases Research at NIH has requested that the process for categorizing and collecting data on spending by category be revised to allow the easier generation of disease-specific totals and totals for all spending on rare diseases research. This would allow a more systematic assessment of current resources and resource allocation.

Categorizing basic research spending by disease is less straightforward than categorizing clinical research, but an informal examination of the RePORTER database of current NIH awards (http://projectreporter.nih.gov/reporter.cfm) indicates that many rare diseases have attracted substantial funding but that funding for specific rare diseases is highly variable. Figure 4-1 presents a scatter plot for 32 rare diseases (selected to be generally representative of different kinds of conditions), with disorder prevalence displayed on the horizontal axis and numbers of awards on the vertical axis. (Limitations of the data source for the prevalence statistics are described in Chapter 2.) The number of NIH awards varies from none for tetralogy of Fallot and one for Ehlers-Danlos syndrome to more than 600 awards for Huntington disease and nearly 800 awards for cystic fibrosis.

Many factors undoubtedly contribute to the variation in the number of awards for this group of diseases. Although a systematic analysis was beyond the committee's resources, several general observations can be made. First, those rare diseases for which a specific gene mutation or set of gene mutations has been identified have generally attracted substantial

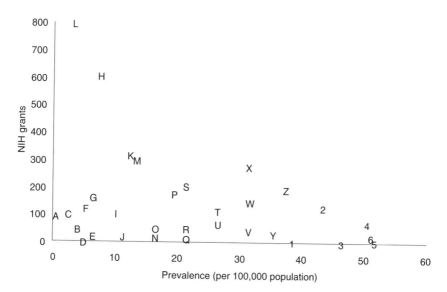

FIGURE 4-1 Plot of NIH grants for illustrative rare diseases by disease prevalence.
NOTE: Prevalence figures come from Orphanet, 2009 (see discussion of data in
Chapter 2). Grant numbers include American Recovery and Reinvestment Act grant
supplements and training grants.
SOURCE: NIH Reporter (http://projectreporter.nih.gov/reporter.cfm).

A — Progeria
B — Niemann-Pick disease
C — Fanconi anemia
D — Ehlers-Danlos syndrome (classic)
E — Primary ciliary dyskinesia
F — Rett syndrome
G — Duchenne muscular dystrophy
H — Huntington disease
I — Tuberous sclerosis
J — Leber congenital amaurosis
K — Sickle cell anemia
L — Cystic fibrosis
M — Acute myeloid leukemia
N — Congenital diaphragmatic hernia
O — Sarcoidosis
P — Familial dilated cardiomyopathy
Q — Hereditary spherocytosis
R — Turner syndrome

S — Gastric cancer
T — Neurofibromatosis (type 1)
U — Alpha$_1$-antitrypsin
V — Marfan syndrome
W — Amyloidosis
X — Acute respiratory distress syndrome (adult)
Y — Cryptosporidiosis
Z — Non-Hodgkin lymphoma
1 — Albright hereditary osteodystrophy
2 — Scleroderma
3 — Tetralogy of Fallot
4 — Narcolepsy (cataplexy)
5 — Melanocortin-4 receptor deficiency
6 — Noonan syndrome

numbers of NIH awards. Second, those disorders for which robust, high-profile patient advocacy groups have been established also tend to be the ones garnering more federal funding. Third, one feature of research on a rare disease, especially an extremely rare disease, is that only one or two investigators may be funded to study the condition, which means that the loss of funding can bring research virtually to a halt. Few advocacy groups have the resources to step into the funding breach.

Table 4-1 presents data on NIH awards for four very rare disorders, progeria, Neiman-Pick disease, Fanconi anemia, and primary ciliary dyskinesia. The numbers of awards for these conditions range from approximately 20 to 100. The variation is fivefold and does not appear to be related to knowledge of genetic or molecular causation, which the committee believes is similar for all four. Most of the awards are directed to basic science exploration of biological mechanisms that are related to the gene(s) of interest for that disorder. A much smaller number of awards fund preclinical (animal models) research examining both pathogenesis and therapeutic interventions.

For these four rare disorders, NIH is funding very few clinical trials. This may reflect the time lag between scientific discovery and clinical therapeutics research, the difficulties of conducting clinical research on very rare conditions, NIH's traditional emphasis on basic research, and the dominance of industry in funding clinical trials of drugs or other thera-

TABLE 4-1 Active NIH Awards for Four Rare Diseases by Number, Funding Total, and Type as of April 2010

Condition	Disease Prevalence (per 100,000)	Total Grants Listed	Annual Total Funding (millions of dollars)	Number of Grants Directly Targeting the Disorder	Pre-clinical Studies	Clinical Trials	Other Clinical Studies
Progeria	0.2	44	22.6	18	3	1	3
Niemann-Pick	0.5	46	17.8	20	7	1	0
Fanconi anemia	1.0	103	45.5	51	15	1	0
Primary ciliary dyskinesia	5.0	23	8.0	13	0	0	3

NOTES: A committee member (TFB) categorized grants directly targeting a disorder by reading the abstract for each grant to judge whether it directly addressed pathogenetic or clinical dimensions of the disorder or was focused on questions that were related only tangentially to the disorder. Likewise, this reader also evaluated whether the research involved preclinical (largely animal model) research, a clinic trial, or other clinical research (e.g., a natural history study). Supplementary grants under the American Recovery and Reinvestment Act are counted as separate awards.
SOURCE: NIH RePORTER (http://projectreporter.nih.gov/reporter.cfm). Prevalence data were taken from Orphanet, 2009 (see discussion of these data in Chapter 2).

peutic agents. Ongoing attention to the balance between basic and applied research for rare diseases will be critical to the acceleration of diagnostic and therapeutic product development.

Beyond those cited above, other factors contributing to the variation in federal funding of rare diseases research may include the number of scientific issues raised by a particular rare disease, the potential broader relevance of those issues, the availability of pilot grants from disease-specific foundations, the extent to which clinical care and clinical research are focused in disorder-specific clinics or centers, and workforce issues such as numbers of trained basic and clinical investigators.

Federal agencies beyond NIH also fund some biomedical research on rare diseases, particularly clinical studies. Chapter 3 describes the small orphan products grant program at FDA. Also within the Department of Health and Human Services, agencies such as the Centers for Disease Control and Prevention, the Bureau of Maternal and Child Health, and the Agency for Healthcare Research and Quality (AHRQ) support some research on rare conditions, particularly clinical, population-based, and health services research. For example, AHRQ has supported a review of the effectiveness of specific screening options to prevent neonatal encephalopathy owing to hyperbilirubinemia (Trikalinos et al., 2009). Chapter 1 cited the Congressionally Directed Research Program at the U.S. Department of Defense, which has been mandated to conduct research on several rare conditions.

Advocacy Groups and Foundations

An increasing number of disease-specific foundations and advocacy groups provide funding for research. The aim of many of these foundations is to attract investigators with skills and research track records in other areas to devote their attention to a particular rare disease. Several also support research training and career development in an attempt to engage future investigators in research efforts that advance their medical scientific agendas. This has worked well for foundations such as CFF, which over the years has committed $50 million to $100 million a year in the support of research. Other groups such as the Fanconi Anemia Research Fund have more recently entered the research funding arena and have been successful in attracting substantial but smaller numbers of investigators. (Appendix F presents several illustrative examples of elements of research support strategies pursued by advocacy organizations.)

Traditionally, disease-specific foundations have recognized that support across the entire continuum—basic research through clinical development—is necessary. In some cases, advocacy groups have been responsible for funding the fundamental scientific breakthroughs that were necessary for progress toward new therapies. Examples include CFF's support for work leading to the discovery of the CF gene (Riordan et al., 1989) and, much earlier, the National Foundation for Infantile Paralysis (now March of Dimes), which funded the work that produced the fundamental scientific insights needed for the development of the polio vaccine.

As part of their strategic planning, some rare diseases research foundations have undertaken analyses of public and private research spending on specific conditions. For example, the International Rett Syndrome Foundation determined that NIH accounted for 72 percent of funding of research on the syndrome, with foreign governments contributing 3 percent and nonprofit organizations 23 percent (IRSF, 2008; see also Appendix F). Of the funding, 94 percent was directed to basic research, with the largest share of both public and private funds devoted to finding and validating potential drug targets. Their conclusion was that a "bottleneck" existed in the translation of basic research findings into new therapies.

A number of foundations sponsor annual research meetings at which investigators share their research results and discuss opportunities in therapeutic development. In some cases, the foundations provide the impetus for the first gatherings of researchers working on certain rare diseases (e.g., the Chordoma Foundation, which jointly sponsored a workshop in 2007 with the NIH Office of Rare Diseases Research). Foundations have also partnered with federal agencies to promote research or launch clinical trials (e.g., the National Marfan Foundation and the Pediatric Heart Network of the National Heart, Lung, and Blood Institute, which launched the first clinical trial for Marfan syndrome [Lacro et al., 2007]).

Although disease-specific foundations do fund important research, private foundations collectively account for less than 10 percent of all support for biomedical research (Dorsey et al., 2010). When this support is divided into research on particular diseases and weighed against the cost of clinical trials, the amount available from private nonprofit sources for development of therapies is typically quite small. Individual foundations often seek to leverage relatively limited funds through the use of seed grants that help investigators develop the data needed to support competitive NIH grant proposals.

Investigator Training and Recruitment

A decision to pursue basic or translational rare diseases research is inherently risky, especially for young investigators. It is important that this reality be appreciated, both by funding agencies and by host academic institutions. Although academic investigators are attracted to the intellectual challenge of a rare diseases puzzle, they confront numerous vulnerabilities, including the scarce funding for research on most rare diseases, the limited number of potential collaborators, the limited access to biospecimens that are necessary for basic research, and the substantial uncertainty about industry interest in translating discoveries into products for rare diseases. All of these factors add to the difficulties normally confronted by academic researchers trying to establish research careers. Other issues, which are not confined to research on rare diseases in the university setting, include the complexities of negotiating contracts and materials transfer and other intellectual property agreements and the need to identify and manage or eliminate conflicts of interest that may arise from financial relationships with industry (e.g., research funding, consulting).

The review process at NIH also raises concerns. Existing study sections may be predisposed toward more common diseases, may not appreciate the critical importance of natural history studies for rare diseases, or may lack expertise to evaluate proposals that involve innovative trial designs and analytic methods for small populations. Possible responses include creating special NIH review mechanisms for rare diseases research proposals or developing guidance for existing study sections on the review of rare diseases proposals.

Specialized incentives to attract young investigators to the field include loan repayment, targeted requests for proposals from young investigators, and fellow-to-faculty transition awards. These mechanisms are useful in attracting young investigators into all disease areas and could be targeted specifically to investigators in areas of rare disease.

Areas of training particularly relevant to the development of rare diseases-oriented basic science careers include research in clinical genetics, tissue engineering and cell therapies, gene therapy, and bioinformatics. Training of clinicians in medical genetics, pediatric cardiology, or adult hematology-oncology represents a possible entry point to careers focused on a number of rare diseases encountered in these subspecialty areas. In addition to programs associated with the Rare Diseases Clinical Research Network (see Chapter 5), a few other training programs focused on rare diseases exist, for example, in juvenile rheumatoid arthritis, cystic fibrosis, muscular dystrophy, and sickle cell disease.

The basic science foundation needed for investigators in rare diseases is not distinct from that required for all biomedical research. Where the training needs diverge is at the point when an identified target is used to discover a potential drug and, from there, to move that drug into candidacy for clinical testing in humans and for therapeutic product development. At this point, the prospects for success begin to be affected by small patient populations and the relative lack of development interest from industry.

A few special programs aim to train individuals in the development of diagnostic or therapeutic products for rare diseases—for example, the SPARK program at the Stanford University School of Medicine (http://sparkmed.stanford.edu/). The program is institutionally funded (in part by an NIH Clinical and Translational Science Award) and seeks to create opportunities for medical and graduate students to build and execute a product development plan for new chemical entities and other discoveries generated by Stanford faculty that are not far enough advanced to attract industry interest. The program provides faculty and industry-experienced mentors for competitively selected projects. One emphasis is product development targeted to rare and neglected diseases, including through the repurposing of old drugs or the reconsideration of abandoned ideas or projects. Several products have been licensed and are in clinical development, which suggests that the goals of this program—education, stimulation of applied research, and commercialization of intellectual property—are being achieved. This is one example of an innovation platform that could accelerate future orphan products development.

Among particular needs for clinical-translational investigators in rare diseases is training in trial designs that can be applied to studies of small populations of patients with rare diseases. These investigators will also have to recognize when they need consultants to give them more expert guidance. Clinical subspecialists who work with both children and adults with rare diseases should be trained to collect data that will lead to standardized and detailed phenotyping and the elucidation of clinical natural histories, two potentially important contributions to research progress related to rare diseases. Training in systems biology and bioinformatics will also be key for future investigators working in rare diseases areas because these disciplines hold the potential to rapidly advance knowledge and its application to rare diseases. Beyond scientific training, successful investigators must know how to build and sustain productive collaborations and must be comfortable communicating their work to interdisciplinary audiences.

Training of young investigators or retraining of experienced investigators to conduct research on specific rare diseases will depend on the existence of productive and funded programs in rare disorders-specific research that can serve as training sites for both basic and clinical research. Thus, adequate funding for rare diseases research is an important first step in establishing training environments. Funding from NIH, other federal agencies, and disease-specific advocacy groups serves the dual purpose of fostering research progress and exposing investigators-in-training or young investigators to the relevant research activities.

The federal government through NIH and other agencies provides training grants, which may focus on individuals or programs (an example of the latter is the T-32 grants from NIH). These grants target specialty fellows in relevant medical subspecialties and graduate students or postdoctoral graduate fellows. Some disease-specific foundations also support training and young investigator grants.

Targeted career development awards for young faculty are particularly important in promoting and sustaining interest in and activity related to rare diseases. Examples of such awards include the K series grants from NIH and young investigator grants from CFF (e.g., the Leroy Matthews and Harry Shwachman Awards). The Dana Foundation's competitive grants programs in brain and immunoimaging and neuroimmunology primarily support new investigators with innovative clinical research hypotheses to develop pilot data on brain or spinal cord diseases, most of which are rare. Some of these new investigators have NIH K-08 (or K-23) mentored grants, which provide up to 75 percent of their salaries, and Dana funds support the remaining 25 percent. Both Dana and the NIH training grants support the new investigators' salaries, and other research-related costs often are supported by the investigators' institutions. The Burroughs Wellcome Fund offers a postdoctoral fellow-to-faculty transition grant for physician scientists, a model for the NIH K99-R00 awards. This approach is particularly effective at establishing early independence for fellows (Pion and Ionescu, 2003), and it could be employed more broadly for researchers in rare diseases areas.

The committee did not locate any compilation of resources for training related to rare diseases. Thus, it was difficult to judge the current amount of training or its content as a basis for identifying specific gaps. The emphasis here is therefore more generally on the need for training in basic and translational or clinical research areas that will be relevant to many rare diseases.

INNOVATION PLATFORMS FOR TARGET AND DRUG DISCOVERY

The high costs and low success rates associated with drug discovery and development, combined with the absence, in the case of rare diseases, of a large market for approved therapies, have stimulated the development of innovation platforms on a number of levels. One typical characteristic of these emerging approaches involves the sharing of the data, biological specimens, chemical compounds, and other resources that are needed at various stages to move from discovery to product approval and marketing.

Another characteristic is the involvement of funding organizations beyond their traditional roles of supporting research projects and training. Some patient-led foundations have taken on the task of "de-risking" the early stages of drug discovery through early-stage clinical trials, for example, by combining an infusion of philanthropic capital with the development of research tools and organized access to patients. For example, CFF has assembled drug discovery tools of potential interest to the scientific community working on the disease: an antibody distribution program, primary human epithelial cells harvested from lung transplants, a purified CFTR (cystic fibrosis transmembrane conductance regulator) protein supply, and validated assay services. These efforts of CFF and others are summarized in Chapter 5. NIH has also created new internal capacities and new partnership mechanisms for facilitating drug discovery, which are described in this section.

Public-Private Partnerships and Other Coordinating Strategies

Public-private partnerships have been a standard approach when the needs of the public sector converge with goals of the private sector, prompting the joint provision and management of resources for targeted projects. Examples include the delivery of services or facilities in the energy, transportation, education, or urban development sectors. NIH defines a public-private partnership as an agreement for the agency "to work in concert with a nonfederal party or parties to advance mutual interests to improve health" (NIH, 2007, p. 2). Although gifts, clinical research contracts and other contracts, and technology transfer agreements involve relationships with a nonfederal party or parties, NIH does not consider these arrangements to be partnerships. Other groups may have more expansive interpretations of the concept.

The formation of public-private partnerships involving government, industry, and nonprofit organizations has been a successful model for the infrastructure gaps in the area of neglected tropical diseases, which share with rare diseases the lack of commercial incentives for product development. For example, the multilateral Special Programme for Research and Training in Tropical Diseases (Morel, 2000; Ridley, 2003) and, more recently, the Medicines for Malaria Venture (Ridley, 2002) combine government, philanthropic, and industry funding[2] and enlist the expertise of an external scientific advisory board to select projects for support. These initiatives coordinate activities between industry and academic centers (e.g., sharing of compound libraries) to discover new molecules for the treatment of tropical diseases and shepherd them through the subsequent stages along the discovery-development pipeline, thereby acting as "virtual biotech" companies. Projects not meeting specified milestones are dropped and replaced with others, such that each organization manages a portfolio

---

[2] The malaria venture was, for example, initially cosponsored by the World Health Organization, the International Federation of Pharmaceutical Manufacturers Associations (IFPMA), the World Bank, the Dutch government, the Department for International Development in the United Kingdom, the Swiss Agency for Development and Cooperation, the Global Forum for Health Research, the Rockefeller Foundation, and the Roll Back Malaria Partnership.

of projects with varying degrees of risk (MMV, 2002, 2003; Nwaka and Ridley, 2003; TDR, 2008).

An example of a public-private partnership in the rare diseases area is the Spinal Muscular Atrophy project (http://www.smaproject.org/). Established by the National Institute of Neurological Diseases and Stroke, the pilot project is a multisite drug discovery and development enterprise that is guided by consultants with academic, FDA, NIH, and pharmaceutical industry expertise. The project focuses on optimizing lead compounds and making them available to researchers for preclinical testing.

NIH has initiated several broader programs to support drug discovery for rare diseases. The NIH Chemical Genomics Center (NCGC), which was established as part of the NIH Roadmap, focuses on novel targets as well as roughly a dozen rare and neglected diseases. As described on its website, it will "optimize biochemical, cellular and model organism-based assays submitted by the biomedical research community; perform automated high-throughput screening (HTS); and perform chemistry optimization on confirmed hits to produce chemical probes for dissemination to the research community" (http://www.ncgc.nih.gov/about/mission.html). The NCGC is also building a library of approved drugs so that these compounds can be more easily screened for possible repurposing for new indications; it has undertaken screening related to certain lysosomal storage diseases among other rare conditions (Austin, 2010).

The Therapeutics for Rare and Neglected Diseases (TRND) program, which was established in 2009, will collaborate with the NCGC as well as companies and nonprofit patient groups; it thus can be considered a public-private partnership (NIH, 2009b). The program aims to bring promising compounds to the point of clinical testing and adoption for further development by commercial interests. TRND, which had an initial budget of $24 million a year, is expected to ramp up to work on roughly five projects per year. Its first pilot projects involve sickle cell disease, chronic lymphocytic leukemia, Niemann-Pick Type C, hereditary inclusion body myopathy, and the parasitic diseases schistosomiasis and hookworm (Marcus, 2010b). (The NIH Rapid Access to Interventional Development program, which takes projects through preclinical development, is discussed in Chapter 5.)

TRND is a much-needed and innovative development. However, its scope (five projects per year) is well below the number of rare diseases that need therapies and have researchers positioned to take advantage of this capability. In addition, extension of services to include access to animal models of rare diseases could facilitate preclinical studies, a frequent barrier to therapeutic development. Expansion of both capacity and geographical distribution of TRND activities could advance therapeutics development for more rare diseases.

Sharing Biological Data on Disease Mechanisms

As discussed earlier in this chapter, arriving at a candidate drug requires extensive basic research into the disease mechanism, identification of potential targets for the drug, and generation of extensive molecular and genetic data. Typically, these mechanistic data are held by intrinsically competitive academic or industry labs that may have interests in protecting publication priorities or intellectual property or both. One consequence is that the data are not collected or stored in a way that ensures broad access to the information. This, in turn, has slowed the pace of information dissemination and driven up the cost of drug discovery.

In recent years, several developments have challenged this approach, particularly in the pharmaceutical industry. One development is the growing recognition that many research questions in human diseases are too complex for any one laboratory or any one company (Duncan, 2009). Another development is accumulating research that shows that many common diseases actually consist of subsets of disease based on their molecular characteristics, which often determine how individuals will respond to therapy. As a result, what might once have been a potentially large market of patients for a particular therapy is fragmented into a number of small markets. At the same time, companies have seen increasing costs of drug discovery and development without a corresponding increase in productivity of the industry, as measured by output of new molecular entities (Munos, 2009).

Taken together, these trends are stimulating innovation in the form of initiatives to share data "precompetitively" (see, e.g., Stoffels, 2009; Hunter and Stephens, 2010; Marcus, 2010a; but see also Munos, 2010). A recent workshop at the Institute of Medicine explored the opportunities and challenges of such collaborations, some of which involve only private entities (e.g., several companies or advocacy groups and companies) whereas others also involve the public sector (IOM, 2010b).

One model of precompetitive collaboration outside the health care arena is the development of the Linux operating system, which involved competitors sharing the benefits of increased productivity resulting from joint, voluntary investments in early-stage research. Given the increasing information richness of biology, similar integration of knowledge about biochemical pathways and networks from a wide range of researchers may spur productivity in the identification of molecular targets for diseases and otherwise advancing discovery research and product development. Existing examples of such efforts to share biological information or technology development resources include the following:

- Enlight Biosciences, a private company created in partnership with major pharmaceutical companies to develop enabling technologies that will alter the process of drug discovery and development (Zielinska, 2009); and

• voluntary, open-source sharing of biological data through the Sage Commons, an initiative of Sage Bionetworks, a new, nonprofit medical research organization (http://sagebase.org).

The second example, Sage Bionetworks, uses data shared by pharmaceutical companies and others to develop computational models that predict potential drug targets as well as potential toxicities (Melese et al., 2009). The data shared with Sage will eventually be publicly available and could be particularly valuable for rare diseases research. For example, the organization has already provided a significant amount of clinical data to the Huntington disease research community. The data were generated in a clinical study of Alzheimer disease in which individuals with Huntington disease were used as controls. Without the Sage resource, these data would likely have remained unknown and unavailable to Huntington disease investigations (Marcus, 2010a).

Some rare diseases advocacy groups have made the sharing of research data by grant recipients a prerequisite for funding. For example, through its Accelerated Research Collaboration model, the Myelin Repair Foundation has insisted that those funded in its collaborations share their research findings with one another without awaiting scientific publication (MRF, 2010). To cite another example, in 2007 the Multiple Myeloma Research Consortium launched a Genomics Portal, through which researchers have unrestricted access to prepublication genomic and other molecular data (Kelley, 2009). This approach is not conventional in academic environments where researchers are rewarded for individual achievement, but by mandating data sharing, the consortium has succeeded in significantly expanding the therapies currently under development for multiple myeloma.

Sharing Compound Libraries

A related trend is the opening of what were once proprietary company libraries of chemical compounds to investigators interested in the potential of compounds to interact with drug targets across a wide range of diseases. Compounds and information on their structures have typically been generated and held tightly by pharmaceutical companies. In recent years, companies have begun sharing compound libraries with researchers working in neglected diseases areas. For example,

• Eli Lilly Co. is sharing its compound libraries with researchers seeking therapies for tuberculosis (http://www.tbdrugdiscovery.org/);

- Pfizer Inc. has signed an agreement with the Drugs for Neglected Diseases initiative to share its library of novel chemical entities so that investigators can screen it for potential treatments for human African trypanosomiasis, visceral leishmaniasis, and Chagas disease (DNDi, 2009); and

- GlaxoSmithKline will share the chemical structures of compounds with potential activity against malaria through websites supported by federal, for-profit, and foundation funding (Guth, 2010).

In addition to the compound sharing initiative noted above, Eli Lilly has also established the Phenotypic Drug Discovery Initiative (https://pd2.lilly.com/pd2Web/). The company provides access to a phenotypic assay panel at no cost to external investigators, who can make a confidential compound submission and receive a full data report in return. Promising findings can lead to a collaboration agreement.

In the area of neglected diseases, access to compound libraries and chemical structures can significantly lower the threshold for pursuing drug discovery and development. Similarly, the European Rare Diseases Therapeutic Initiative has worked to bring about such access for academic institutions pursuing treatments for rare diseases (Fischer et al., 2005). To address intellectual property concerns, it has been proposed that compounds with commercial value might be accessed using a trusted intermediary, with initial confidentiality about the compound maintained and companies' reserving the option of first refusal for development (Rai et al., 2008). The experience with these efforts might inform the development of institutional mechanisms to facilitate access to proprietary compound libraries.

RECOMMENDATIONS

Two critical issues for rare diseases research are the small number of patients available to participate in research on rare diseases and the limited sources of funding for discovery and development of potential therapies for these diseases. It is therefore particularly important to make the best use possible of the information and other products that research generates—whether the research is directed specifically at a rare condition or at a more common condition that potentially has relevance for a rare condition. Making the best use of information and resources has several dimensions that target problems created by current practices. These problems include

- institutional and individual interests—economic, reputational, and professional—that can impede collaboration and resource sharing even as they may also stimulate innovation;

- fragmented, proprietary patient registries that have developed in the absence of consistent standards for the creation of accurate, usable information;
- fragmented, poorly preserved, and inaccessible biospecimen collections; and
- other resources such as biological data and research findings that are not broadly accessible to researchers who may then have to collect that information anew.

The committee does not underestimate the diverse barriers to resource sharing and collaboration or the need for creativity and patience in dealing with them. Nonetheless, it believes that the initiatives cited above illustrate promising strategies for either overcoming or coexisting with these barriers.

As components of an integrated policy to accelerate rare diseases research, several steps can be taken to develop a system that will support the sharing of resources, for example, compound libraries, and discourage the creation of a duplicative infrastructure. In some instances, steps may include the required sharing of research resources, for example, tissue specimens and data generated by federally funded or foundation-funded research on rare diseases. What is envisioned is essentially a "research commons" and public-private partnership (or series of partnerships) that has several unlinked or loosely linked elements.

RECOMMENDATION 4-1: NIH should initiate a collaborative effort involving government, industry, academia, and voluntary organizations to develop a comprehensive system of shared resources for discovery research on rare diseases and to facilitate communication and cooperation for such research.

Creating such a system of shared resources for rare diseases research will require a significant developmental effort and commitment of public, commercial, and nonprofit funding and other resources, for example, assistance in creating mechanisms for coordination and oversight and model provisions for public access to the information developed with government and nonprofit grant support. Key elements of this system would include, among other possible features,

- a repository of publicly available animal models for rare disorders that reflect the disease mechanisms and phenotypic diversity seen in humans;
- a publicly accessible database that includes mechanistic biological data on rare diseases generated by investigators funded by NIH, private foundations, and industry;

- common platforms for patient registries and biorepositories (see Chapter 5);
- model arrangements and agreements (e.g., template language on intellectual property) for making relevant portions of compound libraries available to researchers in rare diseases areas; and
- further exploration of precompetitive models and opportunities for developing technologies and tools for discovery research involving rare diseases.

Given the challenges outlined in this chapter and other parts of this report and given the important role that NIH plays in supporting research on rare diseases, the committee believes that a comprehensive NIH action plan on rare diseases would be useful to better integrate and expand existing work. This plan would take into account developments since the 2000 report of a special panel on coordinating rare diseases research programs within NIH (NIH, 2000). The following recommendation spans all phases of research on rare diseases and orphan products. Thus, it supports not only the discovery research discussed in this chapter but also the product development work and recommendations discussed in Chapter 5. It would likewise encompass research and development involving medical devices for people with rare diseases.

> **RECOMMENDATION 4-2: NIH should develop a comprehensive action plan for rare diseases research that covers all institutes and centers and that also defines and integrates goals and strategies across units. This plan should cover research program planning, grant review, training, and coordination of all phases of research on rare diseases.**

The development of an action plan would, at various points, necessarily involve consultation with FDA, advocacy groups, and industry. It likewise would involve consultation with investigators and academic institutions engaged in rare diseases research and product development.

The aspects of the plan that involve training would include incentives to attract new and established academic investigators to the study of rare diseases and orphan products and also support investigators currently studying rare diseases. Such a plan could include a loan repayment program for investigators working on rare diseases, the creation of an award for highly innovative proposals for rare diseases, and the broader use of the K99-R00 (Pathway to Independence) awards to attract outstanding new investigators in rare diseases research. Training opportunities through the NIH intramural research programs could also be identified. In addition, the program could include a mechanism for identifying training opportunities (especially in computational science, small clinical trial design, and orphan products development) that are particularly useful for investigators of rare diseases. Likewise, the program could support the identification, development, and replication of successful training models for investigators in rare diseases.

For all investigators, the creation of an award similar to the NIH Director's Pioneer Awards could provide an incentive and a reward for innovation. It would also draw attention to the opportunities for rare diseases research. These awards are intended to support investigators of outstanding creativity who propose truly innovative and even transforming biomedical research.

With respect to the review of proposals for research on rare diseases, the NIH action plan would include the development of guidance for study sections and institute councils. This guidance would, for example, clarify the potential public health relevance of rare diseases research, the range of appropriate methods for studying rare diseases, and the use of alternative mechanisms to ensure expert review of grant applications on rare diseases. Such mechanisms could include appointing special experts on rare diseases as primary reviewers to existing study sections, including rare diseases experts in the Center for Scientific Review, or creating a study section dedicated to rare diseases grants. More generally, NIH could investigate means of accelerating its decisions about preclinical (and clinical) awards for research on rare diseases.

Further, as discussed in Chapter 3, NIH and FDA should continue to cooperate in developing training and guidance to improve the quality of NIH-funded rare diseases and orphan products research and increase the likelihood that the research—including preclinical studies—will provide acceptable evidence for FDA review of marketing applications for drugs and biologics. For example, one element of the action plan could be a focused Request for Applications for natural history studies of rare diseases to help identify therapeutic targets for rare diseases or build the evidence base to support FDA approval of a specific drug being studied with NIH support. The lack of natural history studies has been identified as a problem in Chapter 3. Such studies are one focus of the Rare Diseases Clinical Research Network, but this network (as described in Chapter 5 and Appendix E) supports only 19 consortia that study approximately 165 rare conditions. NIH also funds a number of studies outside the network, but the natural history of many more rare diseases remains to be studied.

Another element of the action plan would be the development of a systematic, reliable, and comprehensive system for identifying and tracking public and private funding for rare diseases studies to help highlight gaps and opportunities for public and private research sponsors. As more private foundations and research initiatives are created, the lack of integrated information on funding will become a more serious problem and will interfere with the ability of these groups to target their resources and collaborate effectively.

The following chapter shifts the focus from basic research to the preclinical and clinical development investigations that are required to establish safety and efficacy and otherwise meet regulatory standards for approval of pharmaceuticals and biologics. It concludes with additional recommendations for resource sharing and collaboration.

5

Development of New Therapeutic Drugs and Biologics for Rare Diseases

When it is obvious that the goals cannot be reached, don't adjust the goals, adjust the action steps.

Confucius

Once a potential therapeutic drug or biologic has been discovered, the process of developing the therapeutic for a particular disease, whether rare or not, begins with preclinical development and continues through increasingly complex and demanding phases of clinical testing to support approval for marketing. Much of what is done throughout the process of drug development is driven by necessary regulations that require the sponsor of a new drug to demonstrate its safety and efficacy. (Figure 5-1 depicts the process, in simplified form, from the earliest basic investigations through studies undertaken after a product has been approved for marketing.) Although public and nonprofit organizations have sometimes taken a product through this process, this work, which is expensive and risky, has traditionally been done within pharmaceutical and biotechnology companies. Approximately 10 percent of potential therapeutics that effectively pass preclinical development reach the market, and the cost for each is estimated to average from $100 million to more than $1 billion, depending on the disease and other factors and taking the cost of failed drugs into account (see, e.g., DiMasi et al., 2003; PhRMA, 2007; Gassman et al., 2008). According to one study of the 50 largest pharmaceutical firms, about one in six new drugs that entered clinical testing eventually received approval for marketing, but this rate varied widely by therapeutic class and was slightly higher for drugs licensed into a company than for drugs originated by the company (27 percent

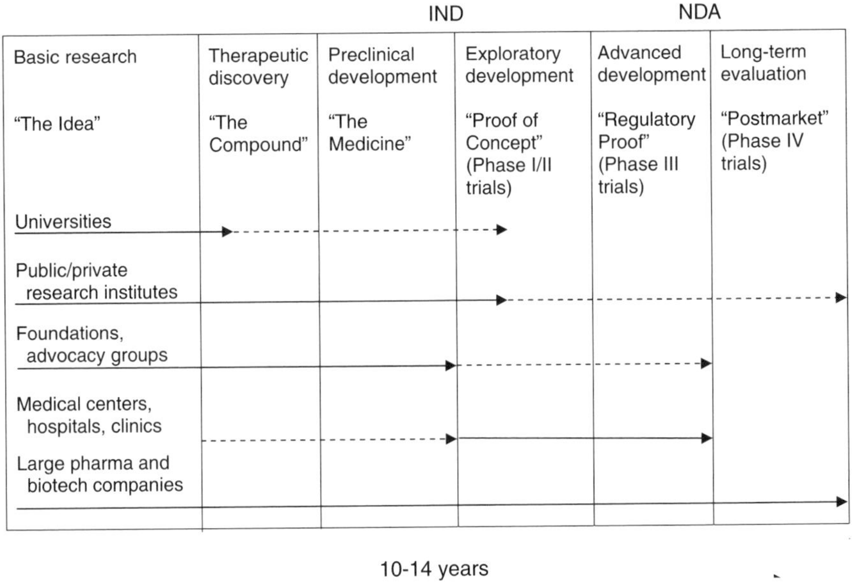

		IND		NDA	
Basic research	Therapeutic discovery	Preclinical development	Exploratory development	Advanced development	Long-term evaluation
"The Idea"	"The Compound"	"The Medicine"	"Proof of Concept" (Phase I/II trials)	"Regulatory Proof" (Phase III trials)	"Postmarket" (Phase IV trials)
Universities					
Public/private research institutes					
Foundations, advocacy groups					
Medical centers, hospitals, clinics					
Large pharma and biotech companies					

10-14 years

FIGURE 5-1 Drug development: from idea to market and beyond.
NOTES: IND = Investigational New Drug application; NDA = New Drug Application; Major emphasis = ⎯⎯⎯▶; Secondary emphasis = ┄┄┄┄▶.
SOURCE: Adapted from Corr, 2008.

versus 16 percent) (DiMasi et al., 2010). The proportion of orphan drug approvals accounted for by large pharmaceutical companies has grown in recent years (Tufts Center, 2010), but the committee found no analysis of the success rate specific to orphan drugs.

Given the relatively low odds of success and the high costs of drug development, pharmaceutical and biotechnology companies usually focus on potential therapies with the highest likelihood of generating a good financial return—as is the case with virtually all companies in any field. This has meant that potential therapies for rare diseases, including therapies for life-threatening conditions, have often languished in the early development pipeline. Moreover, conventional approaches to drug development are often not feasible for rare diseases, which offer not only small markets but also small populations for participation in clinical trials. To paraphrase the adage of Confucius, to achieve the goals of developing effective treatments for rare diseases calls for an adjustment of the action steps.

As described in Chapter 3, the Orphan Drug Act has provided incentives for the development of drugs for rare diseases, and the Food and Drug Administration (FDA) has approved more than 350 applications for the marketing of such drugs. Today, those incentives combined with the increasing expense and difficulty of developing blockbuster drugs have led some major pharmaceutical companies and biotechnology firms to announce that they are launching or considering orphan drug development (Anand, 2005; Dimond, 2009; Pollock, 2009; Whalen, 2009). In addition, charitable foundations linked to advocacy groups have made significant progress during the past 15 years in strategically filling the investment gap for orphan products and in pushing therapies for rare diseases through the development pipeline. The National Institutes of Health (NIH) is also supporting programs to help translate research discoveries into successful products, and innovative strategies for the conduct and analysis of studies involving small populations are allowing sound research when conventional trials designs are not possible or not feasible. At FDA, the recently created position of Associate Director for Rare Diseases at the Center for Drug Evaluation and Research (CDER) is a positive step (see Chapter 3).

This chapter begins with a description of the traditional approach to preclinical and clinical development as it applies to drug therapies for common or rare diseases. Later sections of this chapter examine the infrastructure for drug development (including biomarkers, patient registries, and clinical research training) and adjusted action steps such as alternative models of organizing and funding orphan product development. Some of these models build on public-private partnerships and other innovative strategies that have emerged from initiatives to speed the development of products for neglected tropical diseases.

PRECLINICAL DEVELOPMENT

Once a single promising compound is selected based on the kinds of basic research and therapeutic discovery reviewed in Chapter 4, companies initiate preclinical studies both in vitro and in animals to evaluate a drug's safety and potential toxicity. These preclinical studies are also used to assess potential effectiveness. Sponsors design additional studies to provide convincing evidence that a drug is not mutagenic (i.e., it does not cause genetic alterations) or teratogenic (i.e., it does not cause fetal malformations). Because a patient's ability to excrete a drug can be just as important as the patient's ability to absorb the drug, other preclinical studies focus in detail on those factors.

The following discussion of therapeutics focuses on drugs but also notes certain special features of preclinical studies for biologics. As described earlier in this report, drugs are chemicals—small-molecule medicines that can be taken orally or that may be administered in various other forms, such as injection, infusion, transdermal patch, or dermal application. Biologics are proteins, antibodies, peptides, and some vaccines that are usually injected or infused because they cannot be absorbed orally. For purposes of this discussion, they are usually encompassed under the term drug.

The safety and other data from preclinical studies are crucial in determining whether a drug will move on to studies in humans. Preclinical studies also guide researchers in designing phase I clinical trials. For example, preclinical studies with animals help determine the range of dosing of a test drug to be evaluated in a phase I clinical trial. They also help to identify criteria for evaluating safety in humans, including signs and symptoms that should be monitored closely during early clinical trials. Unfortunately, preclinical studies in animals are not precise predictors of what will happen with humans.

In addition, companies often must undertake carcinogenicity studies in animals to help assess whether a potential therapy might cause tumors. Because carcinogenicity studies require considerable time and resources, FDA guidance advises that "they should be performed only when human exposure warrants the need for lifetime studies in animals" (FDA, 1996, p. 1; see also CDER, 2002). The guidance therefore recommends carcinogenicity studies for any pharmaceutical for which clinical use is expected to be continuous over at least 6 months or to involve intermittent but frequent use in the treatment of chronic or recurring conditions (FDA, 1996). Long-term carcinogenicity studies might not be required when the potential therapy is intended for patient populations for whom life expectancy is predicted to be short (e.g., 2 to 3 years, as for some cancer therapies).

FDA's guidance on carcinogenicity studies also states that rodent carcinogenicity studies usually are not required to be completed prior to conducting large clinical trials in humans, unless a special concern is identified. If studies are required, they ordinarily must be completed before a sponsor applies for marketing approval. However, for drugs intended to treat life-threatening or debilitating diseases, the guidance advises that carcinogenicity testing can be conducted after rather than before a drug is approved for marketing. Thus, FDA required a postmarketing carcinogenicity study for the orphan drug carglumic acid (Carbaglu), a drug that must be used long term (Beitz, 2010) (see also Box 3-3). In addition, the agency generally will not require carcinogenicity studies for endogenous substances such as enzymes that are given as replacement therapy, particularly if previous clinical experience exists with similar products. Thus, FDA has not required pre- or postmarketing carcinogenicity studies for such orphan biologics as galsulfase (Naglazyme) (Weiss, 2005). In at least one case (pentosan polysulfate sodium [Elmiron], approved in 1996), FDA nominated an orphan drug for carcinogenicity testing by the National Toxicology Program (NTP, 2004). The test results allowed the drug's label to be revised in 2006 to report no clear evidence of carcinogenic risk.

One focus of the analysis of CDER reviews as recommended in Chapter 3 would be how the carcinogenicity guidance is being implemented for orphan drugs across FDA review divisions. Depending on the results of that analysis, CDER might develop additional guidance on this topic.

Preclinical work generates a pharmacologic profile of a drug that will be beneficial long into the drug's future. For example, researchers can use the profile to develop the initial manufacturing process and the pharmaceutical formulation to be used for testing with humans. Industry has particular strengths in these areas. Researchers can also use specifications assigned in the preclinical stage to evaluate the chemical quality and purity of the drug, its stability, and the reproducibility of the quality and purity during repeat manufacturing procedures. (This is sometimes referred to as "chemistry, manufacturing, and controls [CMC] information." CMC requirements and CMC activities evolve during the entire development process.) The FDA repurposing initiative described below emphasizes the value of this preclinical work if sponsors see a possible new use of an already-approved drug for a rare disease.

Preclinical studies, as well as manufacture of the drug at small scale, can be very expensive (several million dollars) and time-consuming (1 to 2 years). These studies also require specific expertise, both in the proper design and execution of the studies and in the proper interpretation of the results. Most studies need to be done under good laboratory practice (GLP) conditions to qualify for regulatory submission (21 CFR Part 58). GLP conditions apply not only to specified instrumentation, record keeping, and analysis, but also to specific laboratory conditions that, in most cases, require special facilities. More generally, meeting regulatory requirements for the approval of a drug requires expert knowledge and meticulous documentation. At the stage of drug production, companies must conform to what FDA refers to as current good manufacturing practice, or cGMP, requirements (21 CFR 210, 211).

For biologics (excluding vaccines) the development pathway is similar in many respects to that for small-molecule drugs. Two major differences stand out. First, the production of sufficient quantities of a biologic for preclinical and clinical development studies requires unique approaches for expression of the proteins and their purification to regulatory standards. As is the case for injected drugs, extensive studies are done to formulate the protein for injection under sterile conditions. Second, biologics can potentially elicit an immune response in the recipient. This response must be monitored very closely because it is not always predictable. Thus, biologics may present special issues to be addressed in preclinical studies, such as immunogenicity (i.e., induction of an antibody response) and immunotoxicity (agents intended to stimulate or suppress the immune system may cause cell-mediated changes) (CDER-CBER, 1997).

Preclinical development of biologics is also quite unpredictable. For example, experimental animals are very likely to develop endogenous antibodies against the human wild-type protein that could complicate interpretation of the results related to toxicology, distribution, and metabolism. In many cases, the ease of development of a biologic depends on whether it is a true "wild-type" (i.e., normal) human protein or whether it is a variant protein. As a general rule, the use of wild-type protein as a replacement therapy for a particular rare disease simplifies preclinical as well as clinical development, but there are exceptions. For example, a patient who produces none of a normal human protein because of an underlying genetic defect might easily produce antibodies against replacement wild-type protein, whereas a second patient, who has a different genetic defect and produces low levels of the normal protein, would not recognize the biologic as "foreign" and usually would not mount an immune response to the protein.

By their very nature, studies in preclinical development are major hurdles in the development of therapeutics for all diseases—but especially those that are rare. A later section of this chapter discusses ways in which these hurdles are being or might be addressed by NIH, FDA, companies, and advocacy groups.

The next several sections of this chapter are organized around the clinical trial phases that are conventionally used to develop evidence of safety and efficacy for drugs intended for common conditions. For drugs intended for quite rare diseases, the delineation among phases I, II, and III trials is often not as clear. As discussed in Chapter 3, FDA may not require the usual sequence of trials. The agency strongly encourages sponsors of drugs for rare diseases to seek meetings with FDA to discuss development strategy prior to submission of an Investigational New Drug (IND) application (Pariser, 2010).

PHASE I CLINICAL TRIALS: SAFETY

Before clinical studies can begin, sponsors must submit an IND application to FDA. This application must include the results of the preclinical studies discussed above. Given the generally small numbers of patients available for the study of rare diseases, sponsors benefit particularly from regulatory guidance on the extent of phase I analysis that CDER considers sufficient prior to the start of phase II clinical trials.

Phase I trials initiate the testing of drugs in humans. They often involve small numbers (20 to 100) of healthy volunteers but sometimes include research participants with a rare or other specific condition for which targeted pathways have been identified as potentially relevant to disease pathogenesis.[1] A phase I study may last for several months. Drug doses usually start at very low levels, and research participants are monitored very carefully as the dose is escalated. In some circumstances and depending on the study protocol, individual participants may receive only one dose.

Phase I studies focus on the evaluation of a new drug's safety, the determination of a safe dosage range, the understanding of the drug's clinical pharmacology, the identification of side effects, and sometimes the detection of early evidence of effectiveness if the drug is studied in patients with the target disease. From phase I clinical trials, researchers gain important information about

- the drug's effect;
- the drug's pharmacokinetics (absorption, distribution, metabolism, and excretion) to better understand a drug's properties in the body;
- the acceptability of the drug's balance of potency, pharmacokinetic properties, and toxicity or the specificity of the drug (i.e., its ability to hit its desired target without altering another biological process); and
- the tolerated dose range of the drug.

In January 2006, CDER issued guidance on exploratory IND studies (CDER, 2006). It defined such studies (which some refer to as phase 0 clinical studies) as occurring early in the initial phase of clinical studies, having no diagnostic or therapeutic purposes, and involving very limited exposure of humans to the investigational drug. The guidance urged sponsors to consider exploratory IND studies, in particular, for drugs intended for patients with serious, life-threatening diseases, which is often the case for rare diseases. Such studies involve fewer resources than conventional approaches and thus allow sponsors to "move ahead efficiently with the development of promising candidates" (p. 2). For example, during such an exploratory study, sponsors can test one or more related compounds at very low doses that are sufficient to determine the half-life, absorption, metabolism, and excretion of a drug. Such testing is particularly useful in guiding the selection of one compound among several to take to a full phase I study and in providing more early information when concerns exist about the predictive value of preclinical data from animals. It may be particularly helpful in studies of rare diseases.

---

[1] Among other provisions, government rules on the conduct of research involving human participants require that studies including children either involve no more than minimal risk or have expected benefits that justify the risk involved (OHRP, 2008). Thus, healthy children would generally not be included in a phase I safety study.

The guidance on exploratory IND studies is relatively recent. Such studies will occur long before an application for approval reaches FDA, so it will take time before the effect of this approach on product development for rare conditions can be assessed. In any case, exploratory studies appear a useful option for a company or other sponsor that is nearing the initiation of clinical research for a drug to treat a rare condition.

PHASE II CLINICAL TRIALS: PROOF OF CONCEPT OR EFFICACY

In conventional clinical trials for drugs for common conditions, phase II studies provide an investigational drug's first test of efficacy in research participants who have the disease or the condition targeted by the medication. Even if combined phase I-II trials are performed to obtain initial findings of safety and efficacy, larger phase II trials will normally be needed to determine optimal dosing to maximize efficacy and minimize adverse events. These studies may include up to several hundred participants and may last from several months to a few years.

As described in Chapter 3, for drugs intended for rare conditions, FDA may accept studies involving smaller numbers of research participants than are required for more common conditions. It may also allow the use of historical controls (or possibly no controls) if the rare disease has a defined course in the absence of treatment that will permit comparisons with results for an investigational drug.

Phase II studies help determine the correct dosage, identify common short-term side effects, and define the best regimen to be used in pivotal clinical trials. Conventionally, the initial step is usually a phase IIa clinical trial that is focused on an initial proof of concept. This step is to demonstrate that the drug did what it was intended to do: that is, it interacted correctly with its molecular target and, in turn, altered the disease. Phases I and IIa are sometimes referred to as "exploratory development." Phase IIb trials are larger and may use comparator agents and broader dosages to obtain a much more robust proof of concept and additional guidance on dose selection. They are often done at a regulatory standard that requires conformance with good clinical practice principles and guidelines (see, e.g., CDER-CBER, 1996, and documents at http://www.fda.gov/Science Research/SpecialTopics/RunningClinicalTrials/default.htm).

PHASE III CLINICAL TRIALS: REGULATORY PROOF

Conventional phase III clinical trials are designed to evaluate a candidate drug's benefit in a carefully selected patient population with the disease. These trials are to confirm efficacy, further evaluate safety and monitor side effects, and sometimes compare the candidate drug to commonly used treatments. They provide crucial evidence needed to satisfy regulators that the drug meets the legal requirements for marketing approval and to provide necessary information for product labeling after approval of the drug.

For common conditions, phase III studies are usually conducted with large populations consisting of several hundred to several thousand participants who have the disease or the condition of interest. Specific decisions about the size of the study group will depend on such factors as the magnitude of the effect of interest, characteristics of the study population, and study design. Phase III trials typically take place over several years and at multiple clinical centers around the world. The study drug may be compared with existing treatments or a placebo. Phase III trials are, ideally, double blinded; that is, neither the patient nor the investigator knows which participants are receiving the drug and which are receiving existing treatment or placebo during the course of the trial.

FDA typically requires two phase III clinical trials for approval of a drug, but the law authorizes FDA to approve a drug based on one multicenter study in appropriate circumstances. Because the number of patients available to participate in a clinical trial involving a rare disease is often very small, FDA frequently approves orphan drugs with less extensive requirements for clinical studies (see Chapter 3).

If clinical trials are successful, a New Drug Application (NDA) is submitted to FDA for review. The review process usually takes 10 to 12 months and may include, at the discretion of FDA, an advisory committee review. Drugs for rare conditions may qualify for one of several options for speeding the path to approval (see Chapter 3).

Phase II, and sometimes phase III, trials may fail due to the large heterogeneity of the patient population being studied. As a result of genetic heterogeneity, some research participants may respond well and others may not respond at all to an investigational product. Increasingly, research is subdividing common diseases such as breast or lung cancer into many heterogeneous subtypes that may differ in their responsiveness to different treatments and that may qualify as rare in terms of the number of people who fit a particular subtype.

Because most rare diseases have a more homogeneous genetic pattern than do common diseases and because they are often characterized by similar or identical genetic or epigenetic defects, patients with these diseases could be expected to have a more uniform response to a drug. This should reduce the size of phase II and III studies required to demonstrate efficacy. Indeed, in recognition of this relative homogeneity, CDER has accepted the use of historical controls in phase II trials for extremely rare diseases (see Chapter 3).

PHASE IV POSTMARKETING STUDIES

FDA will frequently specify postmarketing study (phase IV) requirements to further evaluate an approved drug and obtain more information
about safety or effectiveness or both. As described in Chapter 3, such studies are required if the accelerated approval process is used. Approval for one
drug (not for a rare disease) was recently rescinded based on postmarketing
study results that indicated no benefit. Many of the approvals of drugs for
rare diseases reviewed by the committee included provisions for various
kinds of postmarketing studies.

Responding to evidence of the agency's lax monitoring of company fulfillment of postmarketing study requirements, the FDA Modernization Act
of 1997 (P.L. 105-115) required FDA to establish a system for monitoring
and publicly reporting sponsor progress in fulfilling postmarketing study
commitments and requirements. The agency published rules implementing
the legislation in 2000 (65 Fed. Reg. 64607). Although study fulfillment
is important, the committee was not able to investigate this outcome for
orphan drugs.

INFRASTRUCTURE FOR DRUG DEVELOPMENT

The process of drug development, whether it involves a small molecule
or a biologic, is expensive and time-consuming. Invariably, it takes not only
expertise, but robust infrastructure and significant funds to bring a therapy
to market. Almost 70 percent of the total spent in drug development is for
failures at various stages of the drug development process.

Although there are several streams of funding for drug development,
the total amount is inadequate to support investigation of the thousands
of rare diseases profiled earlier in this report—with significant consequences for affected patients, their families, and their communities. Clearly,
innovation—on every level and by all stakeholders—is needed. This section
expands on the discussion begun in Chapter 4 by describing elements of
the infrastructure that are needed for clinical development of therapies, including biomarkers for use as surrogate endpoints in clinical trials, patient
registries, clinical trial consortia, and clinical research training.

Not included in the discussions below are many other infrastructure elements, information sharing initiatives, and collaborations. To cite one example, the Clinical Data Interchange Standards Consortium is a nonprofit
organization to establish standards for acquiring, exchanging, submitting,
and archiving clinical research data (see http://www.cdisc.org/). To cite
another example, Tox21 is a new collaboration involving NIH, FDA, and
the Environmental Protection Agency. It is intended to develop innovative
methods to predict the toxicity of drugs and other chemicals in humans,

speed the testing process by using robotic and informatics technologies to test compounds in cells, and establish priorities for chemicals that require further evaluation (Jones, 2010).

Biomarkers

One important avenue for speeding clinical studies of rare diseases involves the identification of biomarkers to monitor responses to therapy and guide dosing. Biomarkers have multiple uses. As described in a recent Institute of Medicine (IOM) report, they are used "to describe risk, exposures, intermediate effects of treatment, and biologic mechanisms; as surrogate endpoints, biomarkers are used to predict health outcomes" (IOM, 2010a, p. 3). Biomarkers figure significantly in several of the innovative approaches to developing drugs for rare diseases as discussed below.

Developing and validating biomarkers is not a trivial undertaking even for common conditions, but it is highly relevant for rare diseases and warrants concerted attention. Box 5-1 summarizes the recommendations on biomarker evaluation in the IOM report (IOM, 2010a). The IOM report emphasized the importance of context—including disease prevalence and severity—in evaluating biomarkers. It observed that "an intervention meant to treat a rare but life-threatening disease may permit more tolerance of risk than an intervention meant to treat a more common but less serious disease" and that "it may be easier to defend use of a surrogate endpoint for trials of rare and life-threatening diseases than for trials of primary prevention interventions for common but less serious or life-threatening diseases" (IOM, 2010a, p. 113). For biomarkers as well as clinical trial strategies generally, it will be important to consider what constitutes reasonable flexibility in FDA assessments of biomarkers for rare conditions.

Because a validated biomarker can serve as a surrogate endpoint in a clinical trial, this may allow sponsors to reduce the number of research participants and the time required for clinical trials. In addition, the accelerated approval pathway described in Chapter 3 allows FDA to approve a drug based on evidence involving surrogate endpoints that are not considered well established but that are determined to be reasonably likely to predict clinical benefit. FDA then requires postapproval studies to develop further evidence about benefits and risks based on clinical outcomes. (As discussed in Chapter 3, the Government Accountability Office recently expressed concern that FDA did not have an adequate process for monitoring the progress of these studies [GAO, 2009b].)

The Biomarkers Consortium is a public-private partnership that is managed by the Foundation for the National Institutes of Health. It aims to develop biomarkers for use in research, therapeutic and diagnostic development, regulatory approval, and clinical practice (http://www.

BOX 5-1
Summary of Earlier IOM Report Recommendations
for Effective Biomarker Evaluation

The Evaluation Framework

1. The biomarker evaluation process should consist of the following three steps:

  1a. Analytical validation: analyses of available evidence on the analytical performance of an assay;
  1b. Qualification: assessment of available evidence on associations between the biomarker and disease states, including data showing effects of interventions on both the biomarker and clinical outcomes; and
  1c. Utilization: contextual analysis based on the specific use proposed and the applicability of available evidence to this use. This includes a determination of whether the validation and qualification conducted provide sufficient support for the use proposed.

2a. For biomarkers with regulatory impact, the Food and Drug Administration (FDA) should convene expert panels to evaluate biomarkers and biomarker tests.

2b. Initial evaluation of analytical validation and qualification should be conducted separately from a particular context of use.

2c. The expert panels should reevaluate analytical validation, qualification, and utilization on a continual and a case-by-case basis.

SOURCE: IOM, 2010a.

---

biomarkersconsortium.org/). The consortium has several active and approved projects, none of which currently involve rare diseases. However, one of the specific topics mentioned in the recent solicitation of NIH Challenge Grants was the validation of biomarkers for functional outcomes in rare diseases (03-OD(ORDR)-101).

Several research initiatives are investigating biomarkers for rare diseases, for example, Huntington disease (Aylward, 2007) and pulmonary arterial hypertension (Heresi and Dweik, 2010). An example of a generally accepted biomarker for a rare condition is blood phenylalanine level for the rare disease phenylketonuria. Another example is forced expiratory volume (FEV_1), which FDA has accepted as an endpoint to support approval of drugs for cystic fibrosis and other lung disorders (CDER, 2007; Laessig, 2009). The committee heard of at least one example of a CDER review unit's questioning the use of FEV_1 in a clinical area in which its use as a surrogate has been accepted. This is an example of the kind of inconsistency across divisions at FDA that would be evaluated in the analysis proposed in Recommendation 3-1.

Patient Registries

Chapter 4 discusses the importance of patient registries and biorepositories to support basic research on rare conditions. Patient registries are also essential elements in the process of drug development. A patient registry is more than a list of patients with a particular condition, although that is a first step. It involves the systematic collection of uniform information for a specific purpose(s) (see, e.g., Gliklich and Dreyer, 2007; Forrest et al., 2010). Examples include registries created to help describe the natural history of a disease in the absence of treatment and registries to collect additional information about a drug's safety or efficacy after the end of pivotal clinical trials (often as required by FDA as a condition for approving a drug).

The conduct of clinical trials for rare disorders is inherently difficult because of the small number of patients. The problem of small numbers is further complicated when the consequences of a rare condition or its treatment reveal themselves slowly. Patient registries can help with the limitations of small numbers in many ways. First, a comprehensive knowledge of the natural history of disease (e.g., that 80 percent of affected individuals die by 5 years of age) can provide a historic benchmark for judgments about the efficacy of a therapeutic intervention. Such knowledge may then allow the use of a single-arm clinical study without a placebo or other concurrent control group. To cite an example, the evidence submitted to support FDA approval of alglucosidase alfa (Myozyme) for infantile-onset Pompe disease included a comparison of outcomes for 18 pivotal trial participants with outcomes for infants followed in a natural history study (Beitz, 2006). If research participants do not have to be divided into test and control groups, this can significantly increase the number of individuals with a rare condition who can participate in the treatment arm, which may have several advantages (e.g., in allowing informative, planned comparisons of study participant subgroups). Also, patients may be more willing to participate in a trial when they are assured they will receive the test drug, particularly when no standard therapy exists.

A second way that registries can help is when the information collected includes biological specimens or links to specimen data. Such information has the potential to reveal biochemical, histologic, or other markers that may be found to be suitable as surrogate endpoints in clinical trials and that, in turn, can reduce the time required for clinical trials used to support FDA approval, particularly for long-term chronic conditions. In addition, patient registry studies can reveal clinical outcomes that occur prior to but that rigorously predict catastrophic events (e.g., brain damage or death) and so can be used as surrogate measures for clinically relevant outcomes. Ideally, these surrogate clinical markers of disease would occur invariably in advance of the most important clinical outcomes, but their presence (at some reliably measurable level) would not obligate progression to these outcomes, which would allow the productive substitution or modification of experimental therapies in time to make a difference.

Today, an uncounted number of organizations and researchers in this country and around the world maintain rare diseases registries in some form, sometimes for the same condition. No uniform, accepted standards govern the collection, organization, or availability of these data. Organizations and researchers may closely guard their data or may face legal limits (related to patient consent and privacy) on data sharing. At the same time, one estimate is that registries exist for only 20 percent of rare diseases (Wrobel, cited in Forrest et al., 2010). Thus, calls are increasing both for the expanded use of registries and for a more systematic and standardized approach to their creation, maintenance, and accessibility on a national and global basis.

In 2010, the Office of Rare Diseases Research at NIH sponsored a workshop on the intersection of patient registries, biospecimen repositories, and clinical data (see Rubenstein et al., 2010). In 2009, the European organization EPPOSI sponsored a similar workshop on patient registries for rare disorders. As outlined in those workshops and other discussions, features of a systematic, coordinated approach to patient registries for rare diseases would include agreement on minimum common data elements, definitions, and coding protocols and easy access to a common central resource or platform for creating or reconfiguring registries. Not only would these features make the creation or revision of existing registries easier (especially for groups or researchers with limited funds), but also they would facilitate data sharing and pooling. Another feature of a common resource would be the fee-based provision of data management or curation functions. To make the data more widely available for research purposes and to safeguard patient privacy, the common resource would provide for de-identified patient data from registries to be included in an aggregated database. Given the limited resources of many organizations and researchers working on rare diseases, the goal would be for the system to evolve into a self-sustaining, public-private partnership. The specific features of such a system are beyond the scope of this report, but various individuals and groups are working on the elements just described.

A related issue is the absence of standard methods for collecting and categorizing comprehensive patient information and samples during clinical trials for rare disorders, which limits the opportunity for results from one trial to inform another. Given the inherently small sample size and the often restricted time frame available for evaluating the therapeutic effect of an intervention, opportunities to launch or modify clinical trials for rare disorders based upon new insights or hypotheses are limited. Thus, testing all reasonable hypotheses in parallel for rare disorders is wise stewardship of the limited resource of patient information and material. For example, does a therapy for aortic disease in Marfan syndrome also affect musculoskeletal or ocular manifestations? Are there genetic or other biomarkers that predict response to therapy? With standards in place, it would be possible to establish a dedicated and, to an extent, non-hypothesis-constrained effort to establish a rich dataset and sample repository during clinical trials that could be used to test future hypotheses in a retrospective manner.

One potentially comprehensive approach would be for funding agencies to widely advertise the anticipated launch of clinical trials for rare disorders, to request proposals for and prioritize ancillary studies, and to mandate the establishment of or participation by grantees in standardized patient registries and biorepositories. This would depend on a coordinated intellectual, financial, and physical infrastructure (probably including international acceptance and participation) to support such initiatives.

Clinical Research Consortia

Clinical research consortia can be instrumental components of the infrastructure necessary to advance rare diseases research. In general, such consortia provide the underlying infrastructure to conduct clinical trials in a timely manner, including

- supporting research sites that have access to both specialized clinical investigators and relevant patient populations;
- creating a data-coordinating center;
- establishing a protocol development office;
- instituting a data safety monitoring board; and
- providing other components required for clinical investigations.

Consortia can provide a clear pathway for rapidly translating basic research and other discoveries into key trials to evaluate safety and efficacy consistent with FDA expectations. Moreover, they can potentially lower the costs associated with initiating and conducting a clinical trial, which may attract industry partners into the rare diseases clinical research arena.

A spectrum of clinical research consortia currently exists. They include NIH-funded groups, the largest of which is the Children's Oncology Group (COG); a number of very successful, primarily philanthropically supported programs such as the Cystic Fibrosis Foundations' Therapeutics Development Program and the Multiple Myeloma Research Consortium; and a variety of smaller consortia funded by government sources or private foundations. COG is perhaps the preeminent collaborative research organization and was the first to recognize the crucial importance of collaboration in pediatric research. Even common childhood cancers are rare enough that no one center treats the number of children required for large-scale clinical trials. Today, more than 90 percent of the 12,500 children diagnosed with cancer each year in the United States are treated at COG institutions (Liu et al., 2003). COG is thus well positioned to explore adaptive clinical trial designs that have the potential to undergo modification—including imbalancing randomization to favor better-performing treatment arms—while the study is being conducted.

NIH currently funds the Rare Diseases Clinical Research Network (RDCRN), which is in its second cycle of 5-year funding. In addition to their research objectives, another valuable objective of the network consortia is to provide information to patients and families and help patients connect with advocacy groups, clinical experts, and clinical study opportunities. The consortia have to include the following:

- clinical research projects for observational or longitudinal studies and/or clinical trials (at least two projects are required, one of which must be a longitudinal study);
- pilot or demonstration projects (at least one project is required); and
- a training (career development) component.

The RDCRN supports important studies, but disease focus areas studied are quite limited in number—19 consortia that cover more than 135 diseases (see Appendix E). The RDCRN cannot carry out clinical trials for diseases that fall outside the scope of the funded consortia.

Rare diseases investigators do, however, work through other networks to pursue the development of therapeutics. For example, the Pediatric Heart Network (PHN), funded in 2001 by the National Heart, Lung, and Blood Institute (NHLBI) to improve outcomes and quality of life in children with heart disease, allows its eight core sites the flexibility to identify, prioritize, and launch initiatives within their broad domains of expertise in a discretional manner. In 2006, investigators published preclinical findings demonstrating that losartan, an FDA-approved drug for hypertension, prevented aortic aneurysms in a mouse model of Marfan syndrome (Habashi et al., 2006). The network was able to respond to these findings in a timely manner and launched a clinical trial of losartan by February 2007. Network structure and policies allowed the recruitment of 21 auxiliary sites with sizable Marfan patient populations and specific clinical expertise in the management of this disorder.

The committee believes that a similarly flexible network structure for rare diseases research has value as an addition to the RDCRN. Such a structure could utilize NIH U01 or U10 cooperative agreements. Because clinical expertise and relevant patient populations may vary based on the disease, the network would be designed with the flexibility to engage or partner with specific sites or relevant existing networks.

Other components might be considered to support the productivity of an augmented rare diseases clinical research capacity with an overarching goal of maintaining flexibility to meet the diverse research needs of patients with rare diseases. For example, taking into account its experience to date, NIH might consider alternative models for institutional review board (IRB) review of rare diseases research, for example, a central IRB for rare diseases that would assemble the requisite expertise to review protocols while minimizing the duplication and costs associated with multisite reviews by separate IRBs.[2] In addition, it will be important for new rare diseases research to continue the emphasis of the current Rare Disease Clinical Trial Network on active partnerships with relevant advocacy groups and other organizations that are currently committed to rare diseases research.

Innovative Clinical Trial and Data Analysis Strategies

This report has stressed the importance of clinical trial designs and data analysis strategies suited to the challenges of evaluating the safety and efficacy of products for small populations. Chapter 3 discusses the joint education programs of FDA and NIH to familiarize both agency staff and others with these designs. It recommends that the agencies evaluate the extent to which studies submitted in support of orphan drugs are consistent with advances in the science of small clinical trials and associated analytic methods and develop responses based on the findings. It also recommends that the agencies support further work to develop and test innovative clinical research and data analysis strategies for small populations.

An underlying goal of novel clinical trial methodologies is to make better use of available data. To that end, Bayesian statistical methodologies are increasingly being applied in clinical research, which offers the prospect of smaller but more informative trials (see, generally, Berry, 2006). At a basic level, all statistical methods used in clinical research address how to

---

[2] Other NIH groups are investigating ways of dealing with investigator and other concerns about IRBs. Working groups of the Clinical and Translational Science Awards program are considering ways of harmonizing IRB reviews across institutions, educating IRB members about relevant issues, and better assessing the quality of IRB reviews (CTSA, 2010).

deal with uncertainty in research data. Bayesian methodologies define that uncertainty in terms of a probability as opposed to a fixed parameter. Calculations can then ensue at any time during the trial, affording potential advantages of "real-time" modifications in trials. For example, modifications might include imbalancing randomization to favor the better-performing arm of a trial or altering the subpopulation being studied to focus on a better-responding group. It is this continual learning feature that underlies the term "adaptive trial design." Importantly, Bayesian approaches are gaining wider acceptance not only in the medical research community but also in regulatory agencies. (See also the discussion of Bayesian design in medical device trials in Chapter 7.)

Clinical Research Training

Another important foundation for rare diseases research and product development is the training of clinical-translational investigators who understand innovative trial designs that can be applied to drug development-related studies of small populations of patients with rare diseases and who know when they need methodological consultants to give them more expert guidance. In addition, it is important for clinical subspecialists who work with both children and adults with rare diseases to be trained to collect data that will allow standardized and detailed phenotyping and the elucidation of clinical natural histories, two important contributions to research progress in many rare diseases.

A more comprehensive discussion of investigator training is found in Chapter 4. That chapter includes a recommendation for a comprehensive NIH action plan on rare diseases, one element of which would cover research training.

Access to Information on Negative Findings and Decisions

Traditionally, information about failed clinical trials and negative FDA decisions has been limited. With few exceptions, FDA regulations generally prohibit the release of information from or about an IND, NDA, or Biologic Licensing Application (BLA) that does not result in an approval. As a result, FDA does not announce its negative decisions on NDAs, and it does not release information about negative clinical trial findings related to INDs or NDAs that sponsors have withdrawn or abandoned. As part of legal requirements for publicly owned companies, drug and biotechnology companies typically make summary announcements of negative FDA decisions, failed late-stage trials, or company decisions to stop a major drug development effort. These announcements usually do not provide scientific details.

Negative findings are sometimes published in medical journals, but such results are often not submitted for publication or not published if submitted (Fanelli, 2010). Those that are published may not attract as much media and other attention as reports of successful trials.

Although research sponsors may learn from a negative trial, clinical trial results that are not public represent a waste of potentially valuable information. They also are a disservice to the trial's research participants who may have put themselves at risk or forgone participation in more promising research. Withheld findings can be a barrier to progress in product development, which is especially troublesome when a rare disease is involved because research on such diseases is so limited. As observed in Chapter 3, the provision of more information about the reasons that drugs that are not approved by FDA or are withdrawn before approval could be particularly valuable for drugs being considered for the treatment of rare diseases.

In recent years, government, medical journals, advocacy groups, trade associations, and others have taken steps to increase the availability of information about successful and unsuccessful clinical trials. Box 5-2 summarizes some of these.

INNOVATION PLATFORMS FOR DRUG DEVELOPMENT

As discussed in Chapter 4, innovation platforms for research often involve the sharing of resources. Companies, federal agencies, and nonprofit patient groups are taking the initiative to build such new models for drug development for both common and rare diseases. This section highlights such models. More extensive discussions are included in summaries of IOM workshops on innovative business models for drug development for rare and neglected diseases (IOM, 2008), venture philanthropy strategies for translational research (IOM, 2009b), and precompetitive collaboration in oncology research (IOM, 2010b).

Industry

Companies have experimented with different models to achieve greater productivity through a higher success rate for drug approvals or lower costs or both. One approach has been to outsource aspects of drug development as in the case of Eli Lilly's Chorus program. This program, which was developed as a pilot project, has evolved into an alternative research and development unit that focuses on early-stage drug development. It looks for "the most likely winners in a portfolio of molecules (most of which are destined to fail), recommending only the strongest candidates for costly late-stage development" (Bonabeau, 2008, p. 1).

Another industry approach to innovation has been to outsource problem

BOX 5-2
Examples of Initiatives to Increase Information About Clinical Trials and FDA or Company Decisions About Products

Registration of Clinical Trials
    The FDA Modernization Act of 1997 directed the Department of Health and Human Services (DHHS) to create a registry of both federally and privately funded trials, now called ClinicalTrials.gov. It requires sponsors to submit information to a databank about clinical trials conducted under an IND application if the trial is to assess efficacy for a drug to treat a serious or life-threatening disease or condition. Registration information includes basic details about the trial protocol, primary clinical endpoints, and the data analysis plan. The FDA Amendments Act of 2007 expanded the reporting requirements to expressly require the registration of device clinical trials and the reporting of clinical trial results. (See generally 42 USC 282(j).) The reported results are to include basic demographic and baseline information on enrolled participants, findings for primary and secondary outcomes, and a point of contact. In addition, the uniform publication requirements of the International Committee of Medical Journal Editors now specify as a condition of consideration for publication of an article on a clinical trial that the trial be registered in a public trials registry (ICMJE, 2009).

Information About FDA Evaluations and Actions
    In recent years, FDA has made more information available from the reviews associated with the approval of an NDA. It has also posted industry and agency presentations made to advisory committees when they are consulted on an application. These presentations thus can be a source of considerable information if FDA does not approve an NDA. Recently, the agency released for public comment a set of 21 "transparency" proposals (FDA, 2010b). If implemented, these proposals would significantly increase access to information about applications submitted

solving, as in the case of InnoCentive, also an initiative of Eli Lilly. It was born of frustration over certain seemingly intractable aspects of drug synthesis and development (Travis, 2008). Now independent, the company offers public, prize-based challenges to attract a "virtual workforce" to the solution of difficult problems. One example is a set of challenges it organized for a patient group for amyotrophic lateral sclerosis that included a $1 million prize for discovering a validated biomarker to track progression of the disease.

A third approach focuses on precompetitive collaborations across industry. As discussed in Chapter 4 in the context of discovery research, such collaboration might involve several aspects, including that competitors share the costs of early-stage research in rare diseases and also share expertise and findings. Another element might involve cooperation on the development of biomarkers that could be used to monitor therapies for specific diseases and that might ultimately be used as surrogate endpoints

to the agency, for example, whether an IND has been placed on hold or terminated, whether an unapproved NDA or BLA has been withdrawn or abandoned, or whether safety concerns have been identified. With respect to designated orphan drugs specifically, one proposal is that FDA would disclose its determination that a certain product may represent a significant therapeutic advance for a rare disease if an application is withdrawn, terminated, or abandoned for other than a safety reason (e.g., withdrawn solely for business reasons).

Coalition Against Major Diseases

Several major pharmaceutical companies have announced that they will share pooled data from failed clinical trials of drugs for Alzheimer disease. All participating companies will have access to the pooled data as will outside researchers with a valid question. The objective is to identify why the studies fail and use the conclusions to design studies that will be successful. The coalition has similar plans for pooling clinical trials data on Parkinson disease and tuberculosis (Wang, 2010).

Pharmaceutical Research and Manufacturers of America (PhRMA)

For FDA-approved drugs, PhRMA has created an online clearinghouse of results of industry phase III and IV clinical studies completed since October 1, 2002. It includes a bibliography of and links to published articles and results summaries for unpublished clinical studies. References to scientific papers will be posted when they are published. Consistent with FDA regulations on annual reports, companies are encouraged to post summaries of unpublished studies within a year of study completion. The primary audience is physicians. Submissions to the database are voluntary, but the website says that "PhRMA's board of directors . . . agreed that member companies will participate in and support the database and, as with PhRMA's 2002 Principles, communicate all meaningful results, both positive and negative" (http://www.clinicalstudyresults.org/primers/faq.php).

for regulatory approval of a therapeutic. The public-private Biomarkers Consortium administered by the Foundation for NIH was described earlier. Another example of cross-industry collaboration is the Coalition Against Major Diseases, which is cited in Box 5-2. It has announced a public-private initiative to support the development of better treatments for Alzheimer disease and Parkinson disease. In addition to the sharing of information on failed and successful trials, this collaboration among pharmaceutical companies, patient advocacy groups, voluntary health associations, and government agencies will include the development of disease progression models to improve the design of clinical trials to meet FDA standards (C-Path, 2009a). Although drug development research on rare conditions may yield fewer trials than development efforts focused on Alzheimer disease and Parkinson disease, the designations and approvals listed in FDA's orphan drug database illustrate that multiple companies may pursue product development research on a specific rare disease (see listings at http://www.accessdata.fda.gov/scripts/opdlisting/oopd/index.cfm).

Competing companies may also combine insights and work together to solve a particular regulatory problem. A recent example is from the Critical Path Institute (C-Path), an independent, nonprofit organization that brings together FDA, pharmaceutical companies, and others to focus on drug development issues and to support FDA's Critical Path Initiative (see Chapter 3). C-Path's Predictive Safety Testing Consortium involves 16 companies. Recently, as a result of joint efforts across these companies, FDA and its European counterpart, the European Medicines Agency, have both agreed to a new standard for preclinical testing of drugs entering development to predict renal toxicity (C-Path, 2009b). The consortium is now working to qualify and validate new biomarkers in other areas. C-Path was also instrumental in developing the Coalition Against Major Diseases.

Advocacy Groups

Given the challenges and expense that beset the traditional model of pharmaceutical research and development in bringing new drugs to market, developing treatments for rare diseases represents an opportunity to test new paradigms. Led by patients and families, disease-specific foundations have begun to do just that (IOM, 2008). As described in Chapter 4, the strategy includes "de-risking" early-stage research and development for promising products by providing philanthropic capital as well as research tools and access to patients.

Although advocacy groups have traditionally provided support for basic discovery research, many of them have recently assumed a more active role in shepherding the drug development process in their areas of focus. Again, one objective is to minimize the risks associated with the early phases of therapeutic development. For example, building on the promising results of its basic research program, the Muscular Dystrophy Association now supports the preclinical work necessary for an IND application, as well as funding a national patient database, early clinical trials, and associated research infrastructure costs (see information at http://www.mdausa.org/research). Appendix F includes other examples. These novel approaches have begun to bear fruit, increasing the number of promising therapies that proceed to later-stage clinical trials (IOM, 2008).

Another Model: Public-Private Partnerships for Neglected Diseases

Public-private partnerships have played an important role in advancing therapeutics for neglected diseases of the developing world. For example, as mentioned in Chapter 4, the Medicines for Malaria Venture is working with pharmaceutical companies and academic centers to discover promising new molecules; the Special Programme for Research and Training in Tropical Diseases is another example of a public-private partnership. At the end of 2004, about half of the public-private partnerships engaged in research and development for neglected diseases projects involved multinational corporations doing so on a "no-profit, no-loss basis"; the other half involved often smaller firms that found commercial opportunity in these resource-limited markets (Moran, 2005).

Similar kinds of partnerships could be used more effectively to develop therapies for rare diseases. For example, companies could undertake pre-clinical development activities for compounds entering development for a rare disease from NIH or academic institutions. Alternatively, a partnership could, through sheer volume, coordinate these preclinical development activities using specific contract research companies to complete the work at a regulatory standard and at a reduced price. One example is the International Partnership for Microbicides. This approach uses royalty-free licenses for specific compounds from pharmaceutical and biotechnology companies to develop and distribute vaginal gels and other microbicide products to prevent HIV infection (Brooks et al., 2010).

In the realm of clinical development, an example of public-private partnership is the recently announced Critical Path to TB Drug Regimens (Fox, 2010). With C-Path coordinating, this entity will test promising new treatment regimens in collaboration with FDA scientists and 10 pharmaceutical companies. The same approach could be applied to specific rare diseases.

National Institutes of Health

Just as pharmaceutical companies have had reasons to innovate, NIH has, in recent years, been called upon to complement its support for basic biomedical discovery by facilitating the translation of discoveries into therapies for both common and rare diseases. It too is building "innovation platforms" to support such translation.

As part of its Roadmap initiative, NIH launched the Rapid Access to Interventional Development (RAID) program as a pilot activity in 2004. Not a grant program, RAID supports selected aspects of preclinical development, providing expertise and performing required studies at a regulatory level using existing NIH facilities and contract resources (http://nihroadmap. nih.gov/raid/). Academic investigators as well as qualified small businesses are eligible to use the resource. Although not explicitly targeted to rare diseases, the program is meant to facilitate access to preclinical resources for projects that are unlikely to attract private-sector investment. Approved projects have targeted some rare conditions, including beta-thalassemia and Friedreich's ataxia. The online program description notes that several individual NIH institutes offer similar support services. However, the diversity of opportunities and the relatively decentralized structure of NIH may make it difficult for potential grantees to identify the opportunities that best fit their circumstances (Cornetta and Carter, 2010).

In 2006, in recognition of the need to integrate the translational research infrastructure within academic health centers, NIH launched its Clinical and Translational Science Awards (CTSA) program (http://www.ctsaweb.org/). The program now includes 55 institutions; ultimately, NIH plans approximately 60 CTSAs, with total funding of around $500 million per year. Individual CTSA programs are to coordinate clinical research resources within an institution to facilitate involvement in translational research by a greater number of investigators than have traditionally been engaged. The programs are also meant to provide a range of training opportunities and integrate academic medical research with community health. Within the CTSA Child Health Consortium Oversight Committee, a rare diseases work group is seeking to identify gaps in rare diseases research and ways in which the consortium might help fill those gaps.

The CTSA program is also intended to facilitate resource sharing and consortium-wide collaborations, including shared biorepositories and other resources. One example is the Pharmaceutical Assets Portal, which is sponsored by the NIH National Center for Research Resources and Pfizer (http://www.ctsapharmaportal.org/). It allows investigators to learn about compounds that have already been evaluated for specific diseases and might be developed for other conditions.

The networked structure of CTSA institutions would seem to be ideal for facilitating rare diseases research, in which multicenter clinical trials are the rule and investigators are scattered across several institutions. The CTSA program provides a coordinated infrastructure, but funding is still quite limited for the innovative projects it is meant to facilitate.

In 2010, as part of the Patient Protection and Affordable Care Act (Section 10409 of P.L. 111-148), Congress took a significant step to fill the translational research funding gap when it authorized a new Cures Acceleration Network (CAN) to provide up to $500 million annually for conducting and supporting research to develop "high-need cures." These are cures that the Director of NIH determines to be a priority and for which market incentives are not likely to support timely or sufficient development. The program would cover development of drugs, biologics, medical devices, diagnostics, and behavior therapies. One key feature is the provision of assistance to award recipients in devising research protocols so that they will comply with FDA standards throughout all stages of product development.

The program can fund projects through three types of competitive awards, one of which requires the grantee to provide matching funds. Both public and private organizations (including pharmaceutical and biotechnology companies) are eligible for funding.

Although not limited to rare diseases, the program, if funded to its full appropriation, will represent an unprecedented resource for the development of therapies for rare diseases and will offer an important complement to the infrastructure provided by the CTSA program. It is not, however, clear to what extent it will subsume or complement the existing Therapeutics for Rare and Neglected Diseases (discussed in Chapter 4) and RAID programs or whether its activities will be integrated with those of the NIH Office of Rare Diseases Research and the Rare Diseases Clinical Research Network. The existing infrastructure of rare diseases and translational research, although slight in relation to the need, is an important resource. Thus, a recommendation at the end of this chapter emphasizes the importance of coordinating new and existing programs to speed the translation of research discoveries into safe and effective therapies, diagnostics, and preventive interventions for people with rare diseases.

Food and Drug Administration

Critical Path Initiative

In addition to collaborating in some of the initiatives described above, FDA launched the Critical Path Initiative in 2004 to "to find fundamentally faster, more predictable, and less costly ways to turn good biomedical ideas into safe and effective treatments" (FDA, 2004, p. 30). The initiative is intended to help build partnerships involving industry, advocacy groups, and others to share information and expertise and to promote problem solving and innovation in a broad range of areas, including biomarker development, information technology, streamlining clinical trials, and clinical investigator training. The predictive safety effort described above is an example of one such collaborative effort.

The 2009 report on the Critical Path Initiative does not cite any activities focused specifically on orphan products. Nonetheless, a number of the activities should help improve the quality and efficiency of drug trials for rare as well as common conditions. For example, one of the collaborations seeks a better understanding of the genetics of drug-induced liver injury, including Stevens-Johnson syndrome, a serious rare disorder (CPI, 2010).

Repurposing Existing Drugs

In parallel to the concept of precompetitive sharing of compounds or data as discussed in Chapter 4, another avenue for innovation involves repurposing old drugs for potential treatments of rare diseases. That discussion noted that the National Chemical Genome Center is developing a library of approved drugs so that they can be more easily screened for possible repurposing.

Without the need to repeat toxicological or pharmacokinetic assessments, a considerable portion of the costs of bringing a drug through the research and development pipeline can be saved (Chong and Sullivan, 2007). Furthermore, population safety, dosing, and adverse events are already known. In addition, for drugs to treat rare diseases, the marketing protections offered by the Orphan Drug Act provide an incentive to companies that might otherwise not be interested in further work on an old drug for which patent protection had expired.

The Office of Orphan Products Development at FDA recently posted a database of products that already have an orphan drug designation for a rare disease *and* have been approved for the treatment of some other rare disease, for treatment of a common disease, or both. Such products have already gone through preclinical testing and been judged to be pharmacologically active, safe, and effective for some clinical condition (OOPD, 2010).

The repurposing of existing drugs for rare diseases treatments may lead to higher pricing for existing, more common use of the drug. Although the example of colchicine discussed in Chapters 3 and 6 involves a previously unapproved but widely available drug, it may still be suggestive of one consequence of repurposing if patients with the common condition have limited alternatives.[3]

Use of Public and Philanthropic Funding to
Reduce Overall Development Costs

Public and philanthropic funding for drug development and clinical trials for rare diseases, particularly if directed toward nonprofit, patient-led consortia, reduces the need for a high rate of return for the commercial firms that ultimately manufacture and market a new drug. Such funding potentially could attract more industry investment in these therapies. For drugs whose profit margins might be slim or initially nil, public funding such as that proposed in the previously mentioned Cures Acceleration Net-

---

[3] Internationally, pharmaceutical firms have offered preferential pricing for drugs in different countries and for drugs with multiple uses; in the latter situation, customers for one use of a drug pay a higher price so that customers for a different use, typically for a neglected disease, may have closer-to-marginal cost pricing or have access through company donations. The latter kind of dual market requires some serendipity. Examples include a treatment for sleeping sickness that has a secondary cosmetic indication for removing unwanted facial hair for women (eflornithine [brand name Vaniqa]) and a treatment for river blindness that has a lucrative veterinary market for treating heartworm in dogs (e.g., ivermectin [Mectizan]) (see, e.g., Collins, 2004; Torreele et al., 2004).

work initiative may provide the necessary resources to bridge the "valley of death" from preclinical to clinical phases of testing and then fund pivotal clinical trials. One difference between this program and the NIH Small Business Innovation Research program is that the latter excludes nonprofit entities whereas the former extends eligibility to nonprofit research enterprises, such as patient groups that may be particularly effective in recruiting participants for clinical trials.

Examples involving resource sharing arrangements and public and voluntary funding for the development of treatments for neglected diseases offer possible models for rare diseases. One approach involves humanitarian access licensing by universities that offer publicly funded inventions royalty-free in exchange for commitments from companies to produce the drug at no profit or close to marginal cost for those in need in the developing world. For example, the University of California, Berkeley, struck such an arrangement with the Institute for OneWorld Health and Amyris Biotechnologies (see IOM, 2008; and, generally, So and Stewart, 2009). In exchange for a co-exclusive, royalty-free license from the university, Amyris Biotechnologies pledged to use the microbial process of synthesizing artemisinin and to produce the antimalarial at no profit for the developing world. With the support of a $42 million Gates Foundation grant, all three parties benefited (IOWH, 2004). Notably, Amyris Biotechnologies was able to pursue proof-of-concept testing of this technology without diluting shareholder equity. When a company involved in this kind of arrangement seeks to raise second-round venture capital, equity in the firm will be more valuable with this kind of groundwork in establishing proof of concept of the technology.

RECOMMENDATIONS

Chapter 3 includes a number of recommendations for actions by FDA to identify and reduce problems related either to its own performance or to the performance of sponsors of new drugs that may slow or discourage the development of drugs for rare diseases. These recommendations call on FDA to identify areas of inappropriate inconsistency across CDER units in their review of orphan drug applications, develop related guidance on criteria for approval of orphan drugs based on differences in candidate drugs or the associated rare diseases, continue work to expand understanding and appropriate use of small clinical trial designs, and collaborate with NIH to ensure that NIH-funded product development research meets regulatory standards.

The recommendations in this chapter focus primarily on steps that NIH can take in collaboration with industry and advocacy groups to further accelerate development of safe and effective products for people with rare diseases. The first recommendation focuses on the preclinical stage of drug development. The objective is to expand the resources and options for accelerating drug development, including the options available to investigators funded by rare diseases advocacy groups.

RECOMMENDATION 5-1: NIH should create a centralized preclinical development service that is dedicated to rare diseases and available to all nonprofit entities.

The creation of this service could be accomplished through several different models. Within NIH, one possibility would be to expand the capacity of the RAID program, which, although not dedicated to rare diseases, does include them in its project portfolio. Similarly, the TRND program currently overseen by the Office of Rare Diseases Research could be expanded not only in terms of the number of awards but also to provide coverage of preclinical development projects such as the selection and arranging of testing of promising compounds.

Alternatively, to leverage involvement and additional funding from companies and philanthropic organizations, a preclinical development service could be based in an entity such as the Foundation for NIH. This foundation was established specifically to support NIH collaboration with academic institutions, industry, and nonprofit groups without certain constraints that apply to NIH itself (FNIH, 2010). The Biomarkers Consortium is an example of this kind of collaboration. A different and possibly complementary approach would be to establish a consortium of pharmaceutical and biotechnology companies through which selected preclinical development projects would be carried out using the resources provided by consortium members or by individual companies.

As emphasized in this chapter, the development and validation of biomarkers for use as surrogate endpoints in clinical studies of drugs for rare diseases will speed such studies and should reduce their costs. Another IOM committee has recommended a Department of Health and Human Services-wide effort to encourage the collection and sharing of data about biomarkers for drugs, biologics, devices, and foods (IOM, 2010a). In addition, the establishment of clearly defined standards for biomarker validation and application in clinical trials for rare disorders will reduce the possibility that FDA will reject applications for the approval of an orphan drug based on inadequate biomarker validation, a problem noted in Chapter 3.

RECOMMENDATION 5-2: In collaboration with industry, academic researchers, NIH and FDA scientists, and patient organizations, FDA should expand its Critical Path Initiative to define criteria for the evaluation of surrogate endpoints for use in trials of products for rare conditions.

In addition to agreement on criteria for the evaluation of surrogate endpoints for clinical trials, the expansion and improvement of patient registries and biorepositories are other important elements in a strategy to accelerate rare diseases research and product development. Today, an uncounted number of organizations and researchers in this country and around the world maintain rare diseases registries and specimen collections in some form, sometimes for the same condition. No uniform, accepted standards govern the collection, organization, or availability of these resources. An increase in the use of registries and biorepositories and a more systematic approach to their creation, maintenance, and accessibility are needed on a national and global basis. Building on work already begun, NIH can take a lead role in working with industry and private partners to make the creation and maintenance of registries and biorepositories easier and less expensive, to expand information sharing, and to promote standards and processes that yield high-quality data and specimens and protect patients or research participants.

RECOMMENDATION 5-3: NIH should support a collaborative public-private partnership to develop and manage a freely available platform for creating or restructuring patient registries and biorepositories for rare diseases and for sharing de-identified data. The platform should include mechanisms to create standards for data collection, specimen storage, and informed consent by patients or research participants.

For example, features of a systematic, coordinated approach to patient registries for rare diseases would include agreement on minimum common data elements, definitions, and coding protocols and also uniform and widely accepted mechanisms for patient or research participant consent. Partners would have easy access to a common central resource or platform for creating or reconfiguring registries. In clinical trials, the latter might involve a biomarker substudy protocol available with the main study protocol. Study participants would then be asked for consent related to the larger clinical trial and for consent related to future biomarker studies. These features would not only make the creation or revision of existing registries easier (especially for groups or researchers with limited funds), but also facilitate data sharing and pooling. Given the limited resources of many organizations and researchers working on rare diseases, the goal would be for the system to evolve into a self-sustaining, public-private partnership. The committee understands that this would be a complicated undertaking at all stages.

In the realm of clinical research, the Rare Diseases Clinical Research Network is a valuable resource but one with a relatively limited and predetermined scope that constrains its ability to take advantage of unanticipated opportunities presented by scientific discoveries. In some cases, other research networks have greater flexibility as in the Marfan example cited above. These other networks, however, lack a specific focus on rare diseases. The committee believes that it is desirable to enhance existing clinical research activities focused on rare diseases. This enhancement should include a program or programs that are not strictly organized around specific disease areas but rather have the flexibility to partner with or recruit other existing networks or sites to rapidly capitalize on research advances and to achieve common and broadly defined goals in rare diseases research.

> RECOMMENDATION 5-4: NIH should increase its capacity and flexibility to support all phases of clinical research related to rare diseases, including clinical trials of new and repurposed therapeutic agents. Opportunities to be explored include
>
> • expanding the Rare Diseases Clinical Research Network to address opportunities for diagnostic and therapeutic advances for a greater number of rare diseases;
> • setting priorities for rare diseases research within other NIH clinical trials networks;
> • creating a study group approach to rare diseases, modeled after the Children's Oncology Group; and
> • building additional capability for rare diseases clinical research within the Clinical and Translational Science Awards program.

In addition, although the Cures Acceleration Network will not focus exclusively on rare diseases research, such research falls well within the program's intended scope and should benefit from it if appropriations for the network support the goals set for it. For the program to target resources effectively, it is important that it be coordinated with the Office of Rare Diseases Research and that the selection process for network projects include individuals with expertise in rare diseases and the science of small clinical trials.

> RECOMMENDATION 5-5: NIH should establish procedures to ensure coordination of the activities of the Cures Acceleration Network with those of the Office of Rare Diseases Research, FDA's orphan products grants program, and other existing initiatives to promote and facilitate the translation of basic science discoveries into effective treatments for rare diseases. It should build on existing resources when appropriate, avoid creating duplicative research infrastructure, and engage advocacy groups in its work.

A precondition for the network to achieve its goals is the appropriation by Congress of adequate resources. In addition, requiring clinical studies funded through the Cures Acceleration Network to disclose both positive and negative results will underscore the importance of sharing data in accelerating progress toward high-need cures.

The recommendations in this chapter and the preceding one focus on strategies that may directly expand and improve the quantity, quality, and efficiency of rare diseases research and orphan product development. The next chapter turns to a quite different set of considerations that may influence company decisions about research and development activities, that is, health plan policies and practices related to drugs and biologics for rare diseases.

6

Coverage and Reimbursement: Incentives and Disincentives for Product Development

As a person who needs to take the MOST expensive drug in the world to stay healthy . . . I am in my early 30s and looking to take a $400,000/year drug for the rest of my life. . . . I now have to pick jobs based off of their insurance plan, rather than the job itself.
Posted by Billiondollarwoman, 2010

Big companies are starting to get more interested in rare diseases, but the key issue is the high cost of developing a drug and the typically long time it takes to move it from a lab into a clinic as a treatment that gets prescribed. Before starting down this arduous path, a company needs to feel there is a reasonable chance of making a profit.

Marcus, 2010c

A small market is generally viewed as a disincentive for the development of drugs. Many of the costs of developing a new drug are incurred regardless of the size of the potential market. If, however, a company can set a price that is high enough to recover its costs and generate profits because enough public and private health insurance plans and patients and families will pay that price, then a manufacturer may not be deterred by a small target market. Some orphan drugs are among the most expensive drugs in the world, costing as much as $400,000 per year.

Orphan drugs can be very profitable. Wellman-Labadie and Zhou (2009) reported that 43 brand-name drugs with global sales of more than $1 billion had orphan drug designations, and 18 of these had been approved solely as orphan drugs. Most had been approved for the relatively more prevalent rare conditions such as multiple myeloma, but one, imiglucerase (Cerezyme), was approved for Gaucher's disease, which has a U.S. patient population estimated at 3,000 to 6,000.[1] In 2008, about 1,500 patients in the United States were taking the drug, which was priced at more than $300,000 per year (Pollock, 2008).

Biotechnology companies have been prominent in the orphan drug market from the outset, and the Orphan Drug Act has been cited as a key factor in their growth (OIG, 2001b; Ariyanchira, 2008; Grant, 2008). Small- to medium-sized companies have also played a significant role in orphan drug development (Seoane-Vazquez et al., 2008; Villa et al., 2008). Perhaps influenced by challenges in developing traditional blockbuster drugs as well as by the market protection and other incentives provided by the Orphan Drug Act, some major pharmaceutical companies have recently announced that they are considering or pursuing orphan drug development; many already have at least one orphan drug on the market (Anand, 2005; Dimond, 2009; Pollack, 2009; Whalen, 2009).

In addition to incentives for developing orphan drugs provided by the Orphan Drug Act, the potential profitability of orphan versus nonorphan drugs may be affected by several other factors. One is that private health plans generally have little leverage in negotiating prices for expensive biotechnology drugs, many of which are orphan drugs. Even the Kaiser Permanente system in California, which is large and accustomed to negotiating prices, has noted that "opportunities are limited" in this arena (Monroe et al., 2006). In a Government Accountability Office (GAO, 2010b) survey, sponsors of Medicare prescription drug plans cited the lack of competitors in the market for a drug (which gives manufacturers little reason to offer discounts) and the limited volume of a drug used by the plan (which limits a plan's negotiating power) as two primary reasons for a health plan's lack of leverage on drug prices. Orphan drugs often have both of these characteristics.

Colchicine provides an example of the implications for health plans and patients of limited competition. The drug, which had never been approved by the Food and Drug Administration (FDA) because it predated the 1938 Food, Drug, and Cosmetic Act, has long been used to treat gout and has for some time been used to treat familial Mediterranean fever, a rare disease. A company recently received FDA approval for the product as a treatment for gout and, in addition, as an orphan drug to treat familial Mediterranean fever (NDA 022352). It then increased the price of the drug (which is taken two to three times daily) approximately fiftyfold, from about $0.10 a pill to

---

[1] Estimated prevalence range is from 1/50,000 to 1/100,000 population (see, e.g., NHGRI, 2009).

$5 a pill; it also initiated lawsuits to force unapproved competitor products off the market (ACR, 2010; Rockoff, 2010).[2]

When patents and other market protections no longer apply, orphan drugs may still face limited competition because they are less likely than nonorphan products to face competition from generic drugs (see Appendix B). Generic competition results in lower prices and also in large losses in market share for the original brand-name product within 6 to 12 months of generic entry (Grabowski and Vernon, 1992; Frank and Salkever, 1997; Reiffen and Ward, 2005). The small market anticipated by potential generic competitors is one explanation for the lower availability of generics. In addition, many orphan drugs are biologics, which historically have had no clear path for generic approval. The recent Patient Protection and Affordable Care Act of 2010 (P.L. 111-148, hereafter the Affordable Care Act) will change this (see Chapter 3). Nonetheless, it is not clear how much generic competition will arise given that biologics are harder to manufacture and more variable than small-molecule drugs, so FDA may require additional clinical and nonclinical data that are not required for small-molecule drugs.

Also, in markets for ordinary drugs, the initial generic entrant (which is granted a 180-day exclusivity period among generic manufacturers) typically "shadow-prices" (i.e., charges a lower but not a substantially lower price, e.g., 15 percent, than the original brand-name drug) (Reiffen and Ward, 2005). Consistent with this strategy, the chief executive officer of a company with a product that will compete with Cerezyme has said that the company plans to price the product at a 15 percent discount to gain market share (cited in Douglas, 2010). For nonorphan drugs, however, generic prices tend to fall sharply once additional generic competitors enter the market. For orphan products with a small potential market, the entry of multiple generic drugs is less likely; thus limited price competition can be expected to persist.

One factor that could moderate costs for orphan drugs is that manufacturers of orphan products have little need to invest heavily in marketing their drugs because the target populations of physicians and patients are so small. Manufacturers can also often expect that advocacy groups will be active in spreading information about new treatments.

Notwithstanding examples of profitable orphan drugs, companies considering the development of a drug for a disease that affects a small population must evaluate prospects for each potential product individu-

---

[2] For state Medicaid programs, which paid approximately $1 million in 2007 for some 100,000 prescriptions of the drug (most likely for treatment of gout), one estimate is that the added cost for brand-name colchicine could run as much as $50 million per year (Kesselheim and Solomon, 2010).

ally. In addition to market size and costs for research and development, an important consideration is the insurance status of target patients—not only whether they are covered at all but also the scope of coverage and the limits placed on it.

Individuals with serious rare conditions can face a number of problems with health insurance. Insurers, particularly companies that market products directly to individuals rather than indirectly through employer groups, have an understandable concern about covering individuals who do not seek insurance until they or a family member is diagnosed with a serious illness. Companies have therefore screened or underwritten individuals based on their health status and history. As a result, people with both common and rare diseases without access to employment-based health coverage have found it difficult to secure health insurance at an affordable price or at all. For example, an analysis of 2004 Medical Expenditure Panel Survey data found that only 13 of the 7,000 individuals under age 65 who had a disability (broadly defined) reported having nongroup insurance (cited in IOM, 2007). Many restrictive underwriting practices will change as a result of the Affordable Care Act, which should make it easier for some individuals with a rare disorder to obtain coverage in the future.

In response to health care cost increases that have persistently exceeded inflation in the economy overall, insurers have developed an array of strategies to control costs for those they do insure, including transferring more costs to health plan members and adding administrative mechanisms to identify and discourage inappropriate care. Thus, in addition to considering the likelihood that target patients will have insurance, manufacturers may consider

- the processes that different payers use to determine, first, whether to cover a drug and, second, what to pay for it;
- the ways in which payment methods and coverage levels may differ based on the site where the drug is administered;
- the administrative controls that insurers, governments, or other third parties may place on coverage, for example, requirements for prior authorization of very expensive prescription drugs;
- the amounts that insured patients will have to pay out of pocket, which may vary both across and within different categories of drugs; and
- the existence of state or federal mandates that require coverage of certain classes of drugs.

Recent trends in the design and management of prescription drug benefits already include high patient cost sharing for some drug categories, especially expensive drugs. An extensive literature on the effects of patient cost sharing indicates that it reduces both needed and unneeded use of services (see summary in Newhouse et al., 1993) and also that consumers show considerable price sensitivity in making decisions about prescription drug purchases and use, even for drugs that are critical to their health (see, e.g., Frakt and Pizer, 2009; Solomon et al., 2009). As described below, other practices—such as the use of tiered formularies that favor some drugs or drug classes over others—could also affect the use of orphan drugs.

In the next few years, the Affordable Care Act will, if successful, expand access to health insurance for people under age 65. This should benefit companies that develop drugs and biologics as well as patients and families. At the same time, given that health care costs continue to consume a growing share of the Gross Domestic Product and that financial projections for Medicare and Medicaid are alarming, pharmaceutical companies must consider the prospect that governments, employers, and insurers may in the future impose price controls, try to negotiate more vigorously on drug prices, transfer a much higher share of drug costs to patients, or add further administrative barriers to expensive drugs. Pharmaceutical companies may, in addition, contemplate the risks of some kind of backlash against very high prices for orphan drugs, especially if the drugs are also very profitable.

The rest of this chapter examines how the policies and decisions of public and private insurance programs may create incentives or disincentives for companies to develop drugs for small populations. (Chapter 7 discusses policies and practices involving medical devices.) It also examines Medicare and other health plan policies on coverage for certain costs incurred by insured individuals who participate in clinical trials. The chapter concludes with recommendations. Appendix C presents an analysis of coverage of orphan drugs by the private prescription drug plans for Medicare beneficiaries. The focus here is on drugs specifically developed or marketed for people with rare conditions rather than on drugs that are used to relieve pain, respiratory distress, and other symptoms of both common and rare conditions. (As used in this chapter, the term drug includes biologics unless otherwise specified.)

This chapter emphasizes Medicare policies, in part because many adults with debilitating rare conditions are covered by Medicare by virtue of age or qualification for Social Security Disability Insurance (SSDI). In addition, information about Medicare is more readily available than information on private health plans. Although variation is introduced by the contractors that administer various elements of the Medicare program, it is a single program in contrast to the 50-plus Medicaid programs and the thousands of private health plans for which systematic information is limited. The chapter includes brief discussions of Medicaid, private health plans, and company assistance programs and reviews some provisions of recent legislation that may make insurance more available and moderate some limits on coverage, for example, lifetime caps on benefits. The discussion does not examine coverage of genetic testing.[3] It also does not investigate health programs of the Veterans Health Administration or the Department of Defense.

For the most part, this chapter considers health plan coverage and reimbursement policies and practices from the perspective of companies that develop drugs, not from the perspective of patients and families or from perspective of public policy makers considering issues of equity and affordability in the context of escalating government budget deficits. Some of the patient and family stories in Chapter 2 illustrate the importance of insurance to individual and family security. The committee found no analyses of public or private expenditures specifically for orphan drugs.

MEDICARE AND MEDICAID COVERAGE OF FDA-APPROVED DRUGS

Responding to the growing availability of effective medical services and the difficulties that older people faced in paying for these services directly or obtaining health insurance, Congress created Medicare in 1965 to cover people age 65 or over, regardless of income or health status.

Today, Medicare also covers people who qualify for SSDI, although they must generally wait 2 years before they are eligible for Medicare. Congress has provided an exception to this waiting period for SSDI beneficiaries who have amyotrophic lateral sclerosis and has also provided that adults and children with end-stage renal disease are automatically eligible for Medicare whether or not they have qualified for SSDI (SSA, 2010b). In addition, under its compassionate allowances policy, the Social Security Administration has created a mechanism for quickly identifying and processing SSDI applications for individuals with specific conditions that invariably qualify them for benefits. The initial list of conditions included 25 rare diseases and 25 cancers; nearly all of the 38 conditions added in 2010 were rare diseases (SSA, 2010a). Although this procedure does not shorten the Medicare waiting time after SSDI qualification, it does reduce the total waiting time. In 2008, approximately 7.7 million Medicare beneficiaries (about 16 percent of all beneficiaries) had qualified for coverage by reason of disability rather than age (CMS, 2009d).

In 1965, Congress also created the federal-state Medicaid program to insure certain categories of low-income individuals (primarily low-income

---

[3] A 2009 overview of Medicare policy on genetic testing noted that Medicare did not cover genetic testing based only on a family history of disease or in the absence of evidence that the test provided useful information to guide patient care (Straube, 2009). After determining that evidence was insufficient to support genetic testing to guide use of warfarin, the Centers for Medicare and Medicaid Services (CMS) recently announced it would support a clinical study of pharmacogenetic testing to predict patient responsiveness to the drug (Genomeweb. com, 2010).

mothers and children and low-income aged, blind, or disabled people). Certain people ("dual eligibles") qualify for both Medicare and Medicaid. The federal government sets many of the basic rules for Medicaid and subsidizes state programs to varying degrees, but states have some leeway in deciding who and what to cover and how much to pay providers.

Following a model that had been established in private health insurance, Congress initially divided Medicare into two parts: hospitalization insurance (Part A) and supplementary medical insurance for physician and certain other services (Part B). Building on policies initiated in the 1970s, the Medicare Advantage program (Part C) provides Medicare beneficiaries opportunities to enroll in private health plans.[4] In 2003, Congress created a Medicare outpatient prescription drug benefit (Part D), which was implemented in 2006 and is available only through private plans. Medicare is managed by the Centers for Medicare and Medicaid Services (CMS).

For beneficiaries not enrolled in Medicare Advantage plans, how Medicare pays for drugs and what controls it places on payments varies depending on where the drug is administered, for example, hospital, physician office, or home. Although the committee did not find any systematic analysis, a review of the list of approved orphan drugs suggests that most of them are administered in physician office or outpatient clinic settings or are taken by patients at home. Thus, for most drug companies as well as patients and families, Medicare policies related to Part B and Part D are of greater interest than Part A policies.

As discussed below in the section on coverage of certain costs in clinical trials, Medicare does not cover investigational drugs. CMS and FDA recently signed a memorandum of understanding to share data, including FDA data on drugs and medical devices that have not yet been authorized for marketing (75 Fed. Reg. 48699). The agencies are also considering a process of parallel review of products that would reduce the lag between FDA marketing authorization decisions and CMS national coverage determinations (75 Fed. Reg. 57045).

Medicare Part A

Medicare Part A covers inpatient services provided in hospitals. It also covers certain short stays in skilled nursing facilities, hospice services, and

---

[4] The Medicare Modernization Act of 2003 (P.L. 108-173) expanded the private plan options and the financial incentives for these plans under the Medicare Advantage label. The primary private health plan options under Medicare Advantage now include two types of local managed care plans (health maintenance organizations and local preferred provided organizations), fee-for-service plans, regional preferred provider organizations (mainly for rural areas), and special needs plans (mainly for people dually eligible for both Medicare and Medicaid or people with certain chronic health conditions) (KFF, 2009a).

certain home health services. Payment methods vary for each of these categories. Medicare pays for inpatient hospital care on the basis of prospectively determined rates for specified diagnosis-related, severity-adjusted bundles of services (OIG, 2001a). Oversimplified, each diagnosis-related group (DRG) payment has a weight assigned to it based on the average amount of resources used in caring for Medicare patients in that group. (In addition to diagnosis, assignment to a group takes into account other factors, including procedures, age, and comorbidities or complications.) Resources include facilities and services such as routine nursing care, laboratory tests, imaging services, intensive care, and all medications administered during the hospital stay. Within a payment category, payments generally will not vary based on which drugs are included in a hospital's formulary or other details of how hospitals manage services to beneficiaries.[5] The objective of this payment method is to control Medicare expenditures for hospital care by encouraging hospitals to provide care efficiently and economically.

CMS revises DRGs annually based on analysis of past inpatient claims data. In 2000, Congress provided that CMS could make an additional payment for certain new technologies on an interim basis until claims data were available to guide a normal revision in rates (Clyde et al., 2008). In general, Medicare pays half of the incremental cost to the hospital associated with the new technology on a case-by-case basis. To qualify for an add-on payment,

- the technology must be new (generally meaning that it was approved by FDA within the preceding 2 to 3 years);
- it must offer a substantial clinical benefit over existing options; and
- it must not be adequately covered by the existing DRG payment.

In the first 9 years after the policy was implemented in 2001, CMS rejected more than 20 applications for add-on payments and approved 9 applications, 8 of which were for medical devices (Clyde et al., 2008; Berger, 2009; CMS, 2009c; Hill, 2010; see also Chapter 7). The one drug for which an add-on payment was approved was not for an orphan drug.

Medicare Part B

Medicare Part B covers physician services, hospital outpatient care, certain home health services, certain clinical laboratory services, some preventive services, durable medical equipment, and certain drugs. Covered

---

[5] Although not a part of Medicare decision making as such, hospital formularies—like the formularies of private prescription drug plans—reflect hospital financial and quality management judgments and have economic implications for pharmaceutical companies.

drugs include drugs administered in physician offices that usually are not self-administered, drugs used as part of durable medical equipment (e.g., nebulizers), and in some cases, immunosuppressive drugs used after organ transplants and other drugs as authorized by Congress (CMS, 2010; see also, MedPAC, 2008; Cassidy, 2009). Under these provisions, Part B covers certain orphan drugs that are administered by infusion or injection in a physician's office or clinic, for example, galsulfase (Naglazyme), a treatment for Maroteaux-Lamy syndrome, a rare metabolic disorder. Likewise, Part B typically covers certain orphan drugs that are administered at home using equipment that is covered by Part B. An example is dornase alfa (Pulmozyme), a medication for cystic fibrosis that is inhaled using a neubulizer.

In addition, Part B also covers drugs provided as part of hospital outpatient services. These services are covered by a prospective payment system that includes inexpensive drugs and diagnostic radiopharmaceuticals as part of the packaged payment to an outpatient facility for a service such as a surgical procedure. More expensive drugs and biologics are reimbursed separately (MedPAC, 2008).

The Medicare Prescription Drug Improvement and Modernization Act of 2003 changed the way that Medicare pays physicians for Part B drugs and drug administration services. Before 2005, the Medicare payment rate for Part B-covered drugs was set at 95 percent of the average wholesale price, "which can be thought of as a manufacturer's list price" (MedPAC, 2007, p. 4). Policy makers agreed that the payment rates for Part B drugs were too high, but some providers argued that the high rates for the drugs were needed to offset payment rates for administering the drugs that were lower than the costs of administration. Since 2005, physicians who provide Part B drugs to their patients are reimbursed for those drugs at 106 percent of the average sales price, which is computed as the average transaction price for all sales in the United States. The law provided that new biologics and single-source drugs (brand-name drugs with no generic version) would be paid based on an individually determined average sales price so that payment would not be coded or averaged with other products. At the same time that Congress reduced reimbursement for Part B drugs, it increased the payment to physicians for administering the drugs.

A 2007 report by the Medicare Payment Advisory Commission (MedPAC) concluded that the change to the new payment system resulted in lower Part B expenditures for almost all covered drugs, largely due to lower prices (MedPAC, 2007). For example, from 2004 to 2005, the drop in drug expenditures ranged from 1 percent for rheumatology Part B drugs to 52 percent for urology drugs.

Patients pay a general Part B deductible and then 20 percent of the Medicare-approved payment amount. A patient's Part B coinsurance liability for medications is not capped and stays at 20 percent no matter how expensive the drug. However, as of 2006, just over 90 percent of beneficiaries had some form of public or private supplemental insurance that shielded them from Part B cost sharing requirements (MedPAC, 2010b).

Some drugs may be covered under Part B or Part D depending on the circumstances. The 2007 MedPAC report cited above stated that "physicians may work with patients to determine whether it makes more sense to use a drug that would [could] be covered under Part D or Part B," depending on what out-of-pocket costs a particular patient might face (MedPAC, 2007, p. 17).

A MedPAC analysis (2009) found that the top six biologics covered by Medicare Part B accounted for 43 percent ($7 billion) of the total of $17 billion spent for Part B in 2007 for the approximately 650 drugs that are separately paid under Part B. Several of these products were approved as orphan drugs for at least one, generally several, indications. The analysis also found that biologics accounted for 6 percent ($3.9 billion) of Part D spending but that spending on such products was growing faster for Part D than for Part B.

Medicare Part D

Medicare Part D adds an outpatient prescription drug benefit to the Medicare program. All Medicare beneficiaries have access to the benefit. Although they are not required to enroll, beneficiaries who do not enroll during their initial eligibility period and who do not have equivalent alternative coverage will pay more if they enroll later. As of February 2009, more than 26 million beneficiaries were enrolled in a Part D plan (KFF, 2009b).

The Part D benefit is administered by private plans approved by CMS. Part D benefits are offered through stand-alone prescription drug plans and through Medicare Advantage plans that cover all Medicare benefits including medications. Congress also specified that drug coverage for all individuals dually eligible for Medicare and Medicaid would shift from the Medicaid program to the Part D benefit. As a result, all dual eligibles are now enrolled in private Part D plans.

Beneficiary Financial Responsibilities

In 2010, the average adjusted monthly Part D premium was $38.94 (Q1Medicare.com, 2009). Beneficiaries with low incomes and modest assets receive substantial financial assistance with Part D premiums and cost sharing. For example, full-benefit dual eligibles pay no premiums, pay relatively nominal fixed copayments per prescription, and are not subject to the deductible or the coverage gap described below.

Under the standard Part D benefit offered in 2010, most beneficiaries pay a $310 deductible and then 25 percent coinsurance up to the initial coverage limit ($2,830 in total drug spending during the calendar year). In addition, beneficiaries are currently responsible for 100 percent of expenditures between $2,831 and $6,440 in total drug spending. This gap in coverage is sometimes referred to as the "doughnut hole." Once his or her total drug spending exceeds $6,440, a beneficiary pays the higher of 5 percent of a drug's cost or a copayment of $2.50 for a generic prescription or $6.30 for a brand-name prescription for the rest of the calendar year.

Plans have the option to deviate from this standard benefit by offering an actuarially equivalent benefit or by offering enhanced benefits. However, the vast majority of drug plans (80 percent) offered no benefits in the coverage gap as of January 2010, and most plans that did offer such benefits covered only generic drugs in the coverage gap (KFF, 2009b).

Under the Affordable Care Act, beginning January 1, 2011, Part D beneficiaries in the coverage gap will receive a 50 percent discount (absorbed by the manufacturer) off their plan's negotiated price for brand-name drugs and biologics covered by the plan. Despite the discount, 100 percent of the negotiated price will count toward the beneficiary's out-of-pocket expenses and thus toward the catastrophic coverage threshold ($6,440 in 2010). Over the subsequent 10 years, the beneficiary's coinsurance for brand-name drugs in the coverage gap will drop annually or biannually, down to 25 percent by 2020, and the coinsurance for generic drugs will likewise drop to 25 percent.

Structuring Coverage: General

Within limits specified by the federal government, Part D plans have considerable flexibility in structuring formularies, imposing cost sharing requirements, and establishing procedures for managing drug utilization. Plans are required to cover at least one drug in each therapeutic class, although plans must cover "all or substantially all" medications in six protected classes: anticancer drugs, antidepressants, anticonvulsants, antipsychotics, HIV/AIDS drugs, and immunosuppressants.[6] If a product is the only one available for treating a particular condition, Medicare generally requires plans to cover it.

For companies making orphan drugs or considering development of an orphan drug, several features of Part D plans could significantly affect beneficiary access and costs. These features—which include "tiered" cost

---

[6] However, recent legislation codifying the requirement that plans must list "all or substantially all" drugs in these six classes allows CMS to establish exceptions that permit plans to either exclude a drug in the protected classes from its formulary or impose utilization restrictions (CMS, 2009d).

sharing, requirements for prior authorization of coverage and step therapy, and quantity limits—are explained below. More details about these features as they affect orphan drugs are included in Appendix C.

Structuring Coverage: Tiered Cost Sharing

Most Part D plans use tiered formularies. Generic drugs in tier 1 require the lowest copayment; brand-name drugs preferred by the plan in tier 2 require a somewhat higher copayment; nonpreferred brand-name drugs in tier 3 require a still higher copayment.[7] Virtually all plans with tiered cost sharing also include a additional specialty tier to help manage spending for expensive specialty medications (KFF, 2009d). CMS guidelines specify that all drugs listed on the specialty tier must cost at least $600 a month (CMS, 2009a). Rather than paying a fixed copayment per prescription (e.g., $20) as is typical for less expensive drugs, beneficiaries must typically pay a percentage of the cost of medications in the specialty tier as coinsurance.[8] For the 2010 plan year, the median coinsurance rate for medications in the specialty tier across plans is 30 percent (KFF, 2009d; GAO, 2010b). Although the incentives in tiered formularies for beneficiaries to use generic or preferred drugs can provide leverage for plans to negotiate discounts with drug manufacturers, both the lack of competition for many orphan drugs and the small number of users for these drugs, as noted above, weaken the negotiating position of plans.

For a drug with a price to patients of $4,000 or more per month, coinsurance payments at 30 percent (plus the deductible) would reach the "no-coverage" threshold of $2,831 in total drug spending in 2 to 3 months and would exceed the upper end of the coverage gap ($6,440 in total drug spending) in about 6 months. (This assumes that the patient has no other applicable out-of-pocket costs.) At that point, costs for each prescription would drop to approximately 5 percent (which, if a prescription was for a month's worth of medication, would be approximately $200 in this example). Depending on how the initiation of treatment matched the start of a coverage year, that period of more generous coverage could last as long as 6 months before the coverage cycle started anew.

A recent GAO (2010b) study reported that high-cost drugs (i.e., those

---

[7] Plans must have a formal process for considering requests for formulary "exceptions." If an exception is approved, a beneficiary receiving a nonpreferred drug would be required to pay only the lower cost sharing required for a preferred brand drug. No data are available on the extent to which formulary exceptions are granted by Part D plans.

[8] Although most Part D plans require a copayment for medications on all tiers except the specialty tier, the share of plans requiring coinsurance for brand-name drugs not on the specialty tier has increased since 2006. In 2010, one-quarter of plans charged coinsurance for tier 2 drugs, and one-third charged coinsurance for tier 3 drugs (KFF, 2009d).

eligible for the specialty tier) accounted for 10 percent of total Part D costs. It also reported that 55 percent of beneficiaries who used at least one specialty-tier drug exceeded the upper threshold of the coverage gap. In addition, more than 75 percent of prescriptions for specialty tier-eligible drugs were for subsidized beneficiaries such as dual eligibles who qualify for reduced cost sharing for these and other drugs and who are not subject to the coverage gap. To illustrate the impact of increasing drug prices, the report cited the 46 percent price increase for the drug imatinib (Gleevec) from approximately $31,200 per year in 2006 to $45,500 per year in 2009. The increase meant a corresponding increase in out-of-pocket costs for a nonsubsidized beneficiary (taking the drug for the entire year) from $4,900 to $6,300.

Structuring Coverage: Utilization Management

In addition to patient cost sharing features, Part D plans also employ a variety of utilization management strategies to control the use of drugs and overall costs as well as to promote medication safety in some instances. These include prior authorization, step therapy, and quantity limits. Other things being equal, a pharmaceutical company would expect less use of an orphan drug and lower profits if the drug were a target of the most stringent of these utilization controls.

Plans generally require enrollees to obtain prior authorization from the plan to secure coverage for certain medications, particularly higher-cost medications or drugs with particular safety concerns. The committee found no data on the extent to which plans approve or deny requests for prior authorization.

Plans also may employ what are termed step-therapy requirements for certain medications for which alternatives are available. Under step therapy, enrollees are required to try a lower-cost medication and document a poor response to that drug before coverage of a higher-cost medication would be granted.

Quantity limits (i.e., a limit on the amount of a drug that is covered during a fixed time period) are another commonly used utilization management tool. In general, more frequent prescriptions to obtain the same quantity of a drug mean more costs shifted to patients.

Coverage and Off-Label Use

FDA approval of a drug is for a specific indication or indications based on evidence of safety and effectiveness for each indication. These indications are described in the FDA-approved labeling for the product. FDA regulations restrict companies from promoting unapproved or "off-label" uses, but FDA does not regulate the practice of medicine. Physicians may legally prescribe drugs for off-label indications. For example, a drug approved for use with a common disease may be used off-label for a rare condition, and physicians likewise may prescribe an orphan drug for either a common indication or a rare indication other than the indication(s) for which it has been approved. Some have expressed concern that some companies seeking orphan drug approval and marketing protection are really aiming at off-label use for a common indication and are inappropriately benefiting from the marketing protections attached to orphan drug approval (Fugh-Berman and Melnick, 2008; Wellman-Labadie and Zhou, 2009).

In addition to cost concerns, off-label use raises concerns about patient exposure to drugs that have not been determined to be safe and effective for uses other than those approved by FDA. At the same time, such use may provide options for patients for whom FDA-approved products are limited or nonexistent because physicians can try a medically plausible treatment approach to a disease (Kocs and Fendrick, 2003; Gillick, 2009). If case reports suggest promise from such an off-label use, then this may prompt companies or others to undertake controlled studies to support approval by FDA of a new indication. Alternatively, because systematic research could contradict the promising case reports and thereby curtail off-label sales, companies may choose not to pursue further studies.

Studies have indicated that off-label use is common in oncology (see, e.g., Kocs and Fendrick, 2003; Eastman, 2005; Abernethy et al., 2009). Off-label use is likewise common in pediatrics. Indeed, the lack of testing of drugs for use with children prompted legislation to encourage and in some cases require such testing (see Chapter 3). One study of outpatient prescribing patterns reported that of more than 500 medications covered in the study, 21 percent of uses were off-label and most of these off-label uses (73 percent) lacked clinical evidence of efficacy (Radley et al., 2006). Even when off-label uses are backed by research, companies may not wish to incur the costs of pursuing FDA approval unless they expect such approval to encourage further use that will offset those costs.

The initial CMS regulations for the Part D program denied coverage of medications for off-label uses *unless* the prescribed use was supported by one of three specific medical compendia (Le Masurier and Edgar, 2009).[9] Currently, off-label drug treatments for cancer are covered if they are listed in any CMS-approved compendium that is used to determine coverage of

---

[9] Compendia present comprehensive listings of drugs with descriptions of their clinical properties and recommended uses. The Part D regulations were based on 1993 legislation that predates the creation of the Part D program and that focused on drugs covered under Part B and the use of the compendia to identify medically accepted but unlabeled uses of drugs and biologicals in anticancer treatment (Abernethy et al., 2009).

off-label uses of cancer drugs under Part B. One concern is that questions have been raised about the independence of compendia compilers, the degree to which they cite current evidence (or any evidence), the quality of their methods and their assessments of evidence, and the potential for official acceptance of such compendia to discourage research aimed at FDA approval of off-label uses (Tillman and Gardner, 2004; Abernethy et al., 2009; Butcher, 2009; Mitka, 2009; Sox, 2009; see also ASHP, 1992; Gillick, 2009).

To inform future off-label coverage determinations, CMS commissioned a technology assessment from the Agency for Healthcare Research and Quality (AHRQ) to summarize the process by which anticancer drugs are added to various compendia and to identify methods used to collect evidence for listed drugs and biologics and their indicated uses (Abernethy et al., 2009). The assessment covered six compendia and a sample of 14 anticancer combinations that were selected to include newer and older agents, common and rare cancers, and biologics and drugs. Among the findings was that there was little agreement in the evidence regarding efficacy cited by the compendia and that the compendia were discordant on whether they discussed adverse effects among patients with specific cancers. Moreover, when compendia did not include off-label indications, the analysts could not determine whether a particular omission reflected a conscious editorial decision following the evaluation of available evidence or whether the available evidence was not identified and evaluated. The authors observed that although they could not generalize to other disease areas, the compendia's performance might be expected to be highest in oncology, given their importance for reimbursement. The authors also pointed out the major challenges of managing a near-continuous systematic review of large numbers of drug uses not approved by FDA. They also noted that FDA itself was not authorized or prepared to undertake such a review.

For rare diseases, the volume of drugs and uses is obviously much smaller but so is the research to support evaluations of off-label use. The growing databases from Part D claims could, when linked to Medicare hospital and physician claims data, be a resource for studying the nature and outcomes of some off-label use of orphan and other drugs for patients with rare conditions.

Part D Plans and Drug Prices

Congress has not provided CMS itself with the authority to negotiate prices with pharmaceutical manufacturers. However, as noted above, to the extent that private health plans, including Part D plans, are able to "move market share" across drugs in a class using such financial incentives, then plans have the potential to negotiate sizable rebates or discounts from manufacturers. For many expensive drugs, including many orphan drugs, insurers may have little leverage in negotiating price discounts.

Given the introduction of Part D just 4 years ago, only limited empirical evidence has accumulated on its impact on drug prices. A recent study by Duggan and Morton found that Part D led to a decrease in the average price for brand-name drugs and an increase in overall utilization of Part D drugs among Medicare recipients (Duggan and Morton, 2006). They estimate that each percentage point increase in the pre-Part D Medicare market share for a given drug is associated with a 1.2 to 1.4 percent decrease in a drug's average price relative to other drugs. However, Frank and Newhouse (2008) found some evidence that the shift from Medicaid to Part D of drug coverage for dual eligibles resulted in higher drug prices for this population. (These analyses did not specifically consider orphan or specialty-tier drugs.)

An analysis commissioned by MedPAC reported that prices for Part D drugs rose 11 percent between January 2006 and December 2008 (based on national drug codes as the unit of analysis) (MedPAC, 2010a). However, after taking into account the substitution of generic for brand-name drugs (which is encouraged by Part D plans), the analysis found Part D prices declined by 3 percent over the same period.

Analysis of Part D Plan Coverage of Orphan Drugs

Appendix C presents the results of a commissioned analysis of Part D plan coverage of orphan drugs as reported in the January 2010 CMS Prescription Drug Plan, Pharmacy Network, and Pricing Information Files. For drugs that are not covered by Medicare Part B (or, rarely, Part A) and that thus are eligible for Part D coverage, the analysis found that the great majority are covered by more than half of Part D plans (Table 6-1). Of the handful of orphan drugs that were not covered by any plan as of January 2010, several of these have now been added to the formularies of at least one plan. In addition, several drugs that were included in the analysis because they were not in the CMS price list for Part B-covered drugs have since been added to that price list.

There are some differences in coverage of orphan drugs across different types of Part D plans. For example, overall, orphan drug coverage seems to be somewhat more generous among national stand-alone Part D plans than among nonnational stand-alone plans. For orphan drugs, 27 percent are covered by fewer than half of nonnational plans, while only 9 percent are covered by fewer than half of national plans. Still, Medicare beneficiaries who rely on an orphan drug should be able to find a Part D plan that covers it.

Although nearly all orphan drugs are covered by at least half of Part

TABLE 6-1 Coverage of Part D-Eligible Drugs by Type of Medicare Prescription Drug Plan

Extent of Plan Coverage	All Stand-Alone PDPs	MA-PDPs	Stand-Alone National PDPs	Stand-Alone Non-national PDPs	Stand-Alone Bench-mark PDPs	Stand-Alone Non-bench-mark PDPs
No or very low coverage (<25% plan coverage rate)	4	4	4	10	4	4
Low coverage (25-49% plan coverage rate)	3	0	0	13	7	2
Medium coverage (50-74% plan coverage rate)	19	17	19	8	15	19
High coverage (75-99% plan coverage rate)	29	36	19	25	24	29
Complete coverage (100% plan coverage rate)	44	42	57	43	49	45

NOTES: MA = Medicare Advantage plans; PDP = prescription drug plan.
The number of drugs that fall into each coverage rate category in the analysis is 99; therefore, the numbers and percentages of drugs are identical and percentages have not been included in the table.
SOURCE: January 2010 CMS Prescription Drug Plan, Pharmacy Network, and Pricing Information Files; FDA list of orphan drugs as of December 2008.

D plans, significant limits of the kinds described above typically apply. Almost half (46 percent) of orphan drugs are included in specialty tiers by 50 percent or more of stand-alone Part D plans. One-third of orphan drugs were subject to prior authorization requirements before coverage is granted by 50 percent or more of stand-alone plans.

Medicaid

The Medicaid program, which is jointly financed and administered by the federal and state governments, covers health and long-term care services for approximately 20 percent of Americans under age 65, including eligible low-income children, parents, and individuals with disabilities (EPI, 2009). It also covers eligible low-income individuals over 65 who are covered by Medicare. Under the Affordable Care Act, state Medicaid programs will be required to extend eligibility to all individuals with income up to 133 percent of the federal poverty level. One estimate is that this eligibility expansion could increase Medicaid enrollment by approximately 16 million individuals (Holahan and Headen, 2010).

Although states are not required to cover prescription drugs in their Medicaid programs, all 50 states and the District of Columbia offer a drug benefit (KFF, 2008). As noted above, prescription drug coverage for individuals who are dually eligible for Medicare and Medicaid shifted from Medicaid to the Medicare Part D program as of January 2006. Other Medicaid beneficiaries still receive drug coverage from their state Medicaid program. Medicaid programs typically require copayments for each prescription, which generally range from $0.50 to $5 per prescription depending on the type of drug (generic versus brand name, preferred versus nonpreferred) and the state (KFF, 2008).

Under the Medicaid Rebate Program, manufacturers are required to have a rebate agreement with the Secretary of Health and Human Services in order for states to receive federal Medicaid funding for outpatient prescription drugs dispensed to Medicaid patients. Until 2010, the rebate had been 15.1 percent of the average manufacturer price (AMP, or the average price at which the manufacturer sold it) or the difference between AMP and the best price offered by the manufacturer within the United States, whichever is greater (CMS, 2009b). Under the Affordable Care Act, the minimum rebate for innovator drugs will increase in 2010 to 23.1 percent of AMP, with the exception of clotting factors and drugs with only pediatric indications for which the minimum rebate will be 17.1 percent of AMP. (The rebate for noninnovator drugs will increase from 11 to 13 percent of AMP.) Under the new law, Medicaid rebates must be paid on outpatient drugs dispensed to enrollees of Medicaid managed care plans (close to 70 percent of all Medicaid enrollment), which was not the case before 2010.

Overall, the rebate provisions make orphan drugs more affordable for state Medicaid programs, although very expensive drugs remain very expensive. The committee found no analysis specific to orphan drugs, but some evidence suggests that this rebate approach results in much lower prices for Medicaid than for other payers in the market. For example, the House Committee on Oversight and Government Reform estimated that Medicaid pays prices that are about 30 percent lower than prices paid by Medicare Part D (Outterson and Kesselheim, 2009). However, a study by Duggan and Morton (2006) found that drugs sold disproportionately to Medicaid beneficiaries have higher prices than otherwise similar drugs. Because the Medicaid rebate is based on prices paid for these drugs in the private sector, manufacturers have an incentive to increase prices charged in the private sector, thereby distorting both the private market price and the Medicaid price.

In response to increasing prescription drug utilization and expenditures, states have adopted a variety of cost containment approaches over the past decade. For example, according to an analysis of the 50 states and the District of Columbia, 44 states have state maximum allowable cost programs that set maximum reimbursement levels for generic and multisource brand-name drugs, and 26 states were members of multistate purchasing coalitions intended to increase negotiating power over price with pharmaceutical manufacturers (Smith et al., 2009). Forty-four states negotiate supplemental rebates in addition to rebates negotiated through the national drug rebate program for Medicaid. Almost one-third (16 states) limit the number of prescriptions that are covered per enrollee, and 46 require prior authorization before granting coverage of specific medications as of 2009. Although not specific to orphan products, these policies would affect orphan drugs and the patients who use them.

PRIVATE HEALTH PLAN COVERAGE OF FDA-APPROVED DRUGS

As of 2008, approximately 65 percent of nonelderly individuals had private health insurance (KFF-SHF, 2010). This percentage is expected to increase substantially in the next few years when subsidies for the purchase of private insurance plans become available for lower-income individuals under the Affordable Care Act.

Virtually all individuals (98 percent) with employer-sponsored insurance currently have a prescription drug benefit (KFF, 2009c). Employer-sponsored plans vary substantially with respect to cost sharing requirements, formulary breadth, and utilization management requirements. Many of the practices now found in Medicare Part D plans were initially devised for employment-based plans.

According to a survey for the Kaiser Family Foundation, tiered formularies are common among employer-sponsored plans. More than three-quarters (78 percent) of individuals enrolled in these plans face a formulary with three or more tiers (KFF, 2009c). Average cost sharing requirements per prescription have increased steadily over the past few years. The majority of plans require copayments for each prescription filled rather than coinsurance payments per prescription. In 2009, average copayments were $10 for generic drugs in tier 1, $27 for preferred brand-name drugs in tier 2, $46 for nonpreferred brand-name drugs in tier 3, and $85 for drugs in tier 4. A minority of plans required coinsurance rather than copayments for one or more tiers. In 2009, 29 percent required coinsurance for tier 4 drugs, and the average coinsurance rate was 31 percent. A much smaller subset of plans (6 to 10 percent) required coinsurance for medications in tiers 1, 2, and 3.

Traditionally, a substantial proportion of health plans have limited the total amount the plan would pay for a given enrollee over the course of his or her lifetime, often referred to as a lifetime spending maximum. In 2009, 16 percent of those with employer-sponsored coverage had a lifetime maximum between $1 million and $2 million, and another 43 percent had a lifetime maximum of $2 million or more (KFF, 2009c). An adult who receives twice-monthly injections of alglucosidase alfa (Myozyme) for Pompe disease could run up costs of $300,000 a year just for the drug, and the drug can have serious side effects that require hospitalization and additional expenses. Such a patient could reach a $1 million cap fairly quickly. (By way of comparison, total first-year costs for a heart transplant for the year of the transplant could run $800,000, but costs in subsequent years—assuming no serious complications—would be much lower, perhaps $20,000 to $40,000 [UNOS, 2010].) Only a minority (10 percent) of private health plans had an out-of-pocket maximum specifically for prescription drugs in 2009, which limits an enrollee's financial risk for medication costs.

Effective in 2010, the Affordable Care Act prohibits individual and employer health plans from setting lifetime limits on the dollar value of coverage, and it permits annual caps on coverage only as allowed by the Department of Health and Human Services. The law also prohibits plans from canceling coverage because an individual develops health problems. Effective in 2014, the law provides an array of measures to expand access to insurance, one of which will prohibit insurers participating in newly created insurance exchanges from refusing coverage to people with medical problems and varying premiums based on health status. These and other provisions should benefit individuals who use high-cost orphan drugs, although many details remain unclear. For example, private plans could restrict coverage of drugs used by high-cost patients, unless regulations restrict that strategy.

Private health plans vary in their policies and practices with respect to off-label use of prescription drugs. Some conduct evidence reviews for certain drugs (see, e.g., Monroe et al., 2006), and some have set forth criteria for when off-label use will be considered (RegenceRx, 2010; Wellmark Blue Cross Blue Shield, 2010). An informal review of plan policies for a few orphan drugs likewise showed variation. Some excluded one or more of the drugs on the basis that other alternatives are preferable, some required prior authorization, and a few covered the drugs without restriction except for specialty-tier listing.

OTHER MEANS OF FINANCIAL ACCESS TO ORPHAN DRUGS

Even if drug companies expect that they can set profitable prices for a drug for a rare condition and anticipate that they will have a sufficient market of mostly insured patients able to pay those prices, they may also judge it desirable or prudent to provide assistance in some form to patients who cannot afford the drug. A number of companies that have set high prices for orphan products have established some kind of assistance program for patients without insurance (e.g., without Medicare Part D coverage) or for individuals with insurance who face high out-of-pocket costs.[10] Some companies have also established programs to help patients and families understand and navigate health plan requirements and procedures to secure payment for an expensive drug. Companies presumably factor the cost of assistance programs into their economic projections for a drug and then into the price of an approved drug. In this way, public and private health plans and insured individuals who pay for the drug support some of the cost of company assistance.

Company assistance programs may require considerable financial information from individuals seeking assistance, for example, tax returns, bank statements, and W-2 forms. Assistance may be restricted to people who have no insurance, and programs typically set income and asset limits (e.g., income up to some percentage above the federal poverty level). Types of company assistance may include

- providing a supply of the drug at no or reduced cost for 3 months or some other defined period, after which time patients and families must seek a means of continued access now that use of the product has been initiated;
- assisting with the cost of copayments or other cost sharing requirements for patients with insurance coverage; and
- supplying information to patients and families about Medicaid eligibility, private charities, and other possible routes of financial aid.

A survey by Choudry and colleagues (2009) of 165 company assistance programs (not limited to orphan drugs) found considerable variability across programs. They reported that half the programs would not disclose their income eligibility criteria, and very few (4 percent) disclosed how many patients the programs had helped.[11]

The National Organization for Rare Disorders administers financial

---

[10] The American Society of Health-System Pharmacists includes on its website a list of programs that may help patients get assistance from drug manufacturers (ASHP, 2010). In addition to other resources, an organization called NeedyMeds provides a list of programs and companies, some of which are explicitly identified as having no program (http://www. needymeds.org/program_list.taf).

[11] A 2001 study by the Office of the Inspector General at the Department of Health and Human Services examined the implementation of the Orphan Drug Act (OIG, 2001b). It reported that roughly 3 out of 4 of the 36 companies that it contacted said they either had some kind of assistance program or planned to have one if FDA approved their products.

assistance programs for several medical product companies in connection with at least one of their products (information available at http://www. rarediseases.org/programs/medication). It also has several other programs of assistance for a number of mostly rare conditions, including infantile spasms, Hunter syndrome, and paroxysmal nocturnal hemoglobinuria.

In addition to company programs, advocacy groups for rare diseases and other nonprofit programs may assist some patients and families who lack insurance or cannot afford the cost sharing requirements of their health plan. The smaller the group, the more difficult it is likely to be for it to provide assistance. Another option for some individuals is the Patient Advocate Foundation Co-Pay Relief Program (http://www.copays.org/). It offers financial support to qualified insured patients, including Medicare Part D beneficiaries, who are being treated for one of 21 conditions, a few of which (e.g., pancreatic cancer and multiple myeloma) are rare.

Some families themselves or their relatives and friends create fundraising efforts, for example, to raise enough money for a transplant or to help with costs for a child being treated for a brain tumor. It is doubtful that these kinds of activities factor into company decisions about product development.

In the future, an expansion of access to health insurance and the removal of certain limitations on coverage may reduce but are unlikely to eliminate the role of company assistance programs. Some individuals will remain uninsured, and some of those with insurance will continue to have difficulty with out-of-pocket payments.

PUBLIC AND PRIVATE HEALTH PLAN COVERAGE OF CERTAIN COSTS IN CLINICAL TRIALS

In some cases, health plans may cover certain costs of care for patients involved in clinical trials, thus reducing the burden on participants in the trial and potentially easing recruitment challenges for sponsors, including sponsors of trials of orphan drugs. The legislation that created Medicare provided generally that payment was to be limited to items or services that were "reasonable and necessary" for the diagnosis and treatment of illness or injury or to improve the functioning of a malformed body member" (42 USC 1395y). Historically, those administering the Medicare program interpreted the terms "reasonable and necessary" to mean that a service or item must be safe and effective, medically necessary and appropriate, and not experimental in order to qualify for reimbursement. Medicare coverage was typically denied for drugs or devices being studied under an investigational device exemption (see Chapter 7) or an investigational new drug application (see Chapter 3) that had not yet been approved or cleared by FDA.

Based on directives in an Executive Memorandum in 2000, Medicare now covers, subject to certain qualifications, routine care costs for patients in therapeutic trials to support FDA approval of a drug or device as well as costs of medical complications arising from participation in such trials (CMS, 2000). The cost of the investigational product is usually not covered for these trials (but see Chapter 7 for a discussion of policy on medical devices). In addition, beginning in 2004, CMS may pay for some specific new items or services for which evidence is inadequate on the condition that additional patient data be provided to supplement standard claims data, a process termed "coverage with evidence development" (CMS, 2006, 2007). Many state Medicaid programs cover routine patient care costs in clinical trials under policies similar to those for Medicare (ACS, 2010). In addition, approximately 30 states have mandated that private health plans cover such costs (NCI, 2009b).

The Affordable Care Act of 2010 provides that health plans may not, in general, deny coverage for routine patient costs for items and services provided in connection with participation in a clinical trial for cancer and life-threatening conditions and may not discriminate against individuals based on their participation in clinical trials. The law explicitly mentions coverage for trials conducted under an Investigational New Drug application reviewed by FDA. It does not mention trials of devices under investigational device exemptions, although no language otherwise excludes coverage of routine costs associated with medical device trials. Health plans are not required to cover the cost of the investigational item.

RECOMMENDATIONS

As discussed in Chapter 3, the Orphan Drug Act provides significant incentives to companies to develop drugs for rare diseases. Translating these advantages into sales and profits depends on the availability of buyers. Fortunately for companies and individual patients, many of those in need of expensive orphan drugs have found that if they are insured, their health plans have, in general, been willing to cover the drug, usually at a price unilaterally established by the company. The great majority of orphan drugs eligible for Part D coverage are covered by more than half of Part D plans, and very few are covered by no plan. Plans, however, typically require that patients pay a significant share of the cost of expensive drugs, and many plans impose prior authorization requirements that could limit access for certain orphan medications.

Notwithstanding the generally positive picture for orphan drug coverage by Medicare Part D plans, companies keep an attentive eye on public and private health plan policies and coverage trends, recognizing that escalating health care costs put Medicare, Medicaid, and other health programs under pressure to take actions to manage costs, including costs for prescription medications. Although a number of provisions of the Affordable Care Act of 2010 should reduce the burden of high medication costs for patients (if the provisions are not repealed), the escalating costs of health care will keep or increase the pressure on public and private health plans to transfer more costs to patients within the boundaries of the law. To the extent that personalized medicine and other developments lead to an increase in the proportion of drugs that win approval as orphan drugs and an increase in the share of insured patients who use orphan drugs, concerns specific to orphan drugs can be expected to expand to more drugs and more patients.

Better information about some aspects of health plan policies could help decision makers assess how policies may affect access to orphan drugs. In particular, little is known about the application of prior authorization requirements to orphan drugs. Such requirements could have negative effects by restricting or delaying access to needed drugs. They could also have benefits if they improve physician adherence to evidence-based guidelines for effective drug use and reduce unnecessary or even harmful use of expensive drugs. It would be helpful to have some evidence of what is actually occurring with these requirements in Medicare Part D plans. The recommendation below focuses on Medicare and Medicaid. More information on the policies and procedures of other health plans would also be desirable to gauge the effects on people who depend on orphan drugs.

> **RECOMMENDATION 6-1: The Centers for Medicare and Medicaid Services or the Medicare Payment Advisory Commission should study how the implementation of prior authorization requirements by Medicare Part D and state Medicaid plans affects beneficiary access to orphan drugs. The findings should guide recommendations and actions to improve policies and practices for the Part D program.**

A second area the committee identified for attention involves payment for off-label use of orphan drugs or for off-label use of common drugs for patients with rare conditions. Indiscriminate coverage of off-label uses has the potential to harm patients as well as waste scarce resources. Indiscriminate exclusion of such uses likewise has the potential to harm patients and produce a backlash by policy makers, who have already required selective coverage of off-label uses under Medicare Part B and Part D. This coverage has been linked to information provided in compendia prepared by private companies with little public oversight or evaluation of their practices or analyses. The extent to which these compendia cover off-label uses relevant to patients with rare conditions is unknown, and the quality of such discussions as exist is likewise unknown.

Recommendations about compendia generally are beyond the scope of this report. However, the committee believes that the creation of an evidence-based compendium focused specifically on off-label uses of drugs for rare diseases could inform clinicians, health plans, and potentially patients and families. Such a compendium is not likely to be feasible for commercial publishers but could be undertaken by a public agency such as AHRQ that has experience in similar analyses. Based on experience with the U.S. Pharmacopeia, which developed one of the early compendia but discontinued it because sales did not cover expenses, the estimated potential cost of a pilot project to develop and update a pilot compendium is within the range of current AHRQ grants (Dr. Roger Williams, CEO, U.S. Pharmacopeia, June 2010, personal communication to Carolyn Asbury [Committee member].)

> RECOMMENDATION 6-2: The Agency for Healthcare Research and Quality or a similar appropriate agency should undertake a pilot project to develop an evidence-based compendium to inform health plan decisions on both orphan and nonorphan drugs that may have indications for rare conditions that have not been evaluated or approved by FDA.

Some of the issues that such a pilot effort would confront include determining a focus (e.g., rare cancers, rare metabolic disorders), establishing criteria for evaluating research that involves small numbers of participants and nontraditional research designs, and exploring the use of Medicare or Part D claims data for analyses to supplement the review of published studies. Depending on its experience, AHRQ or another agency could propose a strategy for updating or expanding the compendium.

In the process of developing the compendium, analysts may also identify directions for future research on specific drugs to demonstrate efficacy, side effects, or optimum dosage. If not undertaken by industry, such studies might be supported through National Institutes of Health awards, FDA orphan products grants, AHRQ grants to its Centers for Education and Research on Therapeutics, or other grant programs.

7

Medical Devices: Research and Development for Rare Diseases

The Vertical Expandable Prosthetic Titanium Rib (VEPTR), a device that has saved the lives of 300 infants and young children who otherwise would have died from lack of breath [thoracic insufficiency syndrome], has been approved by the U.S. Food and Drug Administration (FDA). . . . The titanium rib is curved like a ribcage and has holes that allow the surgeons to expand the device in outpatient surgery every six months. The rib is implanted in infants as young as 6 months and in teenagers until skeletal maturity, typically age 14 in girls and age 16 in boys. . . . "It took 13 years to gain FDA approval because it took a long time to accumulate a lot of patients with rare diseases" Dr. [Robert] Campbell [the inventor] said.

UTHSCSA, 2004

For rare diseases, efforts to accelerate research and product development clearly focus on drugs and biological products. Devices and the need for devices are much less frequently mentioned in articles or conversations. When devices for rare conditions are discussed, it is generally in connection with pediatric populations.

To acknowledge the emphasis on drugs for rare diseases is not to imply that devices are not important for many people with rare medical conditions. Some people depend critically on devices targeted at distinctive features of their condition, for example, children who have received the implanted titanium rib described above. No pharmaceutical or biological product can provide the mechanical support afforded by this implant. Genetic tests that are necessary for the diagnosis and treatment of certain rare conditions are, in certain cases, regulated as medical devices. In addition, people with rare conditions benefit from a large number of medical devices that are used generally in connection with complex surgery, anesthesia, respiratory support, nonsurgical cardiac procedures, administration of certain medications, diagnostic and therapeutic imaging of various kinds, laboratory testing, and other services.

Clinical studies of the titanium rib were supported under the orphan products grants program described in Chapter 3. Earlier, the National Organization for Rare Disorders provided a seed grant from its donated research funds. The two companies that were involved in manufacturing the device for research use participated out of interest in children's health rather than expectations of profit (Campbell, 2007). After years of investigation and adaptation, the device was approved by the Food and Drug Administration (FDA) in 2004 through a Humanitarian Device Exemption (HDE). This process was established in the Safe Medical Devices Act of 1990 (P.L. 101-629) to provide incentives for the development of medical devices for small populations. Although medical devices for small populations are grouped under the label orphan products in the grants program created by the Orphan Drug Act and are within the charge of the Office of Orphan Product Development (OOPD), the term orphan medical device does not appear in legislative or regulatory language.

Regulatory requirements and product development pathways differ significantly for medical devices compared to drugs and biologics. Thus, this report devotes a separate chapter to medical device development, regulation, and reimbursement.

This chapter begins with a brief overview of important differences between devices and drugs. It then reviews device regulation and reimbursement with an emphasis on the HDE process and other policies or procedures that are potentially most relevant to complex, high-risk devices intended for small populations. This discussion is followed by an overview of the research and development process for complex devices and a discussion of barriers and opportunities for the development of devices for small populations. As this chapter highlights, the stringency of government regulation of devices is related to the risk presented by the device.

DIFFERENCES BETWEEN MEDICAL DEVICES AND DRUGS

Compared to pharmaceuticals, medical devices are an extremely diverse group of products. Some are as simple as adhesive bandages, tongue depressors, and plastic tubing. Others are complex, for example, various implanted cardiac and neurological devices, stair-walking wheelchairs, robotic surgical systems, and magnetic resonance imaging devices. In contrast to single-molecule drugs, many complex devices involve a number of components that, together, form a system.[1] Table 7-1 summarizes several additional differences between devices and drugs as they relate, in particular, to implants and other complex medical devices.

In addition to the cost-related differences noted in the table, companies that develop medical devices also have to consider other costs that may be only minor considerations for most pharmaceutical companies. One category of such costs involves the support and servicing of complex devices once they are released into the market. Depending on the device, highly skilled company personnel may provide training to physicians, clinical staff, and patients (and their families) on the proper use of the device. Service technicians often must be available promptly in case device-related problems arise. Companies must also consider potential obligations to patients if a decision is made at some point to discontinue the device.[2]

As is true of its products, the medical device industry is likewise quite variable. Some companies are large and have diverse product lines and substantial resources to devote to product development and interactions with government regulators. Compared to the drug industry, a larger proportion of device firms are small, focused on single products and narrow market segments, and limited in their resources (see Gelijns et al., 2006; Linehan et al., 2007).

Entrepreneurs at small start-up companies develop many innovative medical devices, including devices that address needs of small patient populations. Company motivations for taking the start-up path to market vary. In some cases, those involved may see the approach as a focused way to address an unmet need and contribute to society without having to navigate the decision-making processes of a large, complex company. In some cases, the projected business opportunity is too small or too risky to be worth attention from an existing company but is still attractive enough to attract venture capitalists or a small group of entrepreneurs. In exchange for partial ownership of the start-up company, angel investors and venture

---

[1] An example is a left ventricular assist device for children that FDA approved in 2004. The device consists of four major subsystems—a pump, an external controller, a clinical data acquisition system, and a patient home support system—plus accessories, including batteries, a battery charger, and a kit to protect the device during showering (H030003 [the FDA approval number for the device]). Further, the pump subsystem involves multiple elements, including a housing around three additional components—an inflow tube, an outflow element, and a probe to measure blood flow—and a cable connecting the implanted pump to the external battery and controls.

[2] For example, implanted devices usually have a finite service life due to battery exhaustion (if electronic or electromechanical) or simply wear and tear, so patients will need replacements. If no alternative device is available and particularly if the patient depends on the device for survival, then the continued availability of a replacement device is crucial. The total replacement heart is an example of such a device.

TABLE 7-1 Complex Medical Devices Tend to Differ from Drugs

Complex Medical Device	Small-Molecule Compound
Physical, engineering-based object (or set of components)	Chemical formulation
Direct mechanism of action and, usually, readily apparent, near-term response	Indirect biochemical mechanism of action via blood, other body fluids, or tissue diffusion
Site- or organ-specific therapy	Usually systemic treatment
Patient responses to therapy generally similar and not dependent on dose response	Patient responses variable (benefits and adverse effects) and dose dependent
High initial product costs amortized over service life	Costs for product accumulate over the course of treatment
Application often requires professional expertise (e.g., surgical implantation); patient use might involve complex instructions	Application or use is often simple and patient controlled (e.g., taking a pill)
Continuing product refinement and short product life cycle that may improve effectiveness and reduce costs	Product (basic molecule) not modified, long product life cycle
Moderate to high development cost	High development cost
Few basic patents, many incremental patents and products	Basic patent, fewer incremental patents or products

SOURCES: Adapted from Linehan et al., 2007; Citron, 2008; see also Feigal et al., 2003.

capitalists often provide the financing needed to bring nascent innovations to the market. In addition to infusions of capital, venture capitalists who have worked with other new companies may provide management expertise and strategic advice to guide the managers of a start-up company.

As discussed further below, the processes of device development and refinement also differ in significant ways from the processes that characterize the development of drugs and biologics (see generally Linehan et al., 2007; Pietzsch, 2009; Zenios et al., 2010). Because medical device companies are often engaged in a continuous process of product refinement and innovation, patents and similar protections may be less important as a source of competitive advantage for device companies than they are for drug companies. As discussed in Chapter 3, once a new drug is approved by FDA, a pharmaceutical company will have marketplace exclusivity for a specific formulation for a period of time and may also receive patent-term restoration that extends the remaining patent life of the drug. In contrast, several device companies may compete simultaneously in the marketplace with devices for the same indication that differ in only limited respects. This might be because the devices are not patented or because manufacturers have been able to design around the patents that protect a particular competitor's devices. Consequently, although FDA-approved devices are eligible for patent-term restoration, patents may not be as useful in protecting devices from competition as they are for pharmaceutical products. Even in instances when patents could provide an element of protection from market competition, the patent holder may elect to license its patents to one or more competitors in exchange for royalties or to cross-license patents in order to acquire access to patents held by a competitor. Nevertheless, medical device companies are aggressive in defending their intellectual property from infringements by competitors (Budd and Liebman, 2009).

REGULATION OF MEDICAL DEVICES

Basic Framework of Medical Device Regulation

Although the Federal Food, Drug, and Cosmetic Act of 1938 mentioned therapeutic medical devices, devices were a relatively inconsequential component of FDA's jurisdiction. The statute specified that devices be adequately labeled and provide adequate instructions for use but did not give FDA premarket regulatory authority over devices. In the 1970s, following widely publicized problems with the Dalkon Shield (an intrauterine contraceptive device) (Hubacher, 2002), Congress turned to the regulation of medical devices with the Medical Device Amendments of 1976 (P.L. 94-295). The legislation created the basic framework for device regulation. As defined by statute (21 USC 321(h)), a device is

an instrument, apparatus, implement, machine, contrivance, implant, in vitro reagent, or other similar or related article, including a component part, or accessory which is:

• recognized in the official National Formulary, or the United States Pharmacopoeia, or any supplement to them,
• intended for use in the diagnosis of disease or other conditions, or in the cure, mitigation, treatment, or prevention of disease, in man or other animals, or
• intended to affect the structure or any function of the body of man or other animals, and

which does not achieve any of its primary intended purposes through chemical action within or on the body of man or other animals and which is not dependent upon being metabolized for the achievement of any of its primary intended purposes.

Within FDA, the Center for Devices and Radiological Health (CDRH) regulates most medical devices. The Center for Biologics Evaluation and Research regulates devices related to blood and cellular products such as blood collection, screening, and processing devices. The OOPD has roles in designation of devices eligible for HDE approval and in awarding product development grants, which are available for device as well as drug development.

Device Classification and Regulation

A fundamental element of the 1976 law was a risk-related device classification scheme that forms the basis for risk-related regulatory requirements. To simplify, the law designated devices of lowest risk and relatively little complexity as Class I; devices of moderate risk and greater complexity as Class II; and devices that support or sustain life or otherwise present a high risk to the patient as Class III.[3]

In general, Class I and II devices have substantially equivalent predecessor or "predicate" devices that are already on the market. Some new devices may be classified automatically as Class III devices because they have no such predicate device. FDA may reclassify such devices as Class II devices based on an analysis of the risk they present. For example, such a reclassification was requested for the first device available to screen newborn infants for inherited abnormalities of amino acids and deficiencies in certain enzymes (Lloyd, 2004).[4]

Regardless of its complexity, any device can present potential harms to patients if it is misused, mislabeled or poorly labeled, badly designed, poorly manufactured, or misrepresented. Thus, the regulatory framework created by Congress covers all classes of devices and extends, in some cases, to requirements for sponsors to conduct postmarket studies to collect data about safety and effectiveness after a device is approved for marketing.

For Class I devices, manufacturers generally must register with FDA and follow FDA's quality system regulations, including adherence to good manufacturing practices. These devices are usually not subject to premarket notification or review.

Manufacturers of Class II devices usually must get FDA clearance of a "510(k) notification" (named for the relevant section of the law) to legally market these devices. The process requires the submission of considerable technical information and sometimes animal study data related to safety and performance characteristics of the new device, in order to demonstrate its "substantial equivalence" to the predicate device. The 510(k) notifica-

---

[3] As of 2006, Class I, II, and III devices accounted for approximately 43, 45, and 13 percent of classified devices, respectively (Tillman as cited in IOM, 2006, p. 76).

[4] This was the NeoGram Amino Acids and Acylcarnitine Tandem Mass Spectrometry Kit.

tion typically does not require clinical data unless the technology for a new device differs from that of the predicate device and clinical data are necessary to evaluate the potential impact of this difference on safe and effective performance. Clinical data are included in approximately 10 percent of 510(k) notifications (Tillman and Gardner, 2004; Rosecrans, 2010). Both a CDRH working group and an Institute of Medicine (IOM) committee (as requested by FDA) are evaluating aspects of the 510(k) process. The CDRH group issued its preliminary report in August 2010 (CDRH, 2010a).

For Class III devices, which account for a small proportion of all legally marketed medical devices, manufacturers must submit premarket approval (PMA) applications and provide data from clinical trials to demonstrate reasonable assurance that a device is safe and effective (what this report terms efficacy) for the intended use in the intended patient population. Examples of Class III devices include implanted devices such as the titanium rib, some diagnostic test kits, and certain surgical sealants. Securing FDA approval of such a device is usually complex, costly, and time-consuming, taking on the order of several years. The cost will vary depending on the complexity of the device and the kinds of nonclinical and clinical data that the sponsor must submit to demonstrate safety and efficacy.

This report focuses on complex devices intended specifically to treat complex rare conditions. Most will be Class III devices and thus will require formal authorization by FDA, usually through the PMA process or, in some cases, the 510(k) process.

For qualifying devices intended for a small population, approval can also come through the HDE process described below. The committee is not aware of any analysis that attempts to catalog devices that have been cleared under the 510(k) process or approved under a PMA specifically for the treatment of rare conditions defined according to the Orphan Drug Act (i.e., conditions affecting fewer than 200,000 individuals). It has found examples of such devices. For example, for the rare eye condition keratoconus, CDRH has cleared devices under the 510(k) process (K992466 and K024164) and also approved a different type of device for the condition under an HDE (H040002). At least one HDE-approved device, Bioglue, was subsequently approved for broader indications under a PMA (P010003).

For devices that are designated as "significant risk devices" because they have the potential to cause serious harm to research participants, manufacturers must secure an Investigational Device Exemption (IDE) before they can conduct clinical studies in humans with the devices.[5] Similar to the Investigational New Drug application, an IDE application must include

---

[5] "Nonsignificant-risk" device clinical trials require institutional review board approval and informed consent but not an approved IDE application (21CFR 812.2(a), 812.3(m)). They are subject to the "abbreviated IDE" requirements and are considered to have a "deemed approved" investigational device exemption (21 CFR 812.2(b)(1)).

data about preclinical studies and any available clinical information. It must also provide a description of the proposed research and analysis strategy. An IDE may prompt extensive discussions and negotiations between the manufacturer and FDA to arrive at agreement on a research plan that will provide data of acceptable quality to support FDA approval of the device. As described in one review of the process, the "first and arguably most important step in this process is the pre-IDE meeting, in which the company, often accompanied by the lead clinical investigator(s), meets with FDA/CDRH to present data about the device, its clinical development program, and its intended use after approval" (Kaplan et al., 2004, p. 3071).

As is the case for pharmaceuticals, FDA may approve medical devices with requirements for postmarketing studies, including clinical studies. For example, when CDRH approved a transcatheter pulmonary valve system under an HDE, it required two postapproval clinical studies (Tillman, 2010). CDRH now tracks the status of postapproval studies required after January 1, 2005, and posts tracking information on a public web page.

Diagnostic Devices, In Vitro Devices, and Genetic Tests

FDA regulates a range of diagnostic devices under the procedures described above. Diagnostic devices include such diverse items as blood pressure cuffs, vision evaluation instruments, cardiac monitors, and sophisticated imaging equipment. Based on their complexity, diagnostic devices are generally assigned to one of the three classes discussed above and regulated accordingly. CDRH has approved HDEs for three diagnostic testing devices.[6]

Diagnostic devices also include an array of products known as in vitro diagnostic devices, which "are those reagents, instruments, and systems intended for use in diagnosis of disease or other conditions" (21 CFR 809.3(a)). FDA regulates in vitro diagnostic devices that are developed and sold by device manufacturers as test kits. In vitro diagnostic devices include genetic and other tests that are important in diagnosing many rare diseases.[7]

---

[6] These are the Fujirebio Mesomark Assay (H060004, approved in 2007), the Heartsbreath test (H030004, approved in 2004), and the TAS Ecarin Clotting Time Test (H990012, approved in 2000).

[7] FDA recognizes two categories of in vitro devices that are in research stages. "Research use only" products are devices that are used only in the preclinical "laboratory research phase of development, that is, either basic research or the initial search for potential clinical utility" (CDRH-CBER, 2007, p. 12). Such a device may not be used for human clinical diagnostic or prognostic use, and the labeling must state: "For research use only. Not for use in diagnostic procedures" (21 CFR 809.10(c)(2)(i)). "Investigational use only" devices are products that are in "the clinical investigation stage of development" but that may be exempt from IDE requirements (CDRH-CBER, 2007, pp. 12-13. These products must be labeled: "For Investigational Use Only. The performance characteristics of this product have not been established" (21 CFR 809.10(c)(2)(ii)). See also Gibbs (2010).

In addition to using in vitro diagnostic test kits to perform diagnostic testing, some clinical laboratories develop their own in-house assays, known as laboratory-developed tests. These laboratory-developed tests are currently regulated under the Clinical Laboratory Improvement Amendments of 1988 (CLIA) and state laws (Maloney, 2010). With rare exceptions, laboratory-developed tests usually are not regulated by FDA.[8] Recently, however, FDA announced its intention to regulate all laboratory-developed tests as medical devices, as discussed below.

FDA regulations do, however, require that a clinical laboratory that develops a test using an analyte-specific reagent must disclose its regulatory status and must add a statement on test reports that the test has not been cleared or approved by FDA (21 CFR 809.30(e)). Analyte-specific reagents (which include polyclonal and monoclonal antibodies, specific receptor proteins, nucleic acid sequences, and similar reagents) are the building blocks that clinical laboratories use to develop in-house assays. Also, although laboratory-developed tests themselves are not usually regulated by FDA, analyte-specific reagents are regulated as "restricted devices." Manufacturers cannot make any claim of clinical or diagnostic effectiveness for an analyte-specific reagent and can only describe what substance it will identify. If a manufacturer combines analyte-specific reagents into a kit, or otherwise offers them for sale together, then the product must be approved as a medical device.

Because most genetic tests are available only as laboratory-developed tests, they are not regulated by FDA (Huang and Javitt, 2008). In a report on the regulation of genetic tests prepared by the Secretary's Advisory Committee on Genetics, Health, and Society, the group identified shortcomings in several areas, including regulations governing clinical laboratory quality and "oversight of the clinical validity of genetic tests" (SACGHS, 2008, p. 191).

In the past several years, various groups have recommended that FDA should regulate either all genetic tests or all laboratory-developed tests under the medical device authorities (Mansfield and Tezak, 2010). In June 2010, CDRH announced a public meeting and requested comments on issues related to the regulation of laboratory-developed tests (75 Fed. Reg. 34463). Although the agency has indicated that it plans to regulate some of these tests as medical devices, the specifics and priorities have yet to be decided. In noting the challenges of encouraging innovation while assuring

---

[8] In draft guidance, CDRH identified one category of laboratory-developed tests, the in vitro diagnostic mulitvariate index assay, as subject to its regulation (CDRH-CBER, 2007). It stated that such "tests are developed based on observed correlations between multivariate data and clinical outcome, such that the clinical validity of the claims is not transparent to patients, laboratorians, and clinicians who order these tests" and "frequently have a high risk intended use" (p. 4). Included in this category are tests that integrate genetic and other information to predict a person's risk of developing a disease.

the safety and efficacy of laboratory-developed tests, the CDRH announcement specifically cited tests for rare conditions.

Another area of regulatory complexity is co-development of a drug and a companion diagnostic. An example is a diagnostic test kit to assess whether a breast cancer patient has a gene mutation that is targeted by the drug trastuzumab (Herceptin). FDA held up approval of the drug until an approved in vitro diagnostic could be substituted for the laboratory-developed test that was initially used in clinical trials. It approved both the drug and the diagnostic in 1998 (Madsen, 2004). After a 2005 concept paper on the topic generated considerable criticism (see, e.g., PMC, 2009), the FDA Commissioner indicated that a new draft guidance document would be published in 2010 and would reflect public comments and scientific and other developments (Hamburg, 2009; Ray, 2010). In the meantime, FDA has been applying a case-by-case approach to regulation of companion diagnostics (Carver, 2010).

Combination Products

Some medical products combine a medical device and a drug or biologic. Examples include the drug-eluting coronary stent (which adds a drug coating to a metal stent in order to reduce the risk of reocclusion of the coronary artery) and the fentanyl patch (which delivers the drug through the skin). Combinations can take several different forms. For a product such as the drug-eluting stent, the device and drug components are truly combined into a single entity. Two items that are physically distinct but packaged together also qualify as a combination product. The category can also cover a product such as a drug that is packaged separately but is labeled as being for use only with a specific device or type of device (such as a specific diagnostic test).[9]

At least one combination product has been approved by CDRH through the HDE process (OP-1 Putty under H020008).[10] As discussed below, the

---

[9] The Office of Combination Products, which was created in 2002, assigns primary responsibility for regulating combination products to the most appropriate unit of FDA. As a general rule, that assignment is based on the primary mode of action of a combination product. Thus, a drug-eluting stent is intended primarily to open a blood vessel, with the drug activity secondary, so regulation would be assigned to CDRH. In contrast, the Center for Drug Evaluation and Research (CDER) would take the regulatory lead for a drug-eluting disk that is intended to deliver chemotherapy agents for brain tumors. For some combinations, the lead might go to the Center for Biologics Evaluation and Research.

[10] The product is approved under the HDE only for use in the posterolateral (intertransverse) lumbar spine in a limited patient population. It is made from mixture of a genetically engineered human protein powder, bovine collagen, saline solution, and a thickening agent to form a putty-like material that is applied to each side of the spine section that is to be fused. In 2008, FDA notified health care practitioners of reports of life-threatening complications associated with one of these elements, recombinant human bone morphogenetic protein (rhBMP)

different incentives for the development of orphan drugs and for the development of devices for small populations theoretically could complicate collaboration on combination products for small populations.

Alternate Approval Route for Medical Devices for Small Populations

As is true for companies that manufacture drugs and biologics, device companies naturally seek business opportunities in markets of sufficient size and profitability to warrant the investment risk. Particularly if FDA requires extensive clinical data for approval of the device, companies may be discouraged from pursuing devices for small markets by the expense and practical challenges of conducting acceptable trials to demonstrate safety and effectiveness.

The Safe Medical Devices Act of 1990 authorized the Humanitarian Device Exemption to encourage the development and introduction of complex device technologies to meet the needs of small patient populations. Although neither the text nor the title of the 1990 law uses the term "rare disease" or "orphan product," the purpose is broadly similar to the purpose of the Orphan Drug Act. The specifics vary in part because the details of device regulation differ and in part because the incentives (particularly market exclusivity) that were viewed as important for drug manufacturers were viewed as less meaningful for device manufacturers.

An HDE application is the same as a PMA application except that it need not include evidence of effectiveness, a characteristic that also distinguishes the requirements for an HDE from the requirements for FDA approval of an orphan drug. The HDE application must, however, "contain sufficient information for FDA to determine that the device does not pose an unreasonable or significant risk of illness or injury, and that the probable benefit to health outweighs the risk of injury or illness from its use" (CDRH, 2009, unpaged).

To be eligible for an HDE, a manufacturer must first request that the device be designated by the OOPD as a Humanitarian Use Device (HUD). A HUD is a "medical device intended to benefit patients in the treatment or diagnosis of a disease or condition that affects or is manifested in fewer than 4,000 individuals in the United States per year" (21 CFR 814.102(a)(5)). (If a device is for diagnostic purposes, the documentation in an HDE application must demonstrate that fewer than 4,000 patients per year would be subjected to diagnosis by the device in the United States.) The statutory language has caused some confusion about whether it refers to incidence or

---

when used in the cervical spine (Schultz, 2008). The manufacturer was indicted in 2009 on charges of illegal promotion of the product for unapproved uses (DOJ, 2009).

prevalence, but FDA provided the following interpretation in the preamble to the HDE regulations issued in June 1996 (61 Fed. Reg. at 33233):

> The agency believes that defining the criteria on a per year basis is consistent with the intent of section 520(m) of the act . . . , whereas a point prevalence definition would be considerably more restrictive and provide less of an incentive for the development of such devices. In response to comments, FDA also has added "or is manifested" to the definition of a HUD in order to establish that HUD designation may be appropriate in cases where more than 4,000 people have the disease but fewer than 4,000 manifest the condition.

CDRH now interprets the 4,000-individual restriction to allow a company to ship up to 4,000 devices a year (or a higher number if the data show that patients need more than one device within a year). The shipment limit means that substantially expanded use of a device either within the approved indication or off-label is controlled in a way that does not apply for orphan drugs. Sponsors must report data to CDRH on a periodic basis to support the continued appropriateness of the HUD designation. The agency may ask companies to withdraw an HDE if evidence indicates that the population criterion is no longer met. (In contrast, a designated orphan drug may be approved with exclusivity even if the affected population has, during the time between designation and approval, exceeded 200,000.)

CDRH will not approve an HDE if a comparable device has been cleared or approved for the same indication through either the 510(k) notification process or the PMA approval process under the procedures described in the preceding section.[11] It will, however, consider an HDE application if a comparable device has been approved under another HDE or if a comparable device is being studied under an IDE (CDRH, 2009).

Comparison of HDE and Orphan Drug Incentives

Table 7-2 summarizes several ways in which the provisions for HDEs differ from the incentives for the development of orphan drugs. In contrast to the orphan drug policy, the HDE policy has no provisions for market exclusivity. This difference reflects the process of ongoing device refinement described earlier and the less significant role of patent or patent-like protection in the medical device industry. Also in contrast to orphan drugs, Con-

---

[11] FDA guidance states that a comparable device need not be identical to a device that is the subject of an HDE application. "In determining whether a comparable device exists, FDA will consider: the device's intended use and technological characteristics; the patient population to be treated or diagnosed with the device; [and] whether the device meets the needs of the identified patient population" (CDRH-CBER, 2010, p. 4).

TABLE 7-2 Incentive Comparison: Drugs or Biologics Versus Devices

Incentive	Orphan Drug or Biologic	Humanitarian Use Device
Product development assistance	Tax credit for qualified clinical testing expenses	
	FDA orphan products grants	FDA orphan products grants
Market exclusivity	7 years	No equivalent
Pricing discretion	Sponsor sets selling price	Limited to cost recovery Profits allowed for products for pediatric populations up to a specified annual limit
Requirement for demonstration of safety or effectiveness (efficacy)	Clinical evidence of safety and effectiveness (efficacy) similar to nonorphan products	Evidence of safety and data showing that probable benefit exceeds risk
Population size constraint	Fewer than 200,000 people with the condition in the U.S.	Fewer than 4,000 people per year in the U.S. (i.e., 4,000 devices shipped per year, unless a patient uses more than one device a year)
Waiver of fees	NDA submission fees waived for sponsors of orphan drugs	Submission fees waived for sponsors of HDEs
Other		An HDE cannot be granted if a comparable device for the same intended use is available under usual approval procedures. More than one HDE can exist for same intended use

gress did not authorize tax credits for clinical research for an HDE, which perhaps reflects the lack of a requirement for clinical evidence of efficacy.

For device manufacturers, the lack of a requirement for clinical evidence of a device's effectiveness (efficacy) can be viewed as an incentive because clinical trials to support effectiveness claims are expensive and can take years to complete. In general, the costs of clinical trials that are usually needed to support a PMA make small markets unattractive or infeasible, particularly for start-ups and small device companies.

Another HDE incentive (and one that parallels that for orphan drugs) is the waiver of the filing fees normally required under the Medical Device User Fee Act (more than $200,000 per PMA application for FY 2010). In addition, the time period specified for regulatory review of an application is shorter for HDEs (including the time for the HUD designation step) than for regular premarket approval applications.

Like developers of orphan drugs, developers of devices are also eligible for orphan products grants. Seven devices for which grants were awarded have subsequently been approved, five through the HDE process and two through the PMA process (Linda C. Ulrich, M.D., Medical Officer, FDA Office of Orphan Product Development, April 26, 2010, personal communication).

At the same time that the HDE route to approval has some advantages compared to the PMA process, it also comes with a critical restriction in addition to the 4,000-unit limit per year. Specifically, sponsors are not permitted to make a profit on the sale of the HUD if the device is sold for more than $250. They can recover certain costs, for example, those related to research and development, manufacturing, and distribution.[12] The sponsor must provide supporting financial documentation to FDA about the price it proposes to charge. Another complication is that even though the sponsor can charge for the device, the HDE device might not be purchased for use in clinical practice—usually within a hospital—if adequate third-party reimbursement is not available to cover an institution's cost to purchase, as discussed in a later section of this chapter.

One unique feature of the HDE policy is the requirement that use of an HDE device requires approval by an institutional review board (IRB) at the institution where the device is to be used. A clinician can usually request IRB approval in advance for several patients so that emergency procedures do not need to be invoked.

The primary responsibility of IRBs is to protect human research participants through review of proposed research. Their role in approving the use of an HDE device is an anomaly and a potential source of confusion because the purpose in question is not research on the device but use of the device in clinical care. The task of securing IRB approval is often a difficult, costly, and sequential (institution-by-institution) task for the HDE sponsor. In addition, marketing of the device to individual centers (which must seek IRB approval) may be more difficult in the absence of the usual FDA premarket approval. The requirement for IRB approval thus is potentially another factor that may discourage companies from developing products for small markets under HDE procedures.

---

[12] This can make an HDE device costly to a purchaser, even if it does not lead to profits for the company. For example, the CEO of Abiomed indicated that the company expected to charge $250,000 for each unit of its HDE-approved AbioCor implantable replacement heart for end-stage heart disease. He also is quoted as indicating that the price for the unit did not cover additional charges associated with training, associated technologies, and diagnostic and clinical support (Zacks, 2008).

The requirement for IRB approval and monitoring also creates complexities for IRBs. IRBs are charged with the review of research involving human subjects, but an HDE application does not relate to the conduct of research. An HDE holder may, however, conduct research on the device without an IDE if the study involves the approved indications, but IRB approval is still required. This aspect of HDE policy may add to confusion for IRBs and sponsors. A survey of IRB chairs in 2008 (with an 18 percent response rate) found that half reported an HDE review within the preceding 5 years and that many were confused about the process (Gordon, 2008).

In 2008, FDA issued draft guidance for HDE holders, IRBs, clinical investigators, and FDA staff in the form of questions and answers. In 2010, it issued a final guidance document (CDRH-CBER, 2010). Although this guidance is helpful, the process and the guidance are still confusing for device companies and IRBs. For example, the guidance states that the local IRB can defer to another IRB but does not explain whether it transfers all of its obligations to the other IRB (including continuing review) or just the initial review. It would have been useful if the guidance had included a sample letter for such a deferral. To cite another shortcoming of the guidance, it states that IRBs will receive reports of adverse events from the FDA Medical Device Reporting system, but it does not explain what IRBs should do with the information.

As noted above, the different incentives for orphan drugs and HDE devices could potentially create difficulties for an innovative combination product in some situations. If the testing of safety and effectiveness for an innovative drug required simultaneous use of the innovative device, that clinical testing should provide evidence to support both approval of the drug and clearance or approval of the device. For example, one company is simultaneously testing an intrathecal drug delivery device with a drug for Hunter syndrome; if testing shows safety and efficacy, the results should support regular FDA clearance or approval of the device (see description at http://clinicaltrials.gov/ct2/show/NCT00920647). (An intravenous formulation of the drug has orphan drug approval.)

If, however, a device were to be developed separately, for example, as an improved method to deliver an already approved orphan drug, it is possible that the different incentives for drugs and devices for small populations could be mismatched in a way that could discourage device companies from collaborating with drug companies on this type of combination product. (This issue could also arise as the development and regulation of companion diagnostic tests evolves, for example, when the companion diagnostic to predict patient responsiveness to a drug for a rare condition is not tested as part of the clinical trial of the drug itself [Swanson, 2009].) The committee did not find information on combination products that were discouraged or impeded because of the differences between the incentives for orphan drug development and the HDE incentives, but it is theoretically possible and may require FDA response in the future.

HDE Approvals

The regulations implementing the HDE process were issued in June 1996 and became effective in October 1996. Between 1996 and the end of 2009, the OOPD received 232 requests for a HUD designation and granted 146 of these (Lewis, 2010). The first HDE was approved in February 1997. As of April 2010, CDRH had approved 50 therapeutic and diagnostic devices through the HDE process. Three HDEs have been withdrawn by the sponsors after FDA indicated that the patient population served by the device had grown to exceed the limits for HDE devices.[13] Approximately two-thirds of HDE devices are implants, and HDEs have been most commonly approved for vascular, cardiac, neurological, and pediatric indications (Bernad, 2009).

Some HDEs are approved for use with patients who have a rare disease as such. For example, the titanium rib is approved for use with Jeune's syndrome or other rare rib cage conditions. Mostly, however, HDE approvals have cited indications that involve a very severely ill subgroup of a larger patient population or a subgroup that has not benefited from usual therapy. (Orphan drug designations and approvals may likewise specify medically relevant subgroups.) This is illustrated in Box 7-1.

Incentives for the Development of Pediatric Medical Devices

Because children are generally a healthy population, companies often do not find it commercially feasible or attractive to develop devices specific to pediatric diseases or to develop smaller versions of adult devices for relatively small numbers of children who might benefit from them.[14] For devices with indications for pediatric use, Congress acted in 2007 to modify

---

[13] For example, in 2006, FDA contacted the manufacturer of a device that had received HDE approval in 2000 for use in closure of a patent foramen ovale (PFO) in patients with recurrent stroke about changes in the patient population. The company subsequently withdrew the approval application, stating that "the subset of patients who once qualified for consideration for PFO closure has increased beyond 4,000, the limit normally allowed under the HDE indication" (Entrepreneur, 2006). The device has regular premarket approval application for use with ventricular septal defects (P000049).

[14] According to testimony presented to an earlier IOM panel on medical devices for pediatric patients, size reduction of devices available for adults is not always possible (IOM, 2006). For instance, although it is possible to reduce on the "bench" the physical size of prosthetic mechanical heart valves routinely used with adults, fluid flow and pressure change once orifices are reduced below certain diameters. Current designs of mechanical valves also do not accommodate the natural growth of a small child's heart.

BOX 7-1
Examples of Devices Approved Under the
Humanitarian Device Exemption

The Spiration IBV is indicated to control prolonged air leaks of the lung, or signifi-cant air leaks that are likely to become prolonged air leaks, following lobectomy, segmentectomy, or lung volume reduction surgery. An air leak present on postop-erative day 7 is considered prolonged unless present only during forced exhalation or cough. An air leak present on day 5 should be considered for treatment if it is (1) continuous, (2) present during normal inhalation phase of inspiration, or (3) present upon normal expiration and accompanied by subcutaneous emphysema or respiratory compromise. Approved October 24, 2008 (H060002).

TAS Ecarin Clotting Time Test is used to determine the anticoagulant effect of re-combinant hirudin (r-hirudin) during cardiopulmonary bypass in patients who have heparin-induced thrombocytopenia. Approved May 11, 2000 (H990012).

Epicel (cultured epidermal autografts) is for use with patients who have deep dermal or full-thickness burns comprising a total body surface area of greater than or equal to 30 percent. It may be used in conjunction with split-thickness autografts or alone in patients for whom split-thickness autografts may not be an option due to the severity and extent of their burns. Approved October 25, 2007 (H990002).

DeBakey VAD Child Left Ventricular Assist System is to provide temporary left-side mechanical circulatory support as a bridge to cardiac transplantation for pediatric patients (5-16 years old, with BSA $\geq$ 0.7 m^2 and <1.5 m^2) who are in NYHA Class IV end-stage heart failure, are refractory to medical therapy, and are (listed) candidates for cardiac transplantation. Approved February 25, 2004 (H030003).

Abiocor Implantable Replacement Heart is indicated for use in severe biventricu-lar end-stage heart disease patients who are not cardiac transplant candidates and who are less than 75 years old, require multiple inotropic support, are not treatable by left ventricular assist device (LVAD) destination therapy, and are not weanable from biventricular support if on such support. Approved September 5, 2006 (H040006).

Activa Dystonia Therapy is for unilateral or bilateral stimulation of the internal globus pallidus (GPi) or the subthalamic nucleus (STN) to aid in the management of chronic, intractable (drug-refractory) primary dystonia, including generalized and/or segmental dystonia, hemidystonia, and cervical dystonia (torticollis) in patients 7 years of age or older. Approved April 15, 2003 (H020007).

SOURCE: FDA listing of CDRH Humanitarian Device Exemptions. HDE approval numbers are in parentheses.

the incentives associated with an HDE approval (P.L. 110-85). Notably, it removed the general restriction on profits. It also directed the Government Accountability Office (GAO) to assess by 2012 the effects of removing that restriction.

The law requires FDA to specify an annual distribution limit on the number of devices that can be sold at a profit (up to a maximum of 4,000). As described in draft agency guidance, the Pediatric Medical Device Safety and Improvement Act of 2007, this number "is determined by estimating the number of individuals (pediatric and adult patients) affected by the disease or condition and likely to use the device each year multiplied by the number of devices reasonably necessary to treat each individual. If the number calculated is less than or equal to 4,000, then this number is the ADN [annual distribution number]. If the number calculated is more than 4,000, then the ADN is 4,000 because in no case can the ADN exceed 4,000 devices. See section 520(m)(6)(A)(ii) of the Act."

As of January 2010, CDRH has approved one HDE under the pediatric provisions. In the approval order for the Medtronic Melody transcatheter pulmonary valve (H080002), CDRH specified an annual distribution number of 2,996, which includes use with both children and adults,. The order includes no explanation of the number, but on its website, Medtronic, the device manufacturer, states that approximately 34,000 children are born each year with congenital heart disease, of which 20 percent are born with a malformation affecting blood flow between the heart and lungs (Medtronic, 2010). A subset of these infants will have a prosthetic conduit surgically implanted, and some of these devices will malfunction, which will require new surgery. The device is intended to extend the life of the malfunctioning conduit without open heart surgery.

Congress also created a grants program to promote the development of pediatric medical devices. OOPD announced the first awards to three pediatric device consortia in 2009 (OOPD, 2009). Box 7-2 describes the expectations for these consortia. One provision, which is similar to a recommendation in this report, specifies that consortia coordinate with companies and FDA to take approval or clearance processes and requirements into account.

Custom Devices

Perhaps the ultimate in devices for small populations is the custom device, which is not subject to 510(k) or PMA requirements. As described by a former FDA Commissioner, a custom medical device is an "example of individualized therapy . . . that is requested of the device manufacturer by a physician for a specific patient. A custom device is a one-of-a-kind device designed for an immediate need and for which the need is not likely

---

BOX 7-2
Expectations for Consortia to Stimulate
Pediatric Device Development

A consortium receiving a grant or contract under Section 305 will facilitate the *development, production, and distribution* of medical devices by

• Encouraging innovation and connecting qualified individuals with pediatric device ideas with potential manufacturers.
• Mentoring and managing device projects through the development process.
• Connecting innovators and physicians to existing Federal and non-Federal Resources.
• Assessing the scientific and medical merit of proposed pediatric device projects.
• Providing assistance as needed on business development, personnel training, prototype development, post-market needs and other activities.

Each consortium will coordinate with the FDA Commissioner and device companies to facilitate applications for approval or clearance of devices labeled for pediatric use. Each consortium will coordinate with the NIH [National Institutes of Health].

SOURCE: From Pediatric Medical Device Safety and Improvement Act of 2007 (P.L. 110-85, section 305).

---

to reoccur. In essence, a physician and a manufacturer collaborate to design a device for a specific circumstance. For such devices, it would be virtually impossible to conduct a clinical trial, and—assuming the device does meet all the criteria defining it as a custom device—the device would be exempt from premarket approval" (Henney, 2000).

FDA regulations specify several criteria that custom devices must meet. These include that the device (1) necessarily deviates from generally available devices or from a PMA requirement in order to comply with the order of an individual physician; (2) is not generally available to other physicians; (3) is not generally available in finished form for purchase or dispensing; and (4) is not offered for commercial distribution through labeling or advertising (21 CFR 812.3(b)). The agency has narrowly interpreted the custom device exemption and has brought enforcement actions against certain manufacturers who have sought to rely upon it.[15]

---

[15] Early in the development of the titanium rib device, FDA approved several uses based on the custom device provisions (Campbell, 2007). It also advised the physician developer on a sole-site feasibility study that eventually expanded to the multisite study that supported the HDE approval in 2004.

Although the committee did not examine the approval and use of custom devices or investigate possible concerns about these devices, the question arose whether a change in the custom device exemption might assist patients with rare conditions. Specifically, could protections for patients still be maintained if FDA were permitted to authorize the approval of a specific custom device for a very small group of patients (e.g., 5 or 10) who had the same rare problem? If the assessment of unmet needs recommended at the end of this chapter includes needs for custom devices, the assessment could help in determining whether allowing slightly broader approval of custom devices could benefit patients with very rare conditions.

COVERAGE AND REIMBURSEMENT FOR HDE MEDICAL DEVICES

Despite the restriction on profits for devices that have been approved through the HDE process, manufacturers may still set substantial prices for such devices based on the costs that they may legally recover under the law. Thus, in considering whether to pursue development of a device that would fit HDE requirements, manufacturers will also consider whether public and private health plans are likely to cover the device and what they might pay.

Most of the devices that have HDE approval are complex devices that are implanted or otherwise applied in an inpatient hospital setting.[16] For care under Medicare, this means that coverage and payment for a device will be subject to the provisions of the Part A program. As described in Chapter 6, Medicare pays hospitals a bundled or per-case payment for institutional services provided in the course of treatment for a particular diagnosis with payment varying depending on the severity of the diagnosis and other factors. For medical device manufacturers, the key relevant feature of the payment method is that the diagnosis-related group (DRG) payment to a hospital will not necessarily be adjusted to reflect any higher costs should a newly approved HDE or other device be used with a particular patient.

To recognize the added costs of desirable new technologies, Medicare can authorize a temporary "add-on" payment to a DRG if three conditions are met. The technology must be new (generally meaning that it was approved by FDA within the preceding 2 to 3 years); it must not be adequately covered by the existing DRG payment; and it must offer a substantial clinical benefit over existing options. This last requirement may be difficult for manufacturers of HDE devices because approval of the device does not require clinical evidence of effectiveness. Absent the availability of an add-on payment for new-technology HDE devices, a hospital might not make

---

[16] The committee did not investigate potential reimbursement for HDEs used in other settings. A few HDE devices might be used in an outpatient setting (e.g., Intacs, a prescription device approved for treatment of keratoconus, an eye condition).

the device available for use if the device was substantially more expensive than existing technology. (Use of an HDE device still requires IRB approval as described above.)

Moreover, by statute, Medicare generally limits payment to items or services that are "reasonable and necessary" for the diagnosis and treatment of illness or injury or to improve the functioning of a malformed body member" (42 USC 1395y). This has generally been interpreted to mean that a service or item must be safe and effective, medically necessary and appropriate, and not experimental in order to qualify for reimbursement.

The Centers for Medicare and Medicaid Services (CMS) have approved add-on payments for some devices that have HDE approval. One is the artificial implantable heart described earlier (AbioMed, 2005). Another is the device for treatment of pulmonary air leaks mentioned in Box 7-1 (Spiration, 2009). Overall, of the seven applications for add-on payments approved between 2001 and 2008, six were for products classified as medical devices (Clyde et al., 2008).

As this report was being completed, CMS and FDA announced a memorandum of understanding to share information and expertise related to the review and use of FDA-regulated devices and other products (75 Fed. Reg. 48699). The agencies are also considering a process of parallel review that would reduce the lag between FDA marketing authorization decisions and CMS national coverage determinations (75 Fed. Reg. 57045).

The committee did not examine the coverage and reimbursement policies of state Medicaid programs or private health plans, but it did find illustrative examples of variation in health plan policies. Some private health plans have authorized coverage for specific uses of an HDE and rejected it for others. For example, Aetna will cover certain uses of total artificial heart devices and left ventricular assist devices, but it considers other uses experimental and investigational (Aetna, 2010). At least one health plan has posted a general policy on coverage that states Humanitarian Use Devices are subject to individual review and prior approval (Wellmark Blue Cross Blue Shield, 2009).

MEDICAL DEVICE RESEARCH AND DEVELOPMENT

In order to lay the foundation for the committee's recommendations for encouraging the development of medical devices for rare diseases, it is useful to review briefly some features of medical device innovation and development. For example, breakthrough implantable devices were made possible, in part, by scientific and engineering advances in areas outside biomedicine. Creative device ideas have often originated with physicians in the clinic who are trying to address specific problems they encounter or to help a specific patient with the tools at hand. The life cycle of devices includes iterative improvements over time, often involving collaborations between engineering and other disciplines.

Emergence of Complex Medical Devices

I cannot believe that six whole months have soared by since I was given a new lease on life. A tiny device called an ICD [implantable cardioverter defibrillator] was surgically implanted beneath a patch of muscle tissue in my chest . . . and now I have a small metal box in my chest that I affectionately refer to as the iFib . . . [which] is both a pacemaker and defibrillator all boxed up in a compact little package. It is about the same size as an iPod Nano, but it can't play music. All it does is guard against sudden death. Let's see an iPod do that!

Sands, 2010

This man, who has lived for decades with muscular dystrophy, has been assisted by a variety of medical devices. As is the case with many devices used for patients with rare conditions, none were devised specifically for patients with muscular dystrophy but all have helped him survive. The most sophisticated of his devices, the implantable cardioverter defibrillator (ICD), is used with patients who have a number of different conditions that put them at risk of sudden cardiac death. Its development and subsequent refinement were made possible by a number of scientific and engineering advances.

Although medical devices have a long history in the form of basic surgical instruments, braces, medical thermometers, and similar relatively simple objects, the development of technologically sophisticated, complex devices advanced significantly in the 1950s and early 1960s, based in part on technological innovations in other arenas. Notably, the transistor, invented in 1947 at Bell Labs, provided the foundation for solid-state electronics, which in turn made possible the miniaturization of electronic devices and improved capabilities. In 1957, surgeons used the world's first transistorized therapeutic medical device, the external cardiac pacemaker, to maintain an appropriate heart rate and adequate cardiac output following open-heart surgery on a young boy (MMF, 2007).

Other innovation within and outside the medical device industry—led to the availability of durable and biologically compatible materials for use in orthopedic, neurological, cardiac, and other implants. Advances in mechanical valve materials and designs and newly available heart-lung machines made replacement heart valves feasible in the 1960s.

Innovation Process for Complex Medical Devices

Although moving from idea to marketing typically takes many years for both drugs and complex medical devices, the nature of medical device innovation and product development and the underlying technical expertise differ in some significant ways for devices. In simple terms, the innovation pathway for drugs is a laboratory-based discovery process that is led by biomedical scientists, chemists, and pharmacologists. Clinicians assume a primary role toward the end of the process, that is, when drugs undergo clinical testing in humans, which regulations require for all drugs. In contrast, device innovation and development has been primarily an engineering process that combines technical expertise from multiple disciplines. Clinicians may be involved from the outset and may continue to be involved in ongoing refinement once a device is authorized for marketing.

As is true for engineered products generally, the process of device development is iterative and circular. Figure 7-1 depicts the device development life cycle for more complex devices as beginning with a basic concept to address an unmet need, followed by initial prototype development and test-

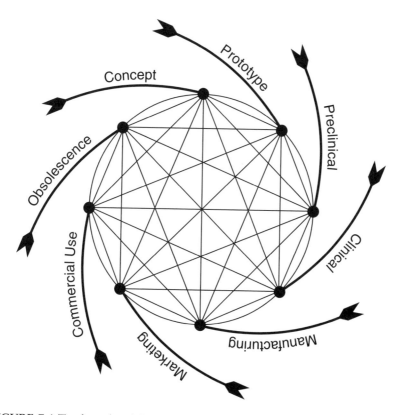

FIGURE 7-1 Total product life cycle for medical devices.
SOURCE: Feigal, 2002.

ing.[17] This latter phase includes consultation with FDA about the evaluative methods and information needed to support FDA decisions to authorize the marketing of the device. After marketing authorization, modifications to the device typically continue for a variety of reasons, sometimes as design enhancements or sometimes in response to safety issues discovered once the device is on the market.

Figure 7-1 draws attention to a key aspect of medical devices, specifically, an "end-of-life" phase. In some cases, a device is supplanted by a radically different product that effectively makes obsolete, or reduces reliance on, the current product. For example, the development of implanted cardiac devices made obsolete the early external devices that often tethered individuals to power sources. In other cases, a device product is altered to make it smaller, safer, more effective, more convenient, or otherwise different in ways that make the older versions less desirable or less cost-effective. In contrast, small-molecule drugs may stay on the market unaltered for decades (except perhaps for additional formulations or methods of administration, e.g., a pill, a time-release capsule, or a liquid).

In addition, in contrast to pharmaceutical development, the process of developing a medical device often is not based on scientific discovery per se. Rather, the process involves the use of existing technological building blocks that are assembled into a "device" that satisfies certain desired performance characteristics related to a clinical need. If an initial approach proves unsatisfactory or clearly has features that can be improved, engineers may create a new design, reconfigure the existing design components, or even invent a new component, for example, one using a novel biomaterial that delivers the performance desired. The titanium rib illustrates a new conceptualization by a physician who had an engineering background. In some cases, an insurmountable performance roadblock is encountered and further development of the device is suspended.

Another distinguishing aspect of device development involves the roles played by clinicians in the innovation process for the most complex and technologically sophisticated therapeutic devices (Citron, 2008). In addition to identifying unmet needs, physicians are sometimes inventors who see the "flash of light" of a new idea and who even take an active role in pursuing it, as did the physician inventor of the titanium rib. Likewise, a clinician

---

[17] Development of in vitro diagnostic devices and tests reflects a more varied approach to innovation. Such devices and tests can be developed based on research by academic medical centers (e.g., many genetic tests), or they may be developed based on needs identified by the clinical laboratories that produce laboratory-developed tests. Public health threats inspired the development of testing for the HIV/AIDS virus and the H1N1 virus, whereas clinical needs are stimulating the development of tests to identify patients likely to respond to particular drugs, for example, as illustrated by tests to determine whether women with breast cancer are likely to respond to the drug trastuzumab.

conceived the fundamental idea for the ICD (Cannom and Prystowsky, 2004).

At other times, physicians provide vital clinical insight regarding the suitability of a proposed technology for their patients, and they also may propose improvements and enhancements for new or developing products. For devices such as the titanium rib or the cardiac pacemaker, they devise surgical techniques necessary for safe implantation. Clinicians also participate in clinical trials to support regulatory submissions, and based on research and clinical practice, they may identify clinical and technical problems and suggest refinements to improve performance. Clinicians involved in product development and testing may also teach their colleagues how to use a new technology correctly. In short, expert physicians are often an integral part of the research and development continuum, not just customers for the end product.

This involvement may add to the challenges of identifying and managing conflicts of interest, particularly if clinicians have an equity interest or other financial stake in the product. Likewise, when clinicians who consult with companies on product refinements also have a role in the choice of implants or other devices used during orthopedic and other surgeries, the potential for the financial interest to bias judgments is a concern. The identification of physician relationships with industry[18] and the management of conflicts of interest[19] have drawn increasing attention in recent years.

The development of deep-brain stimulation provides an example of academic inspiration in the device industry. French professors discovered that they could reduce the effects of movement disorders through neurostimulation using an existing device for an off-label (not FDA approved) indication (Linehan et al., 2007). Although Medtronic, the manufacturer of the device, was not involved in or even initially aware of the early results, later collaboration between the researchers and the company provided a starting point for work that led to FDA approval of the modified device for new uses. The company also learned, largely through the initial investigations of other neurosurgeons, that the device could treat additional neurological

---

[18] Reflecting concerns about inadequate disclosure of such financial relationships, a section in the Patient Protection and Affordable Care Act of 2010 (P.L. 111-148, §602) requires medical product companies to report gifts, consulting fees, research funding, and payments to physicians and teaching hospitals.

[19] Among other recommendations, a recent IOM report recommended that policies of research institutions generally should provide that individuals may not conduct research with human participants involving a product in which they have a significant financial interest (IOM, 2009b). The recommendation provided for an exception for researchers whose participation is essential for the conduct of the research if an effective process for managing the conflict is in place to protect the integrity of the research. As an example of an exceptional situation, the report cited the participation in a pilot study by the surgeon inventor of an implant that requires a complex surgical procedure that has not been mastered by other surgeons.

disorders. Deep-brain stimulators were eventually approved by FDA for several new indications, each involving relatively minor technical changes to the device. The implant received PMA approval for essential tremor in 1997 and advanced Parkinson disease in 2002 and then was granted HDE approval for dystonia in 2003 and chronic, severe, treatment-resistant obsessive compulsive disorder in 2009.

University researchers have been actively involved in developing the technologies used in the genetic and drug discovery research described in earlier chapters. The American Institute for Medical and Biological Engineering cites the development of genomic sequencing and microarrays in its "hall of fame" (AIMBE, 2005). The bioengineering program at Stanford University, summarized in Box 7-3, offers one example of the intersection of device engineering and scientific advances in biological sciences.

Although some technological advances in medical devices have taken advantage of government-supported research and development, direct government investment in accelerating medical device research and development was initially limited. One exception is the total artificial heart

---

BOX 7-3
Stanford University Biodesign Program

About 10 years ago, faculty at Stanford University developed a systematic approach to solving significant medical problems in which invention and innovation were a team activity and were part of a process. The impetus for this initiative, the Stanford Biodesign Program, was the realization that innovations in the medical area involved many technical and scientific disciplines and these disciplines need to collaborate and inform each other.

Biodesign is associated with Stanford's Bio-X program, which promotes interdisciplinary research in biology and medicine. As described on that program's website, "Ideas and methods embodied in engineering, computer science, physics, chemistry, and other fields are being brought to bear upon important challenges in bioscience. In turn, bioscience creates new opportunities in other fields. Significant discoveries and creative inventions are accelerated through formation of new collaborative teams" (http://biox.stanford.edu/about/index.html).

The Biodesign Program creates multidisciplinary collaborative teams composed of graduate students from engineering, medicine, and business. These teams follow a three-stage process or method to create cost-effective, state-of-the-art medical devices for the benefit of patients, industry, and society. The method includes three stages: need identification; concept development; and business or project planning. The program has been emulated both domestically and internationally. Stanford faculty have published a textbook *Biodesign* (Zenios et al., 2010) that describes the process.

program at the National Heart, Lung, and Blood Institute (NHLBI), which began in 1964 (IOM, 1991). Although the program's focus shifted to ventricular assist devices (which have a larger target population than the artificial heart per se), the initial investments provided important knowledge for the development of less ambitious but clinically relevant cardiac support systems. The report of an expert panel convened by NHLBI noted that it "is not probable that development of assist devices would have occurred without the government support that is now being increasingly assumed by industry as clinically effective devices move towards marketing approval" (NHLBI, 2000, p. 3).

During the 1970s, the engineering community sought to increase the visibility of biomedical engineering and to educate the National Institutes of Health (NIH) about the nature and value of research in bioengineering and bioimaging (Hendee et al., 2002). In 2000, after a number of unsuccessful proposals in the 1990s, Congress created the National Institute of Biomedical Imaging and Bioengineering (NIBIB, 2009). NIBIB seeks to advance basic research and improve patient care by integrating the physical and engineering sciences with the life sciences. Relevant disciplines extend beyond biological sciences and various engineering disciplines to include (among others) the information sciences, physics, chemistry, mathematics, materials science, and computer science. The range of NIBIB interests covers, among other areas, biomaterials, bioinformatics, structural biology, drug and gene delivery systems and devices, tissue engineering, microbiomechanics, nanotechnology, sensors, surgical instruments, diverse kinds of imaging, and rehabilitation technology. Some areas of device innovations that illustrate the interaction between innovations in engineering and biological sciences are summarized in Box 7-4. In addition, the discussion in Chapter 4 of discovery research and diagnostic developments identifies other areas in which scientific and technological advances in biomedicine will likely shape innovation in diagnostic devices.

Clinical Studies for Medical Devices

As discussed earlier, FDA clears the majority of medical devices for marketing without requiring formal clinical studies. For a small proportion of devices—in particular, implanted devices or other high-risk devices—FDA requires data from clinical studies. For significant-risk devices, FDA requires formal approval of a request to begin clinical studies.

Under its regulations governing clinical studies to support PMAs, FDA states that the agency relies only on "valid scientific evidence to determine whether there is reasonable assurance that the device is safe and effective" (21 CFR 860.7(c)). The same document goes on to describe valid scientific evidence as

**BOX 7-4
Innovations in Engineering and Biological
Sciences and Medical Device Innovation**

Replacement organs: Using man-made scaffolds and other biomedical techniques, tissue engineering and regenerative medicine discoveries will permit scientists to "grow" organs in the laboratory to replace patients' failed organs. Tissue-engineered urinary bladders have already been implanted in patients. Proof-of-principle laboratory demonstration of a total beating heart (rat) has also been achieved. Such technologies have the potential to overcome the shortage of available donor transplants and to offer patients a biological tissue solution rather than an electromechanical therapy.

Drug delivery: Oral delivery of drugs has significant limitations, including patient compliance, first-pass inactivation by the liver, systemic rather than site-specific effects, and undesirable variability of blood levels between doses. Early generations of implanted drug delivery systems for chronic diseases or symptoms such as spasticity and intractable pain have demonstrated capabilities that address many of the limitations cited for oral delivery. Future generations are expected to provide sensor-based closed-loop operation, delivering drugs only when needed and at appropriate dosages. Delivery will be either site-specific, treating only affected tissue, or systemic. Of particular interest is the development of a fully implanted artificial pancreas that will deliver appropriate amounts of insulin in response to continuous monitoring of diabetic patient's blood glucose levels.

Implanted diagnostics: The concept of an implanted laboratory-on-a-chip has the possibility of revolutionizing how disease is diagnosed and preventing certain diseases or crisis episodes. Biosensors, as described for implanted insulin pumps above, serve as an example of how this might work. Implanted "chips" that contain an array of sensors will continually monitor a patient's condition and, if warranted, communicate to the patient's health care provider that attention is needed. Prototypic versions of rudimentary diagnostic systems have already demonstrated the ability to reduce serious events related to heart failure and also to reduce the number of visits to the emergency room.

Miniaturization: A collection of enabling technologies, some emerging from the field of nanotechnology, will expand possibilities of minimally invasive surgery, produce novel bio-interactive coatings, and reduce the size and expand the service life of implants, making them more suitable for pediatric patients.

SOURCES: AdvaMed, 2004; Braunschweig, 2007; El-Khatib et al., 2010; Trafton, 2010.

evidence from well-controlled investigations, partially controlled studies, studies and objective trials without matched controls, well-documented case histories conducted by qualified experts, and reports of significant human experience with a marketed device, from which it can fairly and responsibly be concluded by qualified experts that there is reasonable assurance of the safety and effectiveness of a device under its conditions of use. The evidence required may vary according to the characteristics of the device, its conditions of use, the existence and adequacy of warnings and other restrictions, and the extent of experience with its use. Isolated case reports, random experience, reports lacking sufficient details to permit scientific evaluation, and unsubstantiated opinions are not regarded as valid scientific evidence to show safety or effectiveness.

The requirements for evidence to support FDA approval of a PMA explicitly provide for more variability (linked to the particular characteristics and uses of a device) than is found in the corresponding expectations outlined in Chapter 3 for the approval of drugs. A recent study examined FDA summaries of the evidence used to support FDA approvals for 78 "high-risk cardiovascular devices" (Dhruva et al., 2009). The analysts reported that nearly two-thirds (65 percent) of the applications were approved based on a single study, that 27 percent of the 123 submitted studies were randomized, that 88 percent of the primary endpoints used were surrogate measures, that 52 percent of the endpoints were compared with controls, and that 31 percent of these controls were historical. Moreover, as described earlier, FDA does not require the same level of evidence for a device approved through an HDE as it does for those approved through a PMA.

For medical devices that require clinical evaluation, a pilot or feasibility study usually involves an initial clinical evaluation of the safety of a prototype device in individuals with the condition for which the device is designed. Such a study may suggest modifications to the prototype device to improve its performance. For a device that requires complex surgery for its implantation or that otherwise is technically demanding to use, the pilot phase may also provide an important period for learning about the process and skills required for the safe and effective clinical use of the device. Experience gained from pilot studies also contributes to the design of pivotal studies, which usually recruit larger numbers of research participants and may involve multiple study sites and centers. If surgical procedures are involved, the process may also require training of investigators at sites not involved in the pilot study.

As is also the case for orphan drugs, the accumulation of sufficient participants may take years for a device that is intended for a small population of patients. For example, clinical testing for the titanium rib (cited at the start of this chapter) occurred over 14 years, a long period that reflected in part the challenges of working with a rare condition and in part the request by FDA for long-term information on the device, which requires repeated adjustment as a child grows (Campbell, 2004).

In addition, many devices present special challenges for the design of clinical trials. Especially for surgically implanted devices, the classic randomized, double-blind comparative study is often not feasible or ethical. A few trials of surgical implant procedures have included sham surgeries for comparison in single-blind studies, but the surgical team obviously had to be aware of which procedure was used (see, e.g., Moseley et al., 2002). Such trials are controversial (see, e.g., Miller, 2003; Mehta et al., 2007). For some electronic devices such as cardiac or neurological stimulators, clinical studies have sometimes used a design that involves implantation of the device in a study population and then comparing a subset of the group in which the device is kept switched on with another subset in which it is switched off for a predetermined period of time (see, e.g., Greenberg et al., 2006).

Staff at CDRH are planning two projects that should provide a better understanding of issues in the design of clinical studies for devices (Linda C. Ulrich, M.D., Medical Officer, FDA Office of Orphan Product Development, April 26, 2010, personal communication). One project is an analysis of the clinical safety and efficacy data submitted in support of PMAs. The other project is preparation of a guidance document on clinical trial design for device trials.

In addition, reflecting the characteristics of device trials, CDRH has developed guidance on the use of Bayesian statistics with clinical trials of medical devices, including situations involving confirmatory trials, device modifications, incomplete data, and opportunities for adaptive design strategies. (FDA released draft guidance in 2006 and final guidance in 2010 [CDRH-OSB, 2010].) FDA development and education efforts in this area date back well over a decade (Campbell, 2008, 2009). Although the Bayesian approach requires companies to have expert statistical advice and to engage in early consultation with FDA, it has the potential to reduce the costs of trials. As of 2009, at least 20 PMAs or PMA supplements using Bayesian analysis were under review (Campbell, 2009). As part of the guidance and education programs on small clinical trials that NIH and FDA are conducting, a commentary examining applications of Bayesian statistics to device trials involving small populations could be useful. In general, recent years have seen a growing appreciation of the special challenges of device trials, the importance of innovative trial and statistical methods, and the opportunities for FDA-industry interaction to improve trial design and analysis techniques and their use (Campbell, 2008).

DEVICE INNOVATION AND THE HDE OPTION

Although individuals and companies may pioneer devices for rare diseases for purely altruistic reasons, such altruism is uncommon because device innovation entails significant costs, protracted time for research and development, and commitment to ongoing support and administrative costs once a device is approved. For complex "new to the world" devices, the research and development costs can run into the tens of millions of dollars, although details of these costs are not readily available. The time lines to produce practical, safe, and reliable implanted devices can be very long, measured in years and even decades.

An HDE approval reduces the time to market because demonstration of effectiveness is not required. Companies can also recover certain costs, for example, research and development costs. Nevertheless, without a reasonable opportunity to make a profit, as provided by the Orphan Drug Act, the costs and investment risks to bring a new technology forward for small markets are substantial and are likely not to appeal to many companies and investors.

These reservations may be moderated if development of a device for a small population is considered a stepping stone for a future application that may serve a larger market. In situations where the technology is truly novel, the HDE can offer a company the opportunity to learn more about it while continuing its development for a broader use. For example, the company Spiration, Inc., received HDE approval for a device to control prolonged air leaks in the lung following lung surgery (H060002). The company is also conducting clinical testing of the device to treat severe emphysema.

In anticipation of additional indications for a broader patient population, a company may view an HDE approval as a way to enter the market more quickly and with a baseline level of revenue. Market entry under an HDE provides a company with an opportunity to further evaluate the technology and identify next-generation design improvements. It also gives surgeons an opportunity to refine surgical techniques and protocols that may benefit future patients. In addition, an HDE could have "good will" value to the sponsor. Nevertheless, as noted above, there remain both the direct costs of supporting the HDE device and the allocation of financial and personnel resources (especially difficult for a small company) to the HDE device in lieu of another IDE device, another indication, or other research and development effort.

Some reservations about the HDE option may be moderated if a company is looking at a new indication for an already approved device. The list of HDE devices includes some devices (e.g., the deep-brain stimulation device) that are modifications of existing products approved under PMAs for other indications. The investment risk to the company for pursuing a new rare diseases indication is moderated in such cases because most of the research and development costs intrinsic to the device have already been incurred. Companies will still incur some additional incremental research and development investments to devise any modifications needed for the rare diseases application and to generate data on safety and probable benefit necessary for the HDE application.

Although the incremental costs may be relatively modest for an HDE based on an already approved product, companies still face the limit on profits for HDE devices and uncertainties about reimbursement. They also still must consider the opportunity cost for pursuing an HDE approval rather than pursuing development of other products or pursuing approval through the regular PMA process. A company's decision about the HDE option could also be influenced by the requirements for IRB approval and the potential for the annual market for the product to be larger than projected and exceed the annual shipment limit. In the latter situation, FDA would likely ask the company to withdraw the HDE device and seek approval through the PMA process.

Interviews conducted by Bernad (2009) suggest that device developers may sometimes decide to pursue HDE approval after the major part of product development has occurred. One company representative noted that the HDE process can save 3 to 4 years in getting a product to market, "which can be the entire product life cycle" (p. 140). An executive for a company with a device that has both PMA and HDE approvals observed that the HDE process was a means of broadening approved indications for the device that "saved 3 years, recovered $10 million from the initial research and development costs, and established good relationships with many physicians in the field" (p. 142). Others interviewed noted that the short-term benefits of the HDE process must be weighed against the negatives of the restriction on profits and the potential for insurers not to cover the device (for lack of evidence of efficacy). One official particularly cited the burdensome IRB process as involving substantial costs for meticulous record keeping, application production, and IRB fees (which could involve hundreds of sites). In addition, in an article summarizing the results of a symposium on the HDE process, Kaplan and colleagues noted that the availability of a device through the HDE process could complicate recruitment for clinical studies to evaluate the safety and efficacy of a device for a more common indication (Kaplan et al., 2005).

As noted earlier, the difference between drug and device incentives could be an issue for a combination product for a small population if the difference in incentives discouraged drug-device company cooperation on a combination product that involved a complex device and that did not intrinsically require simultaneous or coordinated clinical testing of the drug and the device. If such situations arise, Congress or FDA may need to consider a modification in the HDE policy to encourage innovation to meet unmet needs for combination devices while protecting patients from unsafe or ineffective products.

In general, however, rare conditions may be treatment targets for *either* a drug solution *or* a device solution but not both. That is, only one or the other modality holds clinical promise or clinical relevance or presents a reasonable risk-benefit ratio. In such instances, inconsistencies in incentives and regulatory requirements for orphan drugs and Humanitarian Use Devices are not likely to have much practical impact on the development or use of the product. In addition, if a device is one that qualifies for clearance through the 510(k) process, then the HDE process and conditions likely will not be considered.[20]

It is difficult to assess the extent to which the relatively low number of HDE approvals is influenced by the profit disincentive and the limit on yearly shipment or is, rather, a function of limited opportunities for devices—compared to drugs—to meet substantial unmet health needs for small populations. As noted at the beginning of this chapter, the emphasis in discussions of rare diseases is overwhelmingly on drugs.

For devices covered by an HDE, information on the number of device units shipped is not readily available nor are the estimates submitted by companies (in support of their HDE application) of the number of affected individuals. Although indication-specific information is not available, a recent press release by Medtronic recently reported that a cumulative 75,000 patients worldwide had been treated with its implanted deep-brain stimulation technology, including for the four indications described earlier (Medtronic, 2010).

RECOMMENDATIONS

Based on information presented to the committee by representatives of companies and FDA and provided by a review of past proposals for policy change, the committee concluded that the development of reasonable and effective incentives specific to device development for small populations has proven difficult. The incentives relevant for drug development, particularly the protections from market competition, are not well matched to the realities of device development. Although recent initiatives to promote the development of pediatric medical devices modify the HDE process by allowing profits, they do not move toward either the marketing protections or the stricter approval requirements applicable to orphan drugs.

In contrast to pediatric medical devices, relatively little attention has been directed to needs for medical devices for people with rare conditions. (Even the statement to the committee from the Advanced Medical Technology Association focused as much or more on pediatric devices as on devices

---

[20] The committee found one rare condition for which FDA has approved an orphan drug and an HDE, although the approved indication for the device appears considerably more restrictive. In 2000, the agency approved botulinum toxin type A as an orphan drug to decrease the severity of abnormal head position and neck pain associated with cervical dystonia (BLA 103000/1004). In 2003, it approved an implanted deep-brain stimulation device under an HDE for the management of chronic, severe, drug-refractory dystonia, including cervical dystonia (H020007).

for rare diseases [AdvaMed, 2009].) CDRH recently held a meeting to discuss unmet devices needs, but it did not specifically address the needs of people with rare conditions.

Without the time for a very focused examination, the committee found it difficult to assess the possible extent of unmet device needs for adults with rare conditions and the extent to which changes in FDA policies (e.g., an increase in the criterion of 4,000 patients per year for HDE approval) might promote innovation to meet these needs). A first step in understanding the potential areas for device innovation is a needs assessment for adults with rare conditions. Such an assessment, which should involve patient groups, clinicians, biomedical engineers, and device developers, can also illuminate impediments to innovations to meet those needs.

RECOMMENDATION 7-1: FDA and NIH should collaborate on an assessment of unmet device needs and priorities relevant to rare diseases. That assessment should focus on the most plausible areas of unmet need, identify impediments to meeting these needs, and examine options for overcoming impediments and stimulating high priority innovations.

The identification of needs, priorities, and impediments should help inform the consideration by government, private foundations, and others of additional incentives and supports for medical device development for small populations. Beyond simplifying some aspects of the HDE process as suggested in Recommendation 7-4, options to encourage device innovation for rare diseases include

- the provision of additional orphan products grants and NIH awards for the development of devices to meet priority needs;
- the authorization of tax credits for certain research and development costs, similar to those available for companies developing orphan drugs; and
- the creation of inducement prizes for the design and initial testing of novel devices in areas of unmet need.

In addition, the changes in the HDE incentives for pediatric devices, including the relaxation of the restriction on profits, provide an opportunity to examine the case for similar changes to encourage innovative devices for adults with rare conditions. Also, as experience with the revised incentives for pediatric devices is gained, including through the GAO evaluation due in 2010, that knowledge should be applied to the encouragement of devices for adults with rare conditions. One alternative to eliminating the profit restriction altogether would be the development of a cost-plus option that would allow companies to charge a specified amount over certain costs of development. The committee did not examine this idea in depth and recognizes that it would need careful investigation of potential unintended consequences and consideration of safeguards.

> **RECOMMENDATION 7-2:** Congress should consider whether the rationale for its creation of additional incentives for pediatric device development also supports the use of such incentives to promote the development of devices to meet the needs of adults with rare conditions.

A modest step to encourage additional company interest in devices for small populations would involve greater flexibility in the limits on annual shipments of HDE devices. For devices covered by an HDE, information on the number of units shipped is not readily available nor are the estimates submitted by companies (in support of their HDE application) of the number of affected individuals. Such information might help in assessing how often the 4,000-per-year shipment limit is approached and thus how often the limit might restrict access within the existing framework of HDE policy. Such information would not, however, help in determining what applications might be attracted by a higher cap given that the HDE unlike the PMA does not require demonstration of efficacy. Rather than authorizing an increase in the yearly limit of device shipments that are allowed for an HDE device, Congress could provide for the cap to be raised in specific situations when CDRH determined (based on medical, demographic, and scientific information submitted to it) that an increase in the cap or annual distribution number would benefit patients with a rare disease. This policy would require the specification of boundary criteria (e.g., how large a deviation in the cap could be approved). An analysis of experience with company estimates of affected populations and annual shipments could help in evaluating this idea.

> **RECOMMENDATION 7-3:** As a basis for possible congressional action, the Center for Devices and Radiological Health should analyze the supporting justifications offered in successful and unsuccessful Humanitarian Device Exemption applications related to the 4,000-person-per-year limit and should evaluate the subsequent experience with actual device shipments for approved applications, including any communications about projections that a company might exceed the limits. Taking the findings into account, Congress should consider authorizing FDA to permit a small, defined deviation from the yearly limit on shipments for a specific device when the agency determines that such a deviation would benefit patients with a rare disease.

In addition, FDA could take other steps to make the HDE process worth further consideration by potential sponsors. It could offer additional guidance and assistance to make it easier for sponsors and IRBs to manage the requirement for IRB review of HDEs. As discussed earlier, recent CDRH guidance is helpful but still leaves areas of confusion and uncertainty. The agency could also clarify existing guidance on the very specific details of the process for applying for designation of a Humanitarian Use Device. For example, it could provide further guidance on the evidence needed to support claims of probable benefit and the calculation of the size of the target patient population, and it could also offer consultation to help sponsors understand what data will be responsive and justifiable.

> RECOMMENDATION 7-4: FDA should take steps to reduce the burdens on potential sponsors of Humanitarian Use Devices, including
>
> - assigning an ombudsman to help sponsors navigate the regulatory process for these applications;
> - providing more specific guidance and technical assistance on the documentation of the size of the patient population as required for humanitarian use designations; and
> - developing better guidance (including step-by-step instructions and sample documents) for sponsors and IRBs on their roles and responsibilities related to IRB review of HDEs.

In another area, CDRH could also develop new guidance on the use of surrogate endpoints in medical device trials (see discussion in Chapter 5). As noted earlier in this chapter, the planned analysis of the clinical safety and efficacy data submitted in support of PMAs and the planned guidance document on device clinical trials could contribute useful information and perspectives in this area, even though neither activity will focus on HDEs specifically.

8

Toward an Integrated Approach to Accelerating Research and Product Development for Rare Diseases

Rare diseases collectively account for significant unmet health care needs in the United States. As described in this report, rare diseases research and product development is now attracting considerable attention from public and private funders of research, regulatory bodies, industry, advocacy groups, and the academic research community. The genomics era has contributed a rapidly expanding opportunity to describe the molecular basis for individual rare disorders, the targets for therapeutic interventions, and the development of therapies based on these advances. In general, scientific and technological advances are making it easier, faster, and less expensive to study rare diseases, which should aid the development of products to prevent, diagnose, and treat these diseases.

Nonetheless, despite these advances, the molecular basis for many rare diseases is still unknown, and the number of rare diseases for which the Food and Drug Administration (FDA) has approved treatments is small in relation to the total number of rare diseases. Closing the gap between what has been and what can now be accomplished is the challenge for rare diseases research and product development.

A critical question is how to take better advantage of scientific and technological advances and investments in biomedical research in ways that will deliver improved health outcomes for the millions of Americans with rare diseases. Chapter 1 has outlined the elements of an integrated national strategy to accelerate rare diseases research and product development. This chapter begins by briefly reviewing how the analyses and recommendations in preceding chapters relate to these elements. It then presents an additional recommendation for a high-level process to promote greater collaboration and more efficient use of resources, a process that would build on existing initiatives as well as the recommendations discussed in this report. Although many elements of a national rare diseases research policy already exist, they are not integrated or overseen in a way that supports the systematic identification of key research and development gaps or the setting of priorities, even within government.

ELEMENTS OF AN INTEGRATED NATIONAL STRATEGY

Given the broad scope of this report, the analyses and recommendations focus selectively on the range of issues and activities related to rare diseases research and product development. They emphasize actions to be initiated by the National Institutes of Health (NIH) or the Food and Drug Administration (FDA) but also call for participation by advocacy groups, industry, research institutions, and others.

Active Involvement and Collaboration by a Wide Range of Public and Private Interests

A number of recommendations in this report relate to this element of a national policy, including those that explicitly call for cooperative efforts to improve the design and analysis of trials for small populations (Recommendation 3-2); collaborative sharing of resources to facilitate the application of scientific advances in basic and translational research (Recommendation 4-1); an expansion of the FDA's Critical Path Initiative to work on surrogate endpoints for clinical trials in rare diseases (Recommendation 5-2); creation of a public-private partnership on patient registries and biorepositories for rare diseases (Recommendation 5-3); coordination of the Cures Acceleration Network with various rare diseases research initiatives and with advocacy groups (Recommendation 5-5); and the assessment of unmet needs for medical devices for rare diseases and conditions (Recommendation 7-1). In addition, other activities will necessarily involve cooperation, for example, the creation of an action plan for rare diseases research and product development at NIH (Recommendation 4-2) and the expansion of a centralized preclinical development service at NIH that is available to nonprofit organizations (Recommendation 5-2).

At the end of this chapter is another recommendation for a high-level collaboration to promote and monitor the implementation of existing and new initiatives to accelerate rare diseases research and orphan product development (Recommendation 8-1). Although this report does not direct any recommendations narrowly at advocacy groups and companies, it has described increasing interest and involvement from the private sector in public-private and other collaborations. In addition, the report has not systematically considered international collaboration, although it has cited efforts to harmonize certain aspects of national regulatory policies and opportunities to learn from innovative international initiatives, including those directed at neglected diseases.

Timely Application of Scientific Advances: Creative Strategies for Sharing Research Resources and Infrastructure

This report has summarized a number of technological and scientific advances that can speed the pace of some aspects of basic and translational research on rare diseases and, in some cases, lower its cost. It has cited examples of the application of these advances in rare diseases research, but several recommendations should support their more widespread and timely use. These include particularly the recommendation for precompetitive resource sharing for discovery research (Recommendation 4-1), an NIH action plan (Recommendation 4-2), preclinical resource development (Recommendation 5-1), evaluation of surrogate endpoints (Recommendation 5-2), and increasing rare diseases research flexibility and capacity (Recommendations 5-4 and 5-5).

Resource sharing arrangements should support the productive and efficient use of scarce funding, expertise, data, biological specimens, and research participants. As highlighted in the next section, continued efforts to promote the appropriate use of clinical trial designs and analytic methods for small populations (Recommendations 3-2 and 3-3) should likewise support these outcomes. A particular focus of the recommended NIH action plan for rare diseases research (Recommendation 4-2) would be training of researchers on rare diseases and methods particularly applicable to rare diseases. This would attract to the field new investigators who are ready to take advantage of developments in biotechnology and information technology.

Use and Expansion of Trial Designs for Small Populations

Although scientists have unraveled the genetic basis of a number of rare, single-gene conditions more easily than has been the case for more genetically complex conditions, they have often faced special challenges in obtaining biological specimens for basic research and in recruiting patients for clinical studies. For all conditions but especially for rare conditions, it is important that these crucial resources be used to best advantage.

In clinical research, one key is to employ appropriate clinical trial and analytic methods that can guide decisions about trial size and design and minimize the number of participants needed for valid investigations while improving the interpretation of findings. This report stresses the importance of FDA and NIH collaboration to ensure that NIH-funded studies meet FDA standards, including standards for clinical trial design and analysis (Recommendation 3-2). The committee also recommends that FDA and NIH support further work to develop and test clinical research strategies for small populations (Recommendation 3-2). Also important are natural history studies to support valid use of historical controls and efforts to develop acceptable surrogate endpoints for use in rare diseases trials (Recommendation 5-2) and patient registries to facilitate recruitment of study participants (Recommendation 5-3).

Reasonable Rewards and Incentives for Innovation and Prudent Use of Public Resources

The Orphan Drug Act is generally regarded as having created incentives that have attracted new private resources to research and development on products that help people with rare diseases. The nature of medical device innovation and characteristics of the medical device industry have complicated the identification of effective incentives for medical device development for rare diseases. More generally, unmet needs for medical devices for rare diseases have received relatively little attention, and an assessment of such needs and impediments to meeting them would be useful (Recommendation 7-1). Experience with some newly created incentives for pediatric device development—including lifting the restriction on profits for devices approved through the Humanitarian Device Exemption process—may have relevance for policies that could encourage device development for adults with rare conditions.

Incentives for private action sometimes will be viewed as unlikely to be productive or judged to have costs that are disproportionate to the expected benefit. Prudence may then call for the additional use of public funding to support product development (Recommendations 5-4 and 5-5).

In addition to positive incentives, it is also important to reduce or eliminate unreasonable disincentives to research and development involving products for small populations. In particular, uncertainty about the application of FDA standards for product approval can discourage companies from considering orphan product development. The analysis of FDA staff reviews of orphan products may identify inappropriate variation in FDA reviews and other information that will aid the development of guidelines for staff reviews as well as for staff assistance to drug sponsors through consultation beginning with the early stages of product development (Recommendation 3-1). Greater flexibility in yearly shipment limits for devices approved under the Humanitarian Device Exemption process (Recommendation 7-3) and the provision of additional assistance to medical device sponsors on navigating the regulatory process might help make that process less confusing or burdensome (Recommendation 7-4).

Analyses of health plan administrative practices for orphan drugs (Recommendation 6-1) could identify barriers to patient access to these products, for example, high rates of denied requests for prior approval of orphan drug prescriptions. Systematic review of the evidence on the outcomes of off-label use of drugs for rare diseases (Recommendation 6-2) could encourage health plans to reimburse uses that are backed by evidence.

Adequate Organization and Resources

Adequate organizational structures and resources are the foundation for all other elements of a national policy. Chapter 3 discusses the mismatch between FDA's resources and its responsibilities for review, guidance, and consultation. Chapters 3, 4, 5, and 7 describe shortcomings in public and private resources for rare diseases research and product development. The committee recognizes that increasing resources will be more difficult than ever given current and projected budget deficits, but it also notes the potential benefits of modest but well-placed additions of resources, for example, in the orphan products grants program. As described in this report, some of the recommended investments in resource sharing and other infrastructure for rare diseases research will likely produce spillover benefits in the form of better understanding of common diseases.

Resources include not only financing but also infrastructure and other support for rare diseases researchers and sponsors of orphan products. Several aspects of the recommendation for an NIH action plan (Recommendation 4-1) would target infrastructure, as would steps to promote resource sharing (Recommendations 4-1 and 5-1). In addition, it is important that FDA and NIH cooperate to provide those who receive NIH awards for rare diseases product development with the guidance they need to design studies that meet FDA expectations (Recommendation 3-3).

Mechanisms for Weighing Priorities, Establishing Organization-Specific and Collective Goals, and Assessing Progress

As with any complex process or any complex organization, the development of a coherent strategy for setting priorities, establishing goals, and assessing progress is itself complex. None of these activities is cost-free, and as noted above, increases in federal funding face a very difficult environment.

The creation of an NIH action plan (Recommendation 4-2) would focus attention on key aspects of rare diseases research and orphan product development and would draw other parties into the planning process. That action plan proposal is, however, focused on NIH. The recommendation below calls for a task force on rare diseases that would extend beyond NIH and contribute to a broader process of setting priorities and assessing progress.

RECOMMENDATION

The analyses presented in earlier chapters support the emphasis in the policy framework on a coordinated, collaborative approach to rare diseases research and product development. Today, each of the many public and private groups involved in rare diseases research and product development contributes to the common goals of understanding rare diseases and developing more effective means to prevent, diagnose, and treat them. Nonetheless, gaps and duplication of effort are evident. Current collaborations and coordinated efforts are promising but fall short of what is possible.

For example, at NIH, support by the individual institutes for research on rare diseases is difficult to track and therefore to assess and coordinate. The extent to which institute-specific research programs on rare and neglected diseases, unmet needs, and translational research will reinforce each other or work together is unclear. The NIH Office of Rare Diseases Research was established to coordinate and stimulate attention to the study of rare diseases, but it has limited resources and limited influence on the decisions of individual institutes. Other concerns are that NIH study sections sometimes lack the guidance and resources to properly evaluate rare diseases research proposals and that NIH-funded research sometimes fails to meet FDA requirements for the approval of new drugs. Within FDA, the degree of consistency in review unit evaluations of orphan drugs is a concern and an issue for the new Associate Director for Rare Diseases in the Center for Drug Evaluation and Research.

Outside NIH and FDA, the Centers for Disease Control and Prevention and the Department of Defense (under specific Congressional mandates) also independently fund some research on rare diseases. In the private sector, patient advocacy groups often cooperate but also sometimes compete with each other in areas such as the development of patient registries and the pursuit of disease-specific congressional earmarks. Groups also vary in their experience in working with federal agencies, industry, and academic investigators. Pharmaceutical, biotechnology, and medical device companies have not traditionally worked with their peers, although some pharmaceutical companies are now developing precompetitive shared resources as discussed in Chapter 4. The potential for medical devices to treat rare conditions is too often not considered. In an area defined by scarce resources, incremental increases in efficiency can have a disproportionately large impact.

To encourage more collaboration and more efficient use of resources and build on the initiatives and recommendations discussed in earlier chapters, the committee proposes the creation of a time-limited task force on accelerating rare diseases research and product development. This task force would bring together leaders of key groups. Recognizing that mobilizing such a task force might be difficult in the private sector and that high-level backing is crucial, the committee concluded that the responsibility for creating the task force should rest with the Secretary of Health and Human Services. Nearly all of the government agencies discussed here report ultimately to the Secretary.

RECOMMENDATION 8-1: The Secretary of Health and Human Services should establish a national task force on accelerating rare diseases research and product development. The objectives of the task force would be to promote, coordinate, monitor, and assess the implementation of NIH, FDA, and other public- and private-sector initiatives on rare diseases and orphan products and to support additional opportunities for public-private collaboration.

As envisioned here, the task force would bring together a network of stakeholders for accelerating research and development. In the public sector, it would draw on representatives of the National Institutes of Health, the Food and Drug Administration, the Centers for Disease Control and Prevention, the Department of Defense, and other relevant federal agencies. From the private sector, it would recruit senior participants from the pharmaceutical, biotechnology, and medical device industries; patient advocacy groups; private foundations; and academic and other research institutions. International agencies and other relevant parties would be involved as appropriate.

The committee does not envision the task force as open-ended. It might extend for 4 to 8 years, at which point alternatives would be evaluated.

If this approach is to be effective, identifying and engaging the key public- and private-sector stakeholders is an important first step. The involvement of international counterparts of federal agencies and private organizations will also be desirable, especially for many extremely rare diseases for which global research participation is critical. Creating a venue for meaningful interactions and decision making among these groups will require arrangements for convening task force meetings, conducting analyses and developing strategies, following through on recommendations, and creating a scheme for monitoring progress. One major challenge will be identifying and sustaining a stable funding source for these administrative and analytic activities.

The proposed task force would build on existing initiatives and partnerships as well as explore new arrangements. For example, this report recommends that NIH and FDA cooperate to ensure that NIH-funded research for product development meets FDA expectations for regulatory approval. Another example is the potential for new public-private partnerships involving the federal government, industry, and patient advocacy groups to identify high-priority lines of research, jointly fund such research, and otherwise combine resources to accelerate the process of converting basic research findings into therapeutic discoveries and ultimately into effective preventive, diagnostic, and therapeutic measures. Although research on individual disease pathogenesis and treatment is essential, this research can potentially be further accelerated by identifying networks of biological pathways that are common to clusters of rare diseases. The task force can also explore incentives and other strategies beyond those identified in this report to further engage the biopharmaceutical and medical device industry in various stages of the drug and device development process.

Common diseases are increasingly "personalized" as researchers identify a spectrum of genotypes that can cause these diseases and find that patients with different genotypes may respond differently to different treatments. As a result, rare conditions that are actually subsets of common conditions will become more frequent. Researchers and companies studying these subsets will encounter the challenges of conducting research and developing products for small populations. Tensions may arise in health care delivery and financing between current concepts of evidence-based medicine (often promoting the best treatment for the "average" patient with a disease or identifying patient variables that warrant differences in treatment) and an emerging emphasis on personalized medicine (where the use of conventional methods to meet evidence thresholds on outcomes is inherently constrained). Well-organized and appropriately funded collaborative initiatives to accelerate research and product development for rare diseases may provide models for a broader array of diseases in the future.

A task force on rare diseases research and product development will not lessen the need for participants to improve their individual efforts and relationships as outlined in this report. Individual improvement will strengthen the foundation for collaboration.

In summary, the development of more effective drugs and medical devices for people with rare diseases represents an enormous challenge as well as a timely opportunity to improve public health. A successful response depends on further movement toward a more collaborative, coordinated, open, and sustained approach to rare diseases. Although the effort and investment needed are great, the stakes are high. The potential benefits justify a renewed, high-level commitment to accelerating rare diseases research and product development.

References

AAAS (American Association for the Advancement of Science). 2009. *Programs, Science and Policy, R&D Budget and Policy Program*. http://www.aaas.org/spp/rd/guitotal.htm (accessed September 3, 2010).

AAP (American Academy of Pediatrics) Medical Home Initiatives for Children with Special Needs Project Advisory Committee. 2002. The medical home. *Pediatrics* 110(1): 184-186.

Abernethy, A. P., G. Raman, E. M. Balk, J. M. Hammond, L. A. Orlando, J. L. Wheeler, J. Lau, and D. C. McCrory. 2009. Systematic review: reliability of compendia methods for off-label oncology indications. *Annals of Internal Medicine* 150(5):336-343.

AbioMed, Inc. 2005. *ABIOMED Announces Increased Reimbursement from CMS for Successful Recovery of the Native Heart (press release)*. http://www.abiomed.com/news/CMS_Reimbursement.cfm (accessed August 10, 2010).

AbioMed, Inc. 2009. *Form 10-Q*. http://www.faqs.org/sec-filings/091106/ABIOMED-INC_10-Q/ (accessed August 10, 2010).

ACP (American College of Physicians). 2004. *Patient-Centered, Physician-Guided Care for the Chronically Ill: The American College of Physicians Prescription for Change*. Philadelphia, PA: American College of Physicians.

ACR (American College of Rheumatology). 2010. *Summary of January 21 Teleconference with FDA Regarding Colchicine*. http://www.rheumatology.org/advocacy/colchicine_fda.pdf (accessed August 10, 2010).

ACS (American Cancer Society). 2010. *Clinical Trials: State Laws Regarding Insurance Coverage*. http://www.cancer.org/docroot/ETO/content/ETO_6_2x_State_Laws_Regarding_Clinical_Trials.asp (accessed August 10, 2010).

Adams, J. U. 2008. Imprinting and genetic disease: Angelman, Prader-Willi, and Beckwith-Wiedemann syndromes. *Nature Education* 1(1). http://www.nature.com/scitable/topicpage/imprinting-and-genetic-disease-angelman-prader-willi-923 (accessed September 24, 2010).

AdvaMed (Advanced Medical Technology Association). 2004. *Future Trends in Medical Device Innovation*. http://www.advamed.org/MemberPortal/About/NewsRoom/MediaKits/futuretrendsinmedicaldeviceinnovaton.htm (accessed August 10, 2010).

249

AdvaMed. 2009. Statement Presented by Susan Alpert to IOM Committee on Accelerating Rare Diseases Research and Orphan Product Development, Washington, DC. November 23.

Aetna. 2010. *Clinical Policy Bulletin: Heart Transplantation.* http://www.aetna.com/cpb/medical/data/500_599/0586.html (accessed August 10, 2010).

AIMBE (American Institute for Medical and Biological Engineering). 2005. AIMBE Hall of Fame salutes PET as one of 24 achievements in medical, biological engineering. *Molecular Imaging News*, March 10.

Aiuti, A., I. Brigida, F. Ferrua, B. Cappelli, R. Chiesa, S. Marktel, and M. Roncarolo. 2009. Hematopoietic stem cell gene therapy for adenosine deaminase deficient-SCID. *Immunologic Research* 44(1-3):150-159.

Alliance for a Stronger FDA. 2009. *Written Statement of the Alliance for a Stronger FDA, U.S. Food and Drug Administration Regarding FY2011 Appropriations for the U.S. Food and Drug Administration Submitted to the Appropriations Subcommittee on Agriculture, Rural Development, Food and Drug Administration, and Related Agencies, U.S. Senate, March 26, 2010.* http://fdaalliance.files.wordpress.com/2009/11/alliance-statement-senate-appropriations-committee-fy-11.doc (accessed August 10, 2010).

Anand, G. 2005. How drugs for rare diseases became lifeline for companies. *Wall Street Journal*, November 15. http://online.wsj.com/article/SB113202332063297223.html (accessed August 10, 2010).

Anderson, T. 2009. Novartis under fire for accepting new reward for old drug. *Lancet* 373(9673):1414. http://www.thelancet.com/journals/lancet/article/PIIS0140-6736(09)60804-7/fulltext (accessed August 24, 2010).

Anglim, P. P., T. A. Alonzo, and I. A. Laird-Offringa. 2008. DNA methylation-based biomarkers for early detection of non-small cell lung cancer: an update. *Molecular Cancer* 7(81).

Ariyanchira, S. 2008. BioMarket trends: orphan drug arena driven by biologics. *Genetic Engineering and Biotechnology News* 21(1). http://www.genengnews.com/gen-articles/biomarket-trends-orphan-drug-arena-driven-by-biologics/2318/ (accessed August 10, 2010).

Arnon, S. S. 2007. Creation and development of the public service orphan drug human botulism immune globulin. *Pediatrics* 119(4):785-789. http://www.cdph.ca.gov/programs/ibtpp/Documents/Peds-Creatn-Devlpmt-BIG-IV-2007.pdf (accessed August 10, 2010).

Asamoah, A. K., and J. M. Sharfstein. 2010. Transparency at the Food and Drug Administration. *New England Journal of Medicine* 362:25. http://www.nejm.org/doi/pdf/10.1056/NEJMp1005202 (accessed August 20, 2010).

Asbury, C. H. 1985. *Orphan Drugs, Medical Versus Market Value.* Lexington, MA: Lexington Books.

Asbury, C. H. 1991. The Orphan Drug Act: the first 7 years. *Journal of the American Medical Association* 265(7):893-897.

ASH (American Society of Hematology). 2007. *Toward a New Research Paradigm: Building a New Sickle Cell Disease Research Agenda.* http://www.hematology.org/Advocacy/Policy-Statements/2680.aspx (accessed August 10, 2010).

Ashlock, M. 2010. Increasing the therapeutic options for individuals with rare diseases. Presentation to IOM Committee on Accelerating Rare Diseases Research and Orphan Product Development, Washington, DC. February 23.

ASHP (American Society of Health-System Pharmacists). 2010. *Manufacturer PAPs.* http://www.ashp.org/Import/PRACTICEANDPOLICY/PracticeResourceCenters/PatientAssistancePrograms/ManufacturerPAPs.aspx (accessed August 10, 2010).

Atkins, D., J. Siegel, and J. Slutsky. 2005. Making policy when the evidence is in dispute. *Health Affairs* 24(1):102-113.

Austin, C. P. 2010. NIH translational research for rare diseases and orphan products: NCGC and TRND. Presentation to the IOM Committee on Accelerating Rare Diseases Research and Orphan Product Development, Washington, DC. February 4.

Australia. 1989. *Therapeutic Goods Act.* http://www.comlaw.gov.au/ComLaw/Legislation/ActCompilation1.nsf/0/840CB0162B421D54CA256FBF00121547/$file/Therapeutic Goods1989_WD02.pdf (accessed August 10, 2010).

Australian Bureau of Statistics. 2008. *3105.0.65.001 Australian Historical Population Statistics.* http://www.abs.gov.au/AUSSTATS/abs@.nsf/DetailsPage/3105.0.65.0012008? OpenDocument (accessed August 10, 2010).

Aylward, E. H. 2007. Change in MRI striatal volumes as a biomarker in preclinical Huntington's disease. *Brain Research Bulletin* 72(2-3):152-158.

Aymé, S. 2009. From ICD10 to ICD11: proposal for a general approach and incorporation of rare diseases. Presentation to the Committee for Orphan Medicinal Products (COMP), European Medicines Agency, London. April 9. http://www.eurordis.org/IMG/pdf/ICD_revision_S_Ayme_EMEA_March_09.pdf (accessed August 10, 2010).

Azuma, H., N. Paulk, A. Ranade, C. Dorrell, M. Al-Dhalimy, E. Ellis, S. Strom, et al. 2007. Robust expansion of human hepatocytes in Fah-/-/Rag2-/-/Il2rg-/- mice. *Nature Biotechnology* 25(8):903-910. http://kaylab.stanford.edu/manuscripts/NBT07Azuma.pdf (accessed August 10, 2010).

Baily, M. A., and T. H. Murray. 2008. Ethics, evidence, and cost in newborn screening. *Hastings Center Report* 38(3):23-31. http://www.thehastingscenter.org/uploadedFiles/Publications/HCR/Articles/2008_May-June/hcr_2008_may_jun_early_release1.pdf (accessed August 10, 2010).

Bainbridge J. W. B., A. J. Smith, S. S. Barker, S. Robbie, R. Henderson, K. Balaggan, A. Viswanathan, et al. 2008. Effect of gene therapy on visual function in Leber's congenital amaurosis. *New England Journal of Medicine* 358:2231-2239.

Beitz, J. 2006. Approval letter to Genzyme Corporation for BLA 125141/0 [Alglucosidase alfa/Myozyme]. April 28. http://www.accessdata.fda.gov/drugsatfda_docs/appletter/2006/125141s0_LTR.pdf (accessed August 24, 2010).

Beitz, J. 2010. Approval letter to Orphan Europe for NDA 022562 [Carbaglu]. March 18. http://www.accessdata.fda.gov/drugsatfda_docs/appletter/2010/022562s000ltr.pdf (accessed August 19, 2010).

Bellingham, M. C. 2010. A review of the neural mechanisms of action and clinical efficiency of riluzole in treating amyotrophic lateral sclerosis: what have we learned in the last decade? *CNS Neuroscience & Therapeutics* March 10 [e-pub ahead of print].

Benderly, B. L. 2009. *The End of Blinding Trachoma Among The World's Poor Is in Sight.* http://www.dcp2.org/features/75 (accessed August 10, 2010).

Benson, D.A., I. Karsch-Mizrachi, D. J. Lipman, J. Ostell, and D. L.Wheeler. 2008. GenBank. *Nucleic Acids Research* 36 (Database issue):D25-30.

Berger, E. 2009. *Medicare's Inpatient New Technology Add-on: The Trials of InfraReDx, the Triumph of Spiration.* http://larchmontstrategic.blogspot.com/2009/08/medicares-inpatient-new-technology-add.html (accessed August 10, 2010).

Bernad, D. M. 2009. Humanitarian use device and humanitarian device exemption regulatory programs: pros and cons. *Expert Reviews* 6(2):137-145.

Berry, D. A. 2006. A guide to drug discovery: Bayesian clinical trials. *Nature Reviews* 5:27-36.

Beutler, E., T. Gelbart, P. Lee, R. Trevino, M. A. Fernandez, and V. F. Fairbanks. 2000. Molecular characterization of a case of atransferrinemia. *Blood* 96(13):4071-4074.

Billiondollarwoman. 2010. *Comment on: The World's Most Expensive Drugs.* http://rate.forbes.com/comments/CommentServlet?op=cpage&sourcename=story&StoryURI=2010/02/19/expensive-drugs-cost-business-healthcare-rare-diseases.html (accessed August 10, 2010).

Bonabeau, E., N. Bodick, and R. W. Armstrong. 2008. A more rational approach to new product development. *Harvard Business Review*, March. http://people.icoserver.com/users/eric/hbr_NPD.pdf (accessed August 10, 2010).

Boodman, S. G. 2009. Annoying bug turned out to be much more. *Washington Post*, November 3. http://www.washingtonpost.com/wp-dyn/content/article/2009/11/02/AR2009110202432.html (accessed August 10, 2010).

Booz Allen Hamilton Inc. 2008. *Independent Evaluation of FDA's First Cycle Review Performance: Final Report*. http://www.fda.gov/downloads/ForIndustry/UserFees/Prescription DrugUserFee/ucm127982.pdf (accessed August 10, 2010).

Brancati, F., A. Sarkozy, and B. Dallapiccola. 2006. KBG syndrome. *OJRD (Orphanet Journal of Rare Diseases)*. http://www.ojrd.com/content/1/1/50 (accessed August 10, 2010).

Braunschweig, F. 2007. Therapeutic and diagnostic role of electrical devices in acute heart failure. *Heart Failure Reviews* 12(2):157-166.

Brodsky, R. A. 2009. How I treat paroxysmal nocturnal hemoglobinuria. *Blood* 113(26): 6522-6527.

Brooks A. D., W. A. Wells, T. D. McLean, R. Khanna, R. Coghlan T. Mertenskoetter, L. A. Privor-Dumm, et al. 2010. Ensuring that developing countries have access to new healthcare products: the role of product development partnerships. *Innovation Strategy Today* 3:1-5. http://www.ipmglobal.org/pdfs/english/ipm_publications/2010/PDPAccess-InnovationStratToday-Jan2010.pdf (accessed August 23, 2010).

Budd, T. M., and K. A. Liebman. 2009. *Annual Review of Medical Device Patent Litigation*. http://www.faegre.com/showarticle.aspx?Show=9611 (accessed August 10, 2010).

Butcher, L. 2009. When should insurers cover off-label drug usage? *Managed Care*, May. http://www.managedcaremag.com/archives/0905/0905.offlabel.html (accessed August 10, 2010).

Campbell, A. 2004. Appendix B: State regulation of medical research with children and adolescents: an overview and analysis. In *Ethical Conduct of Clinical Research Involving Children*. Washington, DC: The National Academies Press. Pp. 320-383.

Campbell, E. G., B. R. Clarridge, M. Gokhale, L. Birenbaum, S. Hilgartner, N. A. Holtzman, and D. Blumenthal. 2002. Data withholding in academic genetics: evidence from a national survey. *Journal of the American Medical Association* 287(4):473-480.

Campbell, G. 2008. Statistics in medical devices and diagnostics. Presentation at the Ad-vaMed-FDA Statistics Workshop, Bethesda, MD. April 16. http://www.amstat.org/sections/sigmedd/Advamed/Advamed08/presentation/GCampbell_Advamed-FDA_Statistics_4-08.pdf (accessed August 10, 2010).

Campbell, G. 2009. Bayesian statistics at the FDA: The trailblazing experience with medical devices. Presentation at Rutgers Biostatistics Day, New Brunswick, NJ. April 9. http://www.stat.rutgers.edu/iob/bioconf09/slides/Campbell.pdf (accessed August 9, 2010).

Campbell, R. M. 2007. Ensuring safe medicines and medical devices for children. Testimony before the Committee on Health, Education, Labor and Pensions, U.S. Senate, Washington, DC, March 27. http://www.aap.org/advocacy/washing/therapeutics/docs/campbell.pdf (accessed August 27, 2010).

Campeau, P. M., C. R. Scriver, and J. J. Mitchell. 2008. A 25-year longitudinal analysis of treatment efficacy in inborn errors of metabolism. *Molecular Genetics and Metabolism* 95(1-2):11-16.

Cannom, D. S., and E. N. Prystowsky. 2004. The evolution of the implantable cardioverter defibrillator. *Pacing and Clinical Electrophysiology* 27(3):419-421.

Carmichael, M. 2010. Would regulation kill genetic testing? *Newsweek*, June 4. http://www.newsweek.com/2010/06/04/would-regulation-kill-genetic-testing.html (accessed September 1, 2010).

Cartier N., S. Hacein-Bey-Abina, C. C. Bartholomae, G. Veres, M. Schmidt, I. Kutschera, M.Vidaud, et al. 2009. Lentiviral-mediated gene therapy of hematopoietic stem cells delays disease progression in patients with a fatal brain disorder. *Science* 326(5954):818-823.

Carver, K. H. C. 2010. Companion diagnostics: evolving FDA regulation and issues for resolution. In *In Vitro Diagnostics: The Complete Regulatory Guide*, edited by S. D. Danzis and E. J. Flannery. Washington, DC: The Food and Drug Law Institute.

Cassidy, A. 2009. *Coverage and Payment for Prescription Drugs Under Medicare Part B: A Complex Patchwork.* National Health Policy Forum Background Paper. http://www.nhpf.org/library/details.cfm/2755 (accessed August 9, 2010).

Cassidy, S. B., and D. J. Driscoll. 2009. Prader-Willi syndrome. *European Journal of Human Genetics* 17:3-13.

Caves, R. E., M. D. Whinston, and M. A. Hurwitz. 1991. Patent expiration, entry, and competition in the U.S. pharmaceutical industry. Brookings Papers on Economic Activity. *Microeconomics* 1991:1-48.

CBTRUS (Central Brain Tumor Registry of the United States). 2010. *CBTRUS Statistical Report: Primary Brain and Central Nervous System Tumors Diagnosed in the United States in 2004-2006.* http://www.cbtrus.org/2007-2008/2007-20081.html (accessed August 9, 2010).

CDC (Centers for Disease Control and Prevention). 2005. *Marine Toxins.* http://www.cdc.gov/ncidod/dbmd/diseaseinfo/marinetoxins_g.htm (accessed August 9, 2010).

CDC. 2007a. *Hemochromatosis for Health Care Professionals: Epidemiology: Prevalence.* http://www.cdc.gov/ncbddd/hemochromatosis/training/epidemiology/prevalence.htm (accessed August 9, 2010).

CDC. 2007b. Malaria surveillance—United States, 2005. *Morbidity and Mortality Weekly Reports* 56(SS06):23-38. http://www.cdc.gov/mmwr/preview/mmwrhtml/ss5606a2.htm (accessed December 1, 2010).

CDC. 2008a. *Leishmania Infection.* http://www.cdc.gov/ncidod/dpd/parasites/leishmania/factsht_leishmania.htm#get_us (accessed August 9, 2010).

CDC. 2008b. *Nocardiosis.* http://www.cdc.gov/nczved/divisions/dfbmd/diseases/nocardiosis/technical.html (accessed August 9, 2010).

CDC. 2008c. *Schistosomiasis.* http://www.cdc.gov/ncidod/dpd/parasites/schistosomiasis/factsht_schistosomiasis.htm (accessed August 9, 2010).

CDC. 2009a. *Dengue Epidemiology.* http://www.cdc.gov/dengue/epidemiology/index.html (accessed August 9, 2010).

CDC. 2009b. *Fiscal Year 2009: Justification of Estimates for Appropriation Committees.* http://www.cdc.gov/fmo/PDFs/FY09_CDC_CJ_Final.pdf (accessed August 9, 2010).

CDC. 2009c. *HIV/AIDS Surveillance Report: Cases of HIV Infection and AIDS in the United States and Dependent Areas, 2007.* http://www.cdc.gov/hiv/topics/surveillance/basic.htm#hivest (accessed August 9, 2010).

CDC. 2009d. *Newborn Screening Translation Research Initiative.* http://www.cdcfoundation.org/programs/lifestyles/index.aspx#newborn (accessed August 9, 2010).

CDER (Center for Drug Evaluation and Research, Food and Drug Administration). 1998. *The CDER Handbook.* http://www.fda.gov/downloads/AboutFDA/CentersOffices/CDER/UCM198415.pdf (accessed August 9, 2010).

CDER. 2002. *Guidance for Industry: Carcinogenicity Study Protocol Submissions.* http://www.fda.gov/downloads/drugs/guidancecomplianceregulatoryinformation/guidances/ucm078924.pdf (accessed August 9, 2010).

CDER. 2003. *Guidance for Industry: Bioavailability and Bioequivalence Studies for Orally Administered Drug Products-General Considerations.* http://www.fda.gov/downloads/Drugs/GuidanceComplianceRegulatoryInformation/Guidances/ucm070124.pdf (accessed August 24, 2010).

CDER. 2006. *Guidance for Industry, Investigators, and Reviewers: Exploratory IND Studies.* http://www.fda.gov/downloads/Drugs/GuidanceComplianceRegulatoryInformation/Guidances/ucm078933.pdf (accessed August 9, 2010).

CDER. 2007. *Guidance for Industry: Chronic Obstructive Pulmonary Disease: Developing Drugs for Treatment.* http://www.fda.gov/downloads/Drugs/GuidanceCompliance RegulatoryInformation/Guidances/ucm071575.pdf (accessed August 9, 2010).

CDER. 2009. CDER Medical Policy Coordinating Committee. *Manual of Policies and Procedures* November 2. http://www.fda.gov/downloads/AboutFDA/CentersOffices/CDER/ManualofPoliciesProcedures/UCM188694.pdf (accessed August 20, 2010).

CDER-CBER (Center for Biologics Evaluation and Research). 1996. *Guidance for Industry: E6 Good Clinical Practice: Consolidated Guidance.* http://www.fda.gov/downloads/Drugs/GuidanceComplianceRegulatoryInformation/Guidances/ucm073122.pdf (accessed August 24, 2010).

CDER-CBER. 1997. *Guidance for Industry: S6 Preclinical Evaluation of Biotechnology-Derived Pharmaceuticals.* http://www.fda.gov/downloads/Drugs/GuidanceCompliance RegulatoryInformation/Guidances/ucm074957.pdf (accessed August 24, 2010).

CDER-CBER. 1998. *Guidance for Industry: Providing Clinical Evidence of Effectiveness for Human Drug and Biological Products.* http://www.fda.gov/downloads/Drugs/GuidanceComplianceRegulatoryInformation/Guidances/ucm078749.pdf (accessed August 24, 2010).

CDER-CBER. 2002a. *Guidance for Industry: Information Program on Clinical Trials for Serious or Life-Threatening Diseases and Conditions.* http://www.fda.gov/downloads/RegulatoryInformation/Guidances/ucm126838.pdf (accessed August 24, 2010).

CDER-CBER. 2002b. *Guidance for Industry: Special Protocol Assistance.* http://www.fda.gov/downloads/Drugs/GuidanceComplianceRegulatoryInformation/Guidances/ucm080571.pdf (accessed August 24, 2010).

CDER-CBER. 2009. *Guidance for Industry Format and Content of Proposed Risk Evaluation and Mitigation Strategies (REMS), REMS Assessments, and Proposed REMS Modifications.* http://www.fda.gov/downloads/Drugs/GuidanceComplianceRegulatoryInformation/Guidances/UCM184128.pdf (accessed August 24, 2010).

CDER-CBER. 2010a. *Guidance for Industry: Adaptive Design Clinical Trials for Drugs and Biologics (Draft).* http://www.fda.gov/downloads/Drugs/GuidanceComplianceRegulatory Information/Guidances/UCM201790.pdf (accessed August 24, 2010).

CDER-CBER. 2010b. *Guidance for Industry: Non-Inferiority Clinical Trials.* http://www.fda.gov/downloads/Drugs/GuidanceComplianceRegulatoryInformation/Guidances/UCM202140.pdf (accessed August 24, 2010).

CDMRP (Congressionally Directed Medical Research Programs, Department of Defense). 2008. *FY 2008 Annual Report: Contents.* http://cdmrp.army.mil/pubs/annreports/2008 annrep/default.shtml (accessed August 24, 2010).

CDRH (Center for Devices and Radiological Health, Food and Drug Administration). 2009. *Humanitarian Use Device: Overview.* http://www.fda.gov/MedicalDevices/Device RegulationandGuidance/HowtoMarketYourDevice/PremarketSubmissions/Humanitari anDeviceExemption/default.htm (accessed August 9, 2010).

CDRH. 2010a. *CDRH Preliminary Internal Evaluations—Volume 1.* August. http://www.fda.gov/downloads/AboutFDA/CentersOffices/CDRH/CDRHReports/UCM220784.pdf (accessed September 3, 2010).

CDRH. 2010b. *Office of Device Evaluation.* http://www.fda.gov/AboutFDA/CentersOffices/CDRH/CDRHOffices/ucm115879.htm#3 (accessed August 9, 2010).

CDRH-CBER. 2007. *Draft Guidance for Industry, Clinical Laboratories, and FDA Staff: In Vitro Diagnostic Multivariate Index Assays.* http://www.fda.gov/downloads/Medical Devices/DeviceRegulationandGuidance/GuidanceDocuments/ucm071455.pdf (accessed August 24, 2010).

CDRH-CBER. 2010. *Guidance for HDE Holders, Institutional Review Boards (IRBs), Clinical Investigators, and FDA Staff—Humanitarian Device Exemption (HDE) Regulation: Questions and Answers.* http://www.fda.gov/MedicalDevices/DeviceRegulationand Guidance/GuidanceDocuments/ucm110194.htm (accessed August 24, 2010).

CDRH-OSB (Office of Surveillance and Biometrics). 2010. *Guidance for the Use of Bayesian Statistics in Medical Device Clinical Trials.* http://www.fda.gov/downloads/Medical Devices/DeviceRegulationandGuidance/GuidanceDocuments/ucm071121.pdf (accessed August 24, 2010).

Celgene. 2010. *Thalomid®: System for Thalomide Education and Prescribing Safety.* http://www.thalomid.com/steps_program.aspx (accessed August 9, 2010).

CFF (Cystic Fibrosis Foundation). 2008. *Research Milestones.* http://www.cff.org/research/ResearchMilestones/ (accessed August 9, 2010).

CFF. 2009. *Cystic Fibrosis Foundation Patient Registry 2008 Annual Data Report.* http://www.cff.org/UploadedFiles/research/ClinicalResearch/2008-Patient-Registry-Report.pdf (accessed August 9, 2010).

CFF. Undated a. *CF Basic Research Centers.* http://www.cff.org/aboutCFFoundation/Locations/ResearchCenters/ (accessed August 9, 2010).

CFF. Undated b. *CF Foundation-Accredited Care Centers.* http://www.cff.org/treatments/Care CenterNetwork/CFFoundation-accreditedCareCenters/ (accessed August 9, 2010).

CFSAN (Center for Food Safety and Nutrition), Food and Drug Administration. 2007. *Guidance for Industry: Frequently Asked Questions About Medical Foods.* College Park, MD: FDA. http://www.fda.gov/Food/GuidanceComplianceRegulatoryInformation/Guidance Documents/MedicalFoods/UCM054048#q1 (accessed August 9, 2010).

Chamberlain, J. R., U. Schwarze, P. Wang, R. K. Hirata, K. D. Hankenson, J. M. Pace, R. A. Underwood, et al. 2004. Gene targeting in stem cells from individuals with osteogenesis imperfecta. *Science* 303:1198. http://www.sciencemag.org/cgi/reprint/303/5661/1198.pdf (accessed August 23, 2010).

Chan, K., and J. M. Puck. 2005. Development of population-based newborn screening for severe combined immunodeficiency. *Journal of Allergy and Clinical Immunology* 115:391-398.

Chong, C. R., and D. J. Sullivan, Jr. 2007. New uses for old drugs. *Nature* 448:645-646. August 8.

Choudhry, N. K., J. L. Lee, J. Agnew-Blais, C. Corcoran, and W. H. Shrank. 2009. Drug company-sponsored patient assistance programs: A Viable Safety Net? *Health Affairs* 28(3):827-834.

Citron, P. 2008. Medical device considerations. Presentation to IOM Committee on Conflict of Interest in Medical Research, Education, and Practice, Washington, DC. January 21.

Clinton, C., and H. T. Gazda. 2009. *Diamond-Blackfan Anemia.* http://www.ncbi.nlm.nih.gov/bookshelf/br.fcgi?book=gene&part=diamond-b (accessed August 9, 2010).

Clyde, A. T., L. Bockstedt, J. A. Farkas, and C. Jackson. 2008. Experience with Medicare's new technology add-on payment program. *Health Affairs* 27(6):1632-1641.

CMS (Centers for Medicare and Medicaid Services). 2000. *Clinical Trials.* http://www.cms.gov/manuals/downloads/Pub06_PART_35.pdf (accessed August 9, 2010).

CMS. 2006. *Guidance for the Public, Industry, and CMS Staff—National Coverage Determinations with Data Collection as a Condition of Coverage: Coverage with Evidence Development.* July. https://www.cms.gov/mcd/ncpc_view_document.asp?id=8 (accessed August 9, 2010).

CMS. 2007. *CMS Manual System.* http://www.cms.gov/Transmittals/Downloads/R74NCD. pdf (accessed August 9, 2010).

CMS. 2009a. *2010 Combined Call Letter. Prescription Drug Coverage Contracting. March 30.* http://www.cms.gov/PrescriptionDrugCovContra/Downloads/2010CallLetter.pdf (accessed August 19, 2010).

CMS. 2009b. *Medicaid Drug Rebate Program: Overview.* http://www.cms.gov/Medicaid DrugRebateProgram/ (accessed August 9, 2010).

CMS. 2009c. Medicare program; proposed changes to the hospital inpatient prospective payment systems for acute care hospitals and fiscal year 2010 rates and to the long-term care hospital prospective payment system and rate year 2010 Rates; proposed rule. *Federal Register* 74(98):24080-24686. http://edocket.access.gpo.gov/2009/pdf/E9-10458.pdf (accessed August 9, 2010).

CMS. 2009d. *Medicare Enrollment: National Trends 1966-2008.* http://www.cms.gov/ MedicareEnRpts/Downloads/HISMI08.pdf (accessed August 9, 2010).

CMS. 2010. *Medicare & You 2010.* http://www.medicare.gov/publications/pubs/pdf/10050. pdf (accessed August 9, 2010).

Cohen, W. M., and J. P. Walsh. 2008. Real impediments to biomedical research. In *Innovation Policy and the Economy*, edited by A. B. Jaffe, J. Lerner, and S. Stern. Chicago, IL: University of Chicago Press. Pp. 1-30.

Cohn, R. D., C. van Erp, J. P. Habasi, A. A. Soleimani, E. C. Klein, M. T. Lisi, M. Gamradt, et al. 2007. Angiotensin II type 1 receptor blockade attenuates TGF-β-induced failure of muscle regeneration in multiple myopathic states. *Nature Medicine* 13:204-210. E-pub January 21.

Collins, F. S. 2009. Implementing personalized medicine: scientific and translational challenges. Presentation to AAAS Personalized Medicine: Planning for the Future Colloquium, Washington, DC. October 26. http://www.aaas.org/spp/PM/ppts/Collins.pdf (accessed August 9, 2010).

Collins, K. L. 2004. Profitable gifts: a history of the Merck Mectizan donation program and its implications for international health. *Perspectives in Biology and Medicine.* 47(1):100-109.

Cook-Deegan, R. 2008. Gene patents. In *From Birth to Death and Bench to Clinic: The Hastings Center Bioethics Briefing Book for Journalists, Policymakers, and Campaigns*, edited by Mary Crowley. Garrison, NY: The Hastings Center. Pp. 69-72. http://www.thehast ingscenter.org/uploadedFiles/Publications/Briefing_Book/gene%20patents%20chapter. pdf (accessed August 9, 2010).

Coombs, A. 2009. Rare nature of mushroom poisoning means drug trials rarer still. *Nature Medicine* 15(3).

Cornetta, K., and B. Carter. 2010. *Letter on Behalf of the American Society of Gene & Cell Therapy to Francis Collins, Director, NIH. March 10.* http://www.asgct.org/UserFiles/file/ Francis%20Collins%20Letter.pdf (accessed September 24, 2010).

Corr, P. 2008. New business models addressing global health: a framework for private equity. Presentation at IOM Forum on Drug Discovery, Development, and Translation Workshop on Breakthrough Business Models, Washington, DC. June 23.

Cortazar, P. 2007. Clinical review for NDA 22042 [Evista / Raloxifene Hydrochloride]. *CDER Medical Review Part 1 Application Number: 22042.* September 6. p. 16. http://www. accessdata.fda.gov/drugsatfda_docs/nda/2007/022042s000_MedR_P1.pdf (accessed August 19, 2010).

Coté, T. 2009. The state of the Orphan Drug Act. Presentation to IOM Committee on Accelerating Rare Diseases Research and Orphan Product Development, Washington, DC. August 12.

Coté, T. 2010. Orphans at FDA: the fundamentals. Presentation at the American Course on Drug Development and Regulatory Sciences, San Francisco, CA. February 23.

C-Path (Critical Path Institute). 2008. *FDA and EMEA Conclude That New Renal Safety Biomarkers Are Qualified for Specific Regulatory Purposes.* http://www.c-path.org/pdf/ PSTC_nephro_VXDS_summary_final.pdf (accessed August 9, 2010).

C-Path. 2009a. *Coalition Against Major Disease: Workscope 1.1.* http://www.c-path.org/pdf/ CAMDWorkScope.pdf (accessed August 9, 2010).

C-Path. 2009b. *The Predictive Safety Testing Consortium.* http://www.c-path.org/pdf/PSTC_ GeneralInfo_08-28-09.pdf (accessed August 9, 2010).

CPI (Critical Path Initiative). 2010. *The Critical Path Initiative: Report on Key Achievements in 2009.* http://www.fda.gov/downloads/ScienceResearch/SpecialTopics/CriticalPath Initiative/UCM221651.pdf (accessed September 24, 2010).

CTF (Children's Tumor Foundation). 2009. *2008 Annual Report.* http://www.ctf.org/images/ stories/2008_annual_report_final.pdf (accessed August 9, 2010).

CTSA (Clinical and Translational Science Awards, NIH). 2010. *Evaluation—IRB Issues in Evaluation.* http://www.ctsaweb.org/index.cfm?fuseaction=committee.viewCommittee&com_ ID=461&abbr= (accessed August 10, 2010).

CTXinfo.org (Cerebrotendinous xanthomatosis). 2010. *Latest News: February 28.* http:// www.ctxinfo.org/index.html (accessed August 9, 2010).

Dale, D. C., and D. C. Link. 2009. The many causes of severe congenital neutropenia. *New England Journal of Medicine* 360(1):3-5.

D'Andrea, A. D. 2010. Susceptibility pathways in Fanconi's anemia and breast cancer. *New England Journal of Medicine* 362:1909-1919.

Defazio, G., G. Abbruzzese, P. Livrea, and A. Berardelli. 2004. Epidemiology of primary dystonia. *Lancet Neurology* 3(11):673-678.

Delude, C. 2009. Tangier disease: one island's treasure. *Proto Magazine* Fall:16-21. http:// protomag.com/statics/tangiers.pdf (accessed August 9, 2010).

Derbis, J., B. Evelyn, and J. McMeekin. 2008. FDA initiative aims to remove unapproved drugs from market. *Pharmacy Today* August:21-22.

de Siqueira, I. C., J. Dias, H. Ruf, E. A. G. Ramos, E. A. Pires Maciel, A. Rolim, L. Jabur, et al. 2005. *Chromobacterium violaceum* in siblings, Brazil. *Emerging Infectious Diseases* (11)9. http://www.cdc.gov/ncidod/EId/vol11no09/pdfs/05-0278.pdf (accessed August 9, 2010).

Dhruva, S. S., L. A. Bero, and R. F. Redberg. 2009. Strength of study evidence examined by the FDA in premarket approval of cardiovascular devices. *Journal of the American Medical Association* 302(24):2679-2685.

Dietz, H. C. 2009. *Marfan Syndrome.* http://www.ncbi.nlm.nih.gov/bookshelf/br.fcgi?book= gene&part=marfan (accessed August 9, 2010).

Dietz, H. C. 2010. New therapeutic approaches for Mendelian disorders. *New England Journal of Medicine* 363:852-863. http://www.nejm.org/doi/full/10.1056/NEJMra0907180? query=TOC (accessed September 1, 2010).

DiMasi, J. A., R. W. Hansen, and H. G. Grabowski. 2003. The price of innovation: new estimates of drug development costs. *Journal of Health Economics* 22(2003):151-185.

DiMasi, J. A., L. Feldman, A. Seckler, and A.Wilson. 2010. Trends in risks associated with new drug development: success rates for investigational drugs. *Clinical Pharmacology & Therapeutics* 87:272-277.

Dimond, P. F. 2009. Big PhRMA adopting orphan drug strategy. *Genetic Engineering & Biotechnology News.* http://www.genengnews.com/analysis-and-insight/big-pharma-adopting-orphan-drug-strategy/71053206/ (accessed August 9, 2010).

DNDi (Drugs for Neglected Diseases Initiative). 2009. *Pfizer and DNDi Advancing International Research Efforts in the Fight Against Neglected Tropical Diseases* (press release). http://www.dndi.org/press-releases/2009/565-pfizer-and-dndi-advancing-international-research-efforts-in-the-fight-against-neglected-tropical-diseases.html (accessed August 9, 2010).

DOJ (Department of Justice). 2009. *Stryker Biotech and Its Top Management Indicted for Illegal Promotion of Medical Devices Used in Invasive Surgeries* (press release), October 28. http://www.fda.gov/downloads/NewsEvents/Newsroom/PressAnnouncements/UCM188306.pdf (accessed August 24, 2010).

Dorman, D. 2007. Testimony submitted by the National Organization for Rare Disorders before the Social Security Administration Public Hearing on Compassionate Allowances, Washington, DC. December 4.

Dorman, D. 2008. *Statement of Diane Dorman, Vice President for Public Policy National Organization for Rare Disorders (NORD), to FDA Infectious Diseases Planning Committee, Washington, DC. April 28.* http://www.rarediseases.org/pdf/FDA_Infectious_Diseases_Planning_Com_4-22-08.pdf (accessed August 9, 2010).

Dorsey, E. R., J. de Roulet, J. P. Thompson, J. I. Reminick, A. Thai, Z. White-Stellato, C. A. Beck, et al. 2010. Funding of US biomedical research, 2003-2008. *Journal of the American Medical Association* 303(2):137-143.

Douglas, J. 2010. Update: Shire plans to undercut Cerezyme as profit rises. *Dow Jones Newswires*, February 19. http://www.nasdaq.com/aspx/companynewsStoryPrint.aspx?storyid=201002190850dowjonesdjonline000444 (accessed August 9, 2010).

Doulton, D. M. 2010. From cradle to commencement: transitioning pediatric sickle cell disease patients to adult providers. *Journal of Pediatric Oncology Nursing* 27(2):119-123.

Dreifus, C. 2009. Researcher behind the drug Gleevec: a conversation with Brian Druker. *New York Times,* November 2. http://www.nytimes.com/2009/11/03/science/03conv.html (accessed August 9, 2010).

Dudley J. T., R. Tibshirani, T. Deshpande, and A. J. Butte. 2009. Disease signatures are robust across tissues and experiments. *Molecular Systems Biology* 5:307. http://www.ncbi.nlm.nih.gov/pmc/articles/PMC2758720/pdf/msb200966.pdf (accessed August 9, 2010).

Duffner, P. K., V. S. Caviness, R. W. Erbe, M. C. Patterson, K. R. Schultz, D. A. Wenger, and C. Whitley. 2009. The long-term outcomes of presymptomatic infants transplanted for Krabbe disease: report of the workshop held on July 11 and 12, 2008, Holiday Valley, New York. *Genetics in Medicine* 11(6):450-454.

Duggan, M. 2010. The effect of Medicare Part D on pharmaceutical prices and utilization. *American Economic Review* 100(1):590-600.

Duggan, M., and F. M. S. Morton. 2006. The distortionary effects of government procurement: evidence from Medicaid prescription drug purchasing. *Quarterly Journal of Economics* 121(1):1-30.

Duncan, D. E. 2009. Enlisting computers to unravel the true complexity of disease. *New York Times,* August 24. http://www.nytimes.com/2009/08/25/science/25prof.html (accessed August 9, 2010).

Duncan, M. W., and S. W. Hunsucker. 2005. Proteomics as a tool for clinically relevant biomarker discovery and validation. *Experimental Biology and Medicine* 230(11):808-817.

Dykxhoorn, D. M., and J. Lieberman. 2006. Knocking down disease with siRNAs. *Cell* 126(2):231-235.

Eastman, P. 2005. Reimbursement policies discourage off-label drug use. *Oncology Times* 27(20):8, 10.

El-Khatib, F. H., S. J. Russell, D. M. Nathan, R. G. Sutherlin, and E. R. Damiano. 2010. A bihormonal closed-loop artificial pancreas for type 1 diabetes. *Science Translational Medicine* 2(27):27ra27.

Elsas, L. J. 2007. *Galactosemia.* http://www.ncbi.nlm.nih.gov/bookshelf/br.fcgi?book=gene& part=galactosemia (accessed August 9, 2010).

EMEA (European Medicines Agency). 2008. *Annual Report, 2007.* London. http://www. ema.europa.eu/docs/en_GB/document_library/Annual_report/2009/12/WC500016591. pdf (accessed December 1, 2010).

Entrepreneur Newsletter. 2006. NMT medical voluntarily withdraws Cardioseal PFO HDE (Biotech Equipment Update, October 1). http://www.entrepreneur.com/tradejournals/ article/151492685.html (accessed August 9, 2010).

EPI (Economic Policy Institute). 2009. *Employer-Sponsored Health Insurance Erosion Continues: Unabated Declines in Coverage Since 2000 Are Expected to Worsen Through 2009.* http://epi.3cdn.net/6356d48ae59f625af6_xxm6bnyn2.pdf (accessed August 9, 2010).

Escolar, M. L., M. D. Poe, H. R. Martin, and J. Kurtzberg. 2006. A staging system for infantile Krabbe disease to predict outcome after unrelated umbilical cord blood transplantation. *Pediatrics* 118(3):e879-e889.

Eurodis. 2005. Rare diseases in numbers. *European Conference on Rare Diseases,* Luxembourg, June 21-22. http://ec.europa.eu/health/ph_threats/non_com/ev_20050622_co01_ en.pdf (accessed August 6, 2010).

European Commission, Health & Consumer Protection Directorate-General. 2007. *Public Consultation, Rare Diseases: Europe's Challenges.* http://ec.europa.eu/health/ph_threats/ non_com/docs/raredis_comm_draft.pdf (accessed August 6, 2010).

European Union. 1999. *Regulation (EC) No. 141/2000.* http://eur-lex.europa.eu/LexUriServ/ LexUriServ.do?uri=OJ:L:2000:018:0001:0005:EN:PDF (accessed August 6, 2010).

Eurostat. 2010. *Total Population.* http://epp.eurostat.ec.europa.eu/tgm/table.do?tab=table& language=en&pcode=tps00001&tableSelection=1&footnotes=yes&labeling=labels& plugin=1 (accessed August 6, 2010).

Faik, I., E. de Carvalho, and J. Kun. 2009. Parasite-host interaction in malaria: genetic clues and copy number variation. *Genome Medicine* 1(9):82.

Fanelli, D. 2010. Do pressures to publish increase scientists' bias? An empirical support from US states data. *PLoS ONE* 5(4): e10271. http://www.plosone.org/article/info%3Adoi% 2F10.1371%2Fjournal.pone.0010271;jsessionid=EB8BEAAC2BD41631E15776993436 B1B4.ambra01 (accessed August 3, 2010).

Farag-El-Massah, S., M. M. Braun, J. Cloyd, S. Schondelmeyer, K. Xu, M. Thomas, D. Lewis, and T. R. Coté. 2009. Quantitative description of FDA designated and approved orphan drugs and biologics. Poster presentation at annual meeting of the Drug Information Association, San Diego, CA. June 22.

Farmer, J. 2009. Accelerating rare diseases research and orphan product development: a FARA [Friedreich's Ataxia Research Alliance] perspective. Presentation to IOM Committee on Accelerating Rare Diseases Research and Orphan Product Development, Washington, DC. November 23.

Farrell, E., and J. Usuka. 2008. Pharmacogenomics and drug development: the impact of U.S. FDA postapproval tracking on clinical pharmacology. *Personalized Medicine* 5(2):133-139.

Faurisson, F. 2004. *EurordisCare2: Survey of Diagnostic Delays, 8 Diseases, Europe.* http:// archive.eurordis.org/imprimer.php3?id_article=454 (accessed August 6 2010).

FDA (Food and Drug Administration). 1996. *Guideline for Industry: The Need for Long-Term Rodent Carcinogenicity Studies of Pharmaceuticals.* http://www.fda.gov/down loads/Drugs/GuidanceComplianceRegulatoryInformation/Guidances/ucm074911.pdf (accessed August 6, 2010).

FDA. 2004. *Challenge and Opportunity on the Critical Path to New Medical Products.* http:// www.fda.gov/downloads/ScienceResearch/SpecialTopics/CriticalPathInitiative/Critical PathOpportunitiesReports/ucm113411.pdf (accessed September 24, 2010).

FDA. 2009a. *Fast Track, Accelerated Approval and Priority Review.* http://www.fda.gov/ForConsumers/ByAudience/ForPatientAdvocates/SpeedingAccesstoImportantNew Therapies/ucm128291.htm#priorityreview (accessed August 6, 2010).

FDA. 2009b. *Frequently Asked Questions About Therapeutic Biological Products.* http://www.fda.gov/Drugs/DevelopmentApprovalProcess/HowDrugsareDevelopedandApproved/ApprovalApplications/TherapeuticBiologicApplications/ucm113522.htm (accessed August 6, 2010).

FDA. 2009c. *Orphan Products: Hope for People with Rare Diseases.* http://www.fda.gov/Drugs/ResourcesForYou/Consumers/ucm143563.htm (accessed August 6, 2010).

FDA. 2009d. *The Critical Path Initiative: Report on Key Achievements in 2009.* http://www.fda.gov/downloads/ScienceResearch/SpecialTopics/CriticalPathInitiative/CriticalPath OpportunitiesReports/UCM219432.pdf (accessed August 9, 2010).

FDA. 2010a. *FDA Drug Safety Communication: Risk of Progressive Multifocal Leukoencephalopathy (PML) with the Use of Tysabri (Natalizumab).* http://www.fda.gov/Drugs/DrugSafety/PostmarketDrugSafetyInformationforPatientsandProviders/ucm199872.htm (accessed August 6, 2010).

FDA. 2010b. *FDA Transparency Initiative: Draft Proposals for Public Comment Regarding Disclosure Policies of the U.S. Food And Drug Administration.* http://www.fda.gov/downloads/AboutFDA/WhatWeDo/FDATransparencyTaskForce/TransparencyReport/GlossaryofAcronymsandAbbreviations/UCM212110.pdf (accessed August 6, 2010).

FDA. 2010c. *FY 2011 Food and Drug Administration Congressional Justification.* http://www.fda.gov/AboutFDA/ReportsManualsForms/Reports/BudgetReports/ucm202301.htm (accessed August 6, 2010).

FDA. Undated. *FY 2008 Performance Report to the President and the Congress for the Prescription Drug User Fee Act.* http://www.fda.gov/AboutFDA/ReportsManualsForms/Reports/UserFeeReports/PerformanceReports/PDUFA/ucm209305.htm (accessed August 6, 2010).

FDA Science Board. 2007. *FDA Science and Mission at Risk: Report of the Subcommittee on Science and Technology.* http://www.fda.gov/ohrms/DOCKETS/ac/07/briefing/2007-4329b_02_01_FDA%20Report%20on%20Science%20and%20Technology.pdf (accessed August 6, 2010).

Feigal, D. 2002. *CDRH vision—total product lifecycle* (slide). http://www.fda.gov/ohrms/dockets/ac/01/slides/3799s1_11_Feigal/sld002.htm (accessed August 6, 2010).

Feigal, D. W., S. N. Gardner, and M. McClellan. 2003. Ensuring safe and effective medical devices. *New England Journal of Medicine* 348(3):191-192.

Feinberg, A. P., and B. R. Williams. 2003. Wilms' tumor as a model for cancer biology. *Methods in Molecular Biology* 222:239-248.

Filipovich, A. H., J. Johnson, and K. Zhang. 2007. *WAS-Related Disorders.* http://www.ncbi.nlm.nih.gov/bookshelf/br.fcgi?book=gene&part=was (accessed September 7, 2010).

Fischer A., P. Borensztein, and C. Roussel. 2005. The European Rare Diseases Therapeutic Initiative. *PLoS Medicine* 2(9):e243. http://www.plosmedicine.org/article/info%3Adoi%2F10.1371%2Fjournal.pmed.0020243 (accessed August 6, 2010).

Fisher, W. O. 2002. Key disclosure issues for life sciences companies: FDA product approval, clinical test results, and government inspections. *Michigan Telecommunications and Technology Law Review* 8(115):115-193.

Flannery, E. J., and P. B. Hutt. 1985. Balancing competition and patent protection in the drug industry: The Drug Price Competition and Patent Term Restoration Act of 1984. *Food Drug Cosmetic Law Journal* 40:269-309.

Fleming, T. R. 2005. Surrogate endpoints and FDA's accelerated approval process. *Health Affairs* 24(1):67-78. http://content.healthaffairs.org/cgi/content/full/24/1/hits=10&FIRS TINDEX=0&ck=nck&FULLTEXT=surrogate+endpoints+and+FDA%27s+accelerated+ approval+process&SEARCHID=1&gca=healthaff%3B24%2F1%2F67&&eaf (accessed August 6, 2010).

FNIH (Foundation for the National Institutes of Health). 2010. *How We Work.* http://www. fnih.org/about/how-we-work (accessed August 20, 2010).

Forrest, C. B., S. C. Groft, R. J. Bartek, and Y. Rubinstein. 2010. The case for a global rare diseases registry. *Lancet,* published online August 2.

Fox, M. 2010. New collaboration aims to speed TB drugs to market. *Reuters.* March 18.

Frakt, A. B., and S. D. Pizer. 2009. Beneficiary price sensitivity in the Medicare prescription drug plan market. *Health Economics* 19(1):88-100.

Frank, R. G. 2007. The ongoing regulation of generic drugs. *New England Journal of Medicine* 357(20):1993-1996.

Frank, R. G., and J. P. Newhouse. 2008. Should drug prices be negotiated under part D of Medicare? and if so, how? *Health Affairs* 27(1):33-43.

Frank, R. G., and D. S. Salkever. 1997. Generic entry and the pricing of pharmaceuticals. *Journal of Economics and Management Strategy* 6(1):75-90.

Frohnmayer, D., and L. Frohnmayer. 2009. Fanconi Anemia Research Fund. Presentation (by phone) to the IOM Committee on Accelerating Rare Diseases Research and Orphan Product Development, Washington, DC. November 23.

Fugh-Berman, A., and D. Melnick. 2008 Off-label promotion, on-target sales. *Public Library of Science Medicine* 5(10):e210. http://www.plosmedicine.org/article/info: doi%2F10.1371%2Fjournal.pmed.0050210 (accessed August 6, 2010).

GAO (Government Accountability Office). 2009a. *New Drug Approval: FDA Needs to Enhance Its Oversight of Drugs Approved on the Basis of Surrogate Endpoints.* GAO-09-866. http://www.gao.gov/new.items/d09866.pdf (accessed August 6, 2010).

GAO. 2009b. Protecting public health through enhanced oversight of medical products. In *High Risk Series: An Update.* Report No. GAO 09-271. Washington, DC. Pp. 15-21.

GAO. 2010a. *Direct-to-Consumer Genetic Tests; Misleading Test Results Are Further Complicated by Deceptive Marketing and Other Questionable Practices: Testimony before the Subcommittee on Oversight and Investigations, Committee on Energy and Commerce, House of Representatives, July 22.* http://www.gao.gov/new.items/d10847t.pdf (accessed September 1, 2010).

GAO. 2010b. *Medicare Part D: Spending, Beneficiary Cost Sharing, and Cost-Containment Efforts for High-Cost Drugs Eligible for a Specialty Tier.* http://www.gao.gov/new.items/ d10242.pdf (accessed August 6, 2010).

Garnett, C. 2010. New undiagnosed diseases program awash in potential patients. *NIH Record* LXII(1). http://nihrecord.od.nih.gov/newsletters/2010/01_08_2010/story2.htm (accessed August 28, 2010).

Gartner, L. M., and F. R. Greer. 2003. Prevention of rickets and vitamin D deficiency: new guidelines for vitamin D intake. *Pediatrics* 111(4):908-910.

Gassman, O., G. Reepmeyer, and M. v. Zedtwitz. 2008. *Leading Pharmaceutical Innovation: Trends and Drivers for Growth in the Pharmaceutical Industry,* 2nd ed. New York: Springer.

Gelijns, A. C., B. Killelea, M. Vitale, V. Mankad, and A. Moskowitz. 2006. Appendix C: The dynamics of pediatric device innovation: putting evidence in context. In *Safe Medical Devices for Children.* Washington, DC: The National Academies Press. Pp. 302-326.

Genentech. 2010. *Herceptin Development Timeline.* http://www.gene.com/gene/products/ information/oncology/herceptin/timeline.html (accessed August 5, 2010).

Genetic Alliance. 2010. *Genetic Alliance Biobank Executive Summary.* http://www.biobank.org/english/view.asp?x=1364&id=76 (accessed August 5, 2010).

Genomeweb.com. 2010. CMS approves Iverson clinical study of genetic testing for Warfarin. *Genomeweb Daily News.* July 26.

Gessen, M. 2008. *Blood Matters: From Inherited Illness to Designer Babies, How the World and I Found Ourselves in the Future of the Gene.* Orlando, FL: Harcourt.

GHR (Genetics Home Reference). 2007. *Pulmonary Arterial Hypertension.* http://ghr.nlm.nih.gov/condition=pulmonaryarterialhypertension (accessed August 27, 2010).

Gibbs, J. N. 2010. Oversight of research use only products. *Genetic Engineering & Biotechnology News* 30(5).

Gillick, M. R. 2009. Controlling off-label medication use. *Annals of Internal Medicine* 150(5):344-347.

Glaser, C., F. Schuste, S.Yagi, S. Gavali, A. Bollen, C. Glastonbury, R. Raghavan, et al. 2008. Balamuthia amebic encephalitis—California, 1999-2007. *Morbidity and Mortality Weekly Report* 57(28):768-771. http://www.cdc.gov/mmwr/PDF/wk/mm5728.pdf (accessed August 5, 2010).

Gliklich, R. E., and N. A. Dreyer. 2007. *Registries for Evaluating Patient Outcomes: A User's Guide.* Outcome DEcIDE Center, AHRQ Publication Number 07-EHC001-1. http://www.effectivehealthcare.ahrq.gov/repFiles/PatOutcomes.pdf (accessed August 5, 2010).

Glover, G. J. 2007. The influence of market exclusivity on drug availability and medical innovations. *AAPS Journal* 9(3):34. http://www.aapsj.org/articles/aapsj0903/aapsj0903034/aapsj0903034.pdf (accessed August 20, 2010).

Goodman, J. L. 2010. *FDA's Efforts on Rare and Neglected Diseases: Statement to the Senate Appropriations Subcommittee on Agriculture, Rural Development, Food and Drug Administration, and Related Agencies.* Washington, DC. June 23. http://www.fda.gov/NewsEvents/Testimony/ucm216991.htm (accessed August 5, 2010).

Gordon, E. J., and S. Philpott. 2008. The convergence of research and clinical practice: institutional review board review of humanitarian use device applications. *Journal of Empirical Research on Human Research Ethics* 3(4):81-89.

Grabowski, G. A., and R. J. Hopkin. 2003. Enzyme therapy for lysosomal storage disease: principles, practice, and prospects. *Annual Review of Genomics and Human Genetics* 4:403-436. http://arjournals.annualreviews.org/doi/abs/10.1146/annurev.genom.4.070802.110415 (accessed September 7, 2010).

Grabowski, H. 2005. Encouraging the development of new vaccines. *Health Affairs* 24(3): 697-700.

Grabowski, H. G., and J. M. Vernon. 1992. Brand loyalty, entry, and price competition in pharmaceuticals after the 1984 Drug Act. *Journal of Law and Economics* 35(2):331.

Grant, B. 2008. The Orphan Drug Act turns 25. *The Scientist.com* 22(10):67.

Greenberg, B. D., D. A. Malone, G. M. Friehs, A. R. Rezai, C. S. Kubu, P. F. Malloy, S. P. Salloway, et al. 2006. Three-year outcomes in deep brain stimulation for highly resistant obsessive-compulsive disorder. *Neuropsychopharmacology* 31(11):2384-2393. http://www.nature.com/npp/journal/v31/n11/full/1301165a.html (accessed August 5, 2010).

Greibel, D. 2010. Memorandum to Julie Beitz, Director, Office of Drug Evaluation III, Center for Drug Evaluation and Research, FDA RE: Approval Action—NDA 022562. *Summary Review, NDA 022562 [Carbaglu/carglumic acid].* March 16. http://www.accessdata.fda.gov/drugsatfda_docs/nda/2010/022562s000sumr.pdf (accessed August 19, 2010).

Grenier, D., E. J. Elliott, Y. Zurynski, R. Rodrigues Pereira, M. Preece, R. Lynn, R. von Kries, et al. 2007. Beyond counting cases: public health impacts of national paediatric surveillance units. *Archives of Disease in* Childhood 92(6):527-533.

Guth, R. A. 2010. Glaxo tries a Linux approach: drug maker shares its research data online in test of open-source principles. *Wall Street Journal,* May 26. http://online.wsj.com/article/SB10001424052748703341904575266583403844888.html?mod=WSJ_hps_MIDDLE FifthNews (accessed August 5, 2010).

Habashi J. P., D. P. Judge, T. M. Holm, R. D. Cohn, B. L. Loeys, T. K. Cooper, L. Myers, et al. 2006. Losartan, an AT1 antagonist, prevents aortic aneurysm in a mouse model of Marfan syndrome. *Science* 312(5770):117-121.

Hacein-Bey-Abina, S., J. Hauer, A. Lim, C. Picard, G. P. Wang, C. C. Berry, C. Martinache, et al. 2010. Efficacy of gene therapy for X-linked severe combined immunodeficiency. *New England Journal of Medicine* 363(4):355-364.

Haffner, M. E. 1991. Orphan products: origins, progress, and prospects. *Annual Review of Pharmacology and Toxicology* 31:603-620.

Haffner, M. E. 2006. Adopting orphan drugs—two dozen years of treating rare diseases. *New England Journal of Medicine* 354(5):445-447.

Haffner, M. E., and P. D. Maher. 2006. The impact of the Orphan Drug Act on drug discovery. *Expert Opinion on Drug Discovery* 1(6):521-524.

Haffner, M. E., J. Torrent-Farnell, and P. D. Maher. 2008. Does orphan drug legislation really answer the needs of patients? *Lancet* 371:2041-2044.

Haigh, C. 2008. Gut-derived serotonin regulated bone formation. *Endocrine Today,* December 25. http://www.endocrinetoday.com/view.aspx?rid=33535 (accessed August 11, 2010).

Hamburg, M. A. 2009. *Remarks of Margaret A. Hamburg, M.D., Commissioner of Food and Drugs at AAAS—The Future of Personalized Medicine.* http://www.fda.gov/NewsEvents/Speeches/ucm191356.htm (accessed August 5, 2010).

Hamburg, M. A. 2010a. *Remarks of Margaret A. Hamburg, M.D., Commissioner of Food and Drugs at the Announcement of FDA/NIH Collaboration.* http://www.fda.gov/NewsEvents/Speeches/ucm201687.htm (accessed August 5, 2010).

Hamburg, M. A. 2010b. *Statement before the Subcommittee on Agriculture, Rural Redevelopment, Food and Drug Administration, and Related Agencies, U.S. Senate. March 9.* http://www.fda.gov/NewsEvents/Testimony/ucm204379.htm (accessed August 5, 2010).

Han, J. 2007. The optimal scope of FDA regulation of genetic tests: meeting challenges and keeping promises. *Harvard Journal of Law & Technology* 20(2):423-441.

Harris, G. 2010. FDA backtracks and returns drug to market. *New York Times,* September 3. http://www.nytimes.com/2010/09/04/health/policy/04fda.html (accessed September 9, 2010).

Harvey, W. 2006. Letter IX, to John Vlackveld (24 April 1657). In *The Circulation of the Blood.* New York: Cosimo. Pp. 200-201.

Heemstra, H. E., S. van Weely, H. A. Büller, H. G. M. Leufkens, and R. L. A. de Vrueh. 2009. Translation of rare disease research into orphan drug development: disease matters. *Drug Discovery Today* 14(23-24):1166-1173.

Hemsley, K. M., and J. J. Hopwood. 2009. Delivery of recombinant proteins via the cerebrospinal fluid as a therapy option for neurodegenerative lysosomal storage diseases. *International Journal of Clinical Pharmacology and Therapeutics* 47(Suppl 1):S118-123.

Hendee, W. R., S. Chien, C. D. Maynard, and D. J. Dean. 2002. The National Institute of Biomedical Imaging and Bioengineering: history, status, and potential impact. *Annals of Biomedical Engineering* 30:2-10.

Henig, R. M. 2009. What's wrong with Summer Stiers? *New York Times,* February 18. http://www.nytimes.com/2009/02/22/magazine/22Diseases-t.html (accessed August 5, 2010).

Henkel, J. 1999. Orphan Drug Law matures into medical mainstay. *FDA Consumer Magazine.*

Henney, J. 2000. Presentation to Mid-America Coalition on Health Care meeting on managing medical risk, Kansas City, MO. March 27. http://www.fda.gov/NewsEvents/Speeches/ucm054279.htm (accessed August 23, 2010).

Heresi, G. A., and R. A. Dweik. 2010. Biomarkers in pulmonary hypertension. *Pulmonary Vascular Research Institute Review* 2(1):12-16. http://www.pvrireview.org/article. asp?issn=0974-6013;year=2010;volume=2;issue=1;spage=12;epage=16;aulast=Heresi (accessed August 27, 2010).

Herper, M. 2010. The world's most expensive drugs. *Forbes.com*. http://www.forbes.com/2010/02/19/expensive-drugs-cost-business-healthcare-rare-diseases.html (accessed August 5, 2010).

Heubi, J. E., K. D. Setchell, and K. E. Bove. 2007. Inborn errors of bile acid metabolism. *Seminars in Liver Disease* 27(3):282-294.

High, K. A. 2009. The Jeremiah Metzger Lecture: gene therapy for inherited disorders: from Christmas disease to Leber's amaurosis. *Transactions of the American Clinical and Climatological Association* 120:331-359.

Hildebrandt, F., and W. Zhou. 2007. Nephronophthisis-associated ciliopathies. *Journal of the American Society of Nephrology* 18(6):1855-1871.

Hill, N. 2010. Spiration® experience with the humanitarian device exemption (HDE) process. Presentation to the IOM Committee on Accelerating Rare Diseases Research and Orphan Product Development, Washington, DC. February 4.

Hirschhorn, J. N. 2009. Genomewide association studies—illuminating biologic pathways. *New England Journal of Medicine* 360(17):1699-1701.

Hoffman, G. S. 2006. *WG or VF: What's in a Name?* http://www.vasculitisfoundation.org/node/1708.

Holahan, J., and I. Headen. 2010. *Medicaid Coverage and Spending in Health Reform: National and State by State Results for Adults At or Below 133% FPL*. http://www.kff.org/healthreform/upload/Medicaid-Coverage-and-Spending-in-Health-Reform-National-and-State-By-State-Results-for-Adults-at-or-Below-133-FPL.pdf (accessed August 5, 2010).

Hollaway, R. 2007. *Joe Is Not My Son. Alphas, Friends & Family*. http://www.alpha-1foundation.org/alphas/joe-is-not-my-son (accessed August 27, 2010).

Horner, M. D., and L. A. G. Ries. 2007. Leukemia (Chapter 29). In *SEER Survival Monograph: Cancer Survival Among Adults: U.S. SEER Program, 1988-2001, Patient and Tumor Characteristics*, edited by L. A. Ries, J. L. Young, G. E. Keel, M. P. Eisner, Y. D. Lin, and M. D. Horner. NIH Pub. No. 07-6215. National Cancer Institute: Bethesda, MD. http://seer.cancer.gov/publications/survival/surv_leukemia.pdf (accessed September 1, 2010).

Howell, R. R. 2005. *Letter to Michael Leavitt, Secretary, U.S. Department of Health and Human Services, RE: Recommendations to the Secretary of Health and Human Services from the Advisory Committee on Heritable Disorders in Newborns and Children*. September 9. http://www.hrsa.gov/heritabledisorderscommittee/correspondence/sep2005letter.htm (accessed August 19, 2010).

Huang, A., and G. Javitt. 2008. *FDA Regulation of Genetic Tests*. http://www.dnapolicy.org/images/issuebriefpdfs/FDA_Regulation_of_Genetic_Test_Issue_Brief.pdf (accessed August 5, 2010).

Hubacher, D. 2002. The checkered history and bright future of intrauterine contraception in the United States. *Perspectives on Sexual and Reproductive Health* 34(2):98-103.

Hunter, J., and S. Stephens. 2010. Is open innovation the way forward for big pharma? *Nature Reviews Drug Discovery* 9:87-88.

Hyde, J. 2006. Memorandum to Julie Beitz, Office of Drug Evaluation 3, Center for Drug Evaluation and Research, FDA, RE: Summary Supervisory Review of BLA/STN, 125151/0 [Elaprase] Idursulfase for Mucopolysaccharidosis Type II (Hunter Syndrome). Silver Spring, MD. July 24.

Hyman, S. E. 2008. A glimmer of light for neuropsychiatric disorders. *Nature* 455(7215): 890-893.

ICMJE (International Committee of Medical Journal Editors). 2009. *Uniform Requirements for Manuscripts Submitted to Biomedical Journals: Publishing and Editorial Issues Related to Publication in Biomedical Journals: Obligation to Register Clinical Trials.* http://www.icmje.org/publishing_10register.html (accessed August 13, 2010).

IFOPA (International Fibrodysplasia Ossificans Progressiva Association). 2009. *FOP FAQ.* http://www.ifopa.org/index.php?option=com_content&view=article&id=24&Itemid=156&lang=en (accessed August 5, 2010).

Imel, E. A., L. A. DiMeglio, S. L. Hui, T. O. Carpenter, and M. J. Econs. 2010. Treatment of X-linked hypophosphatemia with calcitriol and phosphate increases circulating fibroblast growth factor 23 concentrations. *Journal of Clinical Endocrinology and Metabolism* 95(4):1846-1850.

Interagency Task Force to the Secretary of Health, Education, and Welfare. 1979. *Significant Drugs of Limited Commercial Value.* Rockville, MD: Food and Drug Administration.

IOM (Institute of Medicine). 1991. *The Artificial Heart: Prototypes, Policies, and Patients.* Washington, DC: National Academy Press.

IOM. 2001. *Tuberculosis in the Workplace.* Washington, DC: National Academy Press.

IOM. 2004. *Improving Medical Education: Enhancing the Behavioral and Social Science Content of Medical School Curricula.* Washington, DC: The National Academies Press.

IOM. 2006. *Safe Medical Devices for Children*, edited by M. J. Field and H. Tilson. Washington, DC: The National Academies Press.

IOM. 2007. *Future of Disability in America.* Washington, DC: The National Academies Press.

IOM. 2008. *Breakthrough Business Models: Drug Development for Rare and Neglected Diseases and Individualized Therapies: Workshop Summary.* Washington, DC: The National Academies Press.

IOM. 2009a. *Preventing Mental, Emotional, and Behavioral Disorders Among Young People: Progress and Possibilities.* Washington, DC: The National Academies Press.

IOM. 2009b. *Venture Philanthropy Strategies to Support Translational Research. Workshop Summary.* Washington, DC: The National Academies Press.

IOM. 2010a. *Evaluation of Biomarkers and Surrogate Endpoints in Chronic Disease.* Washington, DC: The National Academies Press.

IOM. 2010b. *Extending the Spectrum of Precompetitive Collaboration in Oncology Research. Workshop Summary.* Washington, DC: The National Academies Press.

IOWH (Institute for OneWorld Health). 2004. *$42.6 Million Five-Year Grant From Gates Foundation for Antimalarial Drug Brings Together Unique Collaboration of Biotech, Academia and Nonprofit Pharma* (press release). December 13. http://www.oneworldhealth.org/documents/DP_%20Malaria%20Release%20121304.pdf (accessed September 7, 2010).

Iribarne, A. 2003. Orphan diseases and adoptive initiatives. *Journal of the American Medical Association* 290:116.

IRSF (International Rett Syndrome Foundation). 2008. *Rett Syndrome Research Landscape.* http://www.rettsyndrome.org/dmdocuments/IRSF_LANDSCAPE%20ANALYSIS_2008-1.pdf (accessed August 20, 2010).

Javitt, G. H. 2007. In search of a coherent framework: options for FDA oversight of genetic tests. *Food and Drug Law Journal* 62(4):617-652.

Johnston, J. J., J. K. Teer, P. F. Cherukuri, N. F. Hansen, S. K. Loftus, NIH Intramural Sequencing Center, K. Chong, et al. 2010. Massively parallel sequencing of exons on the x chromosome identifies rbm10 as the gene that causes a syndromic form of cleft palate. *American Journal of Human Genetics* 86(5):743-748.

Jones, J. A., F. G. Spinale, and J. S. Ikonomidis. 2009. Transforming growth factor-beta signaling in thoracic aortic aneurysm development: a paradox in pathogenesis. *Journal of Vascular Research* 46(2):119-137. http://www.ncbi.nlm.nih.gov/pmc/articles/PMC2645475/ (accessed August 11, 2010).

Jones, M. 2010. *FDA Joins NIH and EPA in Tox21 Effort. July 20.* http://www.genomeweb.com/fda-joins-nih-and-epa-tox21-effort (accessed August 20, 2010).

JPMA (Japan Pharmaceutical Manufacturers Association, E. R. I. T. F). 2008. Pharmaceutical administration and regulations in Japan. *Information in English on Japan Regulatory Affairs.* http://www.nihs.go.jp/mhlw/yakuji/yakuji-e0808.pdf (accessed August 5, 2010).

Justice, R. 2007. *Approval Letter to Bayer Pharmaceuticals Corporation for New or Modified Indication Application Number 021923 [Nexavarto].* Rockville, MD. November 16. http://www.accessdata.fda.gov/drugsatfda_docs/appletter/2007/021923s004,s005,s006,s007.pdf (accessed August 19, 2010).

Kaback, M., J. Lim-Steele, D. Dabholkar, D. Brown, N. Levy, K. Zeiger, and the International TSD Data Collection Network. 1993. Tay-Sachs disease—carrier screening, prenatal diagnosis, and the molecular era: an international perspective, 1970 to 1993. *Journal of the American Medical Association* 270(19):2307-2315.

Kakkis, E. 2010. Accelerating development of treatments for rare diseases. Presentation to IOM Committee on Accelerating Rare Diseases Research and Orphan Product Development, Washington, DC. February 4.

Kaplan, A. V., D. S. Baim, J. J. Smith, D. A. Feigal, M. Simons, D. Jefferys, T. J. Fogarty, et al. 2004. Medical device development: from prototype to regulatory approval. *Circulation* 109(25):3068-3072.

Kaplan, A. V., E. D. Harvey, R. E. Kuntz, H. Shiran, J. F. Robb, and P. Fitzgerald. 2005. Humanitarian use devices/humanitarian device exemptions in cardiovascular medicine. *Circulation* 112(18):2883-2886.

Karst, K. R. 2009a. Outstanding Pre-FDAAA Citizen Petition Causes FDA to Rule Against 180-Day Exclusivity Forfeiture for Generic Skelaxin. http://www.fdalawblog.net/fda_law_blog_hyman_phelps/2010/05/outstanding-prefdaaa-citizen-petition-causes-fda-to-rule-against-180day-exclusivity-forfeiture-for-g.html (accessed August 5 2010).

Karst, K. R. 2009b. The rarely used "cost recovery" path to orphan drug designation and approval. *FDA Law Blog.* http://www.fdalawblog.net/fda_law_blog_hyman_phelps/2009/02/the-rarely-used-cost-recovery-path-to-orphan-drug-designation-and-approval.html (accessed July 15, 2010).

Karst, K. R. 2009c. The unusual case of the "MC-to-PC" orphan drug designation/approval. *FDA Law Blog.* http://www.fdalawblog.net/fda_law_blog_hyman_phelps/2009/01/the-unusual-case-of-the-mctopc-orphan-drug-designationapproval-.html (accessed August 5, 2010).

Karst, K. R. 2010. FDA issues NOOH proposing to withdraw all midodrine HCl approvals. *FDA Law Blog.* http://www.fdalawblog.net/fda_law_blog_hyman_phelps/2010/08/fda-issues-nooh-proposing-to-withdraw-all-mididrine-hcl-approvals.html (accessed September 1, 2010).

Kay, M. A., C. N. Landen, S. R. Rothenberg, L. A. Taylor, F. Leland, S. Wiehle, B. Fang, et al. 1994. In vivo hepatic gene therapy: complete albeit transient correction of factor IX deficiency in hemophilia B dogs. *Proceedings of the National Academy of Sciences* 91(6):2353-2357.

Kelley, S. L. 2009. MMRF and MMRC collaborative research model for a rare disease. Presentation on behalf of the Multiple Myeloma Research Foundation and the Multiple Myeloma Research Consortium to the IOM Committee on Accelerating Rare Diseases Research and Orphan Product Development, Washington, DC. November 23.

Kelly, A. M., B. Kratz, M. Bielski, and P. M. Rinehart. 2002. Implementing transitions for youth with complex chronic conditions using the medical home model. *Pediatrics* 110(6):1322-1327.

Kelly, P. F., S. Radtke, C. Von Kalle, B. Balcik, K. Bohn, R. Mueller, T. Schuesler, et al. 2007. Stem cell collection and gene transfer in Fanconi anemia. *Molecular Therapy* 15(1):211-219.

Kesselheim, A. S., and M. M. Mello. 2010. Gene patenting—is the pendulum swinging back? *New England Journal of Medicine* 362(20):1855-1858.

Kesselheim, A. S., and D. H. Solomon. 2010. Incentives for drug development—the curious case of colchicine. *New England Journal of Medicine* 362(22):2045-2047.

KFF (Kaiser Family Foundation). 2008. *[Medicaid] Benefits by Service: Prescription Drugs (October 2008)*. http://medicaidbenefits.kff.org/service.jsp?gr=off&nt=on&so=0&tg=0&yr=4&cat=5&sv=32 (accessed August 5, 2010).

KFF. 2009a. *Fact Sheet: Medicare Advantage*. http://www.kff.org/medicare/upload/2052-13.pdf (accessed August 5, 2010).

KFF. 2009b. *Fact Sheet: The Medicare Prescription Drug Benefit*. http://www.kff.org/medicare/upload/7044-10.pdf (accessed August 5, 2010).

KFF. 2009c. *Employer Health Benefits: 2009 Annual Survey*. http://ehbs.kff.org/pdf/2009/7936.pdf (accessed August 5, 2010).

KFF. 2009d. *Medicare Part D 2010 Data Spotlight: Benefit Design and Cost Sharing*. http://www.kff.org/medicare/upload/8033.pdf (accessed August 5, 2010).

KFF-SHF (Kaiser Family Foundation, statehealthfacts.org). 2010. *Health Insurance Coverage of Nonelderly 0-64, States (2007-2008), U.S. (2008)*. http://www.statehealthfacts.org/comparetable.jsp?ind=126&cat=3 (accessed August 5, 2010).

Kleta, R., and W. A. Gahl. 2004. Pharmacological treatment of nephropathic cystinosis with cysteamine. *Expert Opinion on Pharmacotherapy* 5(11):2255-2262.

Kocs, D., and A. M. Fendrick. 2003. Effect of off-label use of oncology drugs on pharmaceutical costs: the rituximab experience. *American Journal of Managed Care* 9(5):393-400.

Kramer, D. L. B., E. Mallis, B. D. Zuckerman, B. A. Zimmerman, and W. H. Maisel. 2010. Premarket clinical evaluation of novel cardiovascular devices: quality analysis of premarket clinical studies submitted to the Food and Drug Administration 2000-2007. *American Journal of Therapeutics* 17(1):2-7.

Kuehn, B. M. 2010. Strategy reveals rare disease genes. *Journal of the American Medical Association* 303(24):2463.

Lacro, R. V., H. C. Gietz, L. M. Wruck, T. J. Bradley, S. D. Colan, R. B. Devereux, G. L. Klein, et al. 2007. Rationale and design of a randomized clinical trial of beta-blocker therapy (atenolol) versus angiotensin II receptor blocker therapy (losartan) in individuals with Marfan syndrome. *American Heart Journal* 154(4):624-631.

Laessig, K. 2009. Presentation at Division of Anti-infective Drugs Advisory Committee Meeting, Washington, DC. December 10. http://www.fda.gov/downloads/Advisory Committees/CommitteesMeetingMaterials/Drugs/Anti-InfectiveDrugsAdvisoryCommittee/UCM197009.pdf (accessed August 5, 2010).

Lai, K., M. Tang, X. Yin, H. Klapper, K. Wierenga, and L. J. Elsas. 2008. ARHI: a new target of galactose toxicity in classic galactosemia. *Bioscience Hypotheses* 1(5):263-271.

LeBowitz, J. H. 2005. A breach in the blood-brain barrier. *Proceedings of the National Academy of Sciences* 102(41):14485-14486. http://www.pnas.org/content/102/41/14485.full%5d.

LeMasurier, J. D., and B. Edgar. 2009. MIPPA: first broad changes to Medicare Part D Plan operations. *American Health & Drug Benefits* 2(3):111-118. http://www.ahdbonline.com/docs/april_09/LeMasurier_AprilMay09.pdf (accessed August 5, 2010).

Lerner, B. H. 2009. When diseases disappear: the case of familial dysautonomia. *New England Journal of Medicine* 361(17):1622-1625.

Lewis, D. 2010. Rare diseases update. Presentation to IOM Committee on Accelerating Rare Diseases Research and Orphan Product Development, Washington, DC. February 4.

LGDA (Lymphangiomatosis & Gorham's Disease Alliance). 2009. *About Gorham's Disease.* http://lgdalliance.org/en/aboutGorhamsDisease/Default.aspx (accessed August 5, 2010).

Li, Y., K. Brockmann, F. Turecek, C. R. Scott, and M. H. Gelb. 2004. Tandem mass spectrometry for the direct assay of enzymes in dried blood spots: application to newborn screening for Krabbe disease. *Clinical Chemistry* 50(3):638-640.

Library of Congress. 1994. *Country Studies: Japan.* http://memory.loc.gov/frd/cs/jptoc.html (accessed August 5, 2010).

Lifton, R. P. 2010. Individual genomes on the horizon. *New England Journal of Medicine* 362(13):1235-1236.

Lifton R. P., A. G. Gharavi, and D. S. Geller. 2001. Molecular mechanisms of human hypertension. *Cell* 104(4):545-556.

Lim-Melia, E. R., and D. F. Kronn. 2009. Current enzyme replacement therapy for the treatment of lysosomal storage diseases. *Pediatric Annals* 38(8):448-455.

Linehan, J. H., M. E. Paté-Cornell, P. G. Yock, and J. B. Pietzsch. 2007. *Study on Medical Device Development Models Final Report.* Stanford, CA: Stanford University.

Liu L., M. Krailo, G. H. Reaman, and L. Bernstein. 2003. Childhood cancer patients' access to cooperative group cancer programs: a population-based study. *Cancer* 97:1339-1345.

Llovet, J. M., S. Ricci, V. Mazzaferro, P. Hilgard, E. Gane, J.-F. Blanc, and A. C. de Oliveira. 2008. Sorafenib in advanced hepatocellular carcinoma. *New England Journal of Medicine* 359(4):378-390.

Lloyd, C. 2004. Letter to Carol Benson, Center for Devices and Radiological Health RE: de nova classification of NeoGram Amino Acids and Acylcarnitines Tandem Mass Spectrometry Kit, Model MS-8970. *Dockets Management, Docket # 2004P-0419.* June 30. http://www.fda.gov/ohrms/dockets/dailys/04/sep04/091404/04p-0419-cp00001-vol1.pdf (accessed August 19, 2010).

Long, F. 2008. When the gut talks to bone. *Cell* 135(5):795-796.

Lu, M., D. Z. Vasavada, and C. Tanner. 2009. Lemierre syndrome following oropharyngeal infection: a case series. *Journal of the American Board of Family Medicine* 22(1):79-83.

Lupski, J. R., J. G. Reid, C. Gonzaga-Jauregui, D. Rio Deiros, D. C. Y. Chen, L. Nazareth, M. Bainbridge, et al. 2010. Whole-genome sequencing in a patient with Charcot-Marie-Tooth neuropathy. *New England Journal of Medicine* 362(13):1181-1191.

Madsen, C. A. 2004. Herceptin (Trastuzumab) a real world example of pharmacogenomics—maximizing patient benefit. *WeSRCH Medtech.* July 29. http://medical.wesrch.com/pdf ME1XXFF7UAXKL (accessed September 22, 2010).

Maegawa, G. H. B., and R. D. Steiner. In press. Treating genetic disorders. In *Medical Genetics and Pediatric Practice: A Handbook,* edited by R. A. Saul. Elk Grove Village, IL: American Academy of Pediatrics.

Maestri, N. E., and T. H. Beaty. 1992. Predictions of a 2-locus model for disease heterogeneity: application to adrenoleukodystrophy. *American Journal of Medical Genetics* 44(5):576-582.

Maher, E. R., L. Iselius, J. R. Yates, M. Littler, C. Benjamin, R. Harris, J. Sampson, et al. 1991. Von Hippel-Lindau disease: a genetic study. *Journal of Medical Genetics* 28:443-447.

Majumdar, S. R. 2009. Cost sharing and the initiation of drug therapy for the chronically ill—invited commentary. *Archives of Internal Medicine* 169(8):748-749.

Maloney, P. 2010. Laboratory regulation under the Clinical Laboratory Improvement Amendments of 1988 and state laws. In *In Vitro Diagnostics: The Complete Regulatory Guide*, edited by S. D. Danzis and E. J. Flannery. Washington, DC: The Food and Drug Law Institute.

Manning, E., S. Pham, S. Li, R. I. Vazquez-Padron, J. Mathew, P. Ruiz, and S. K. Salgar. 2010. Interleukin-10 delivery via mesenchymal stem cells: a novel gene therapy approach to prevent lung ischemia-reperfusion injury. *Human Gene Therapy* 21(6):713-727.

Mansfield, E., and Ž. Težak. 2010. FDA regulation of genetic testing. In *In Vitro Diagnostics: The Complete Regulatory Guide*, edited by S. D. Danzis and E. J. Flannery. Washington, DC: The Food and Drug Law Institute.

March of Dimes. 2010. *Fact Sheet: Newborn Screening*. http://www.marchofdimes.com/professionals/14332_1200.asp (accessed August 5, 2010).

Marcus, A. D. 2010a. My data, your data, our data. *Wall Street Journal*, April 13. http://online.wsj.com/article/SB10001424052748703625304575116512173339800.html#printMode (accessed August 5, 2010).

Marcus, A. D. 2010b. NIH takes on new role in fight against rare diseases. *Wall Street Journal*, July 24. http://online.wsj.com/article/NA_WSJ_PUB:SB10001424052748704249004575 385363395104490.html#articleTabs%3Darticle (accessed August 20, 2010).

Marcus, A. D. 2010c. Push to cure rare diseases. *Wall Street Journal*, March 10. http://www.kgi.edu/Documents/In_the_news/FDA%20Pushes%20for%20Cures%20for%20Rare%20Diseases.pdf (accessed August 27, 2010).

Maron, B. J., and N. A. M. Estes. 2010. Commotio cordis. *New England Journal of Medicine* 362(10):917-927.

Maschke, K. J. 2009. Disputes over research with residual newborn screening blood specimens. *Hastings Center Report* 40(2).

Masiello, S. A., and J. S. Epstein. 2003. Correction Letter to Stephen Arnon, Senior Director, Regulatory Affairs, Cato Research, Inc. for October 23, 2003, Approval letter BabyBIG. December 9. http://www.fda.gov/BiologicsBloodVaccines/BloodBloodProducts/ApprovedProducts/LicensedProductsBLAs/FractionatedPlasmaProducts/ucm117164.htm (accessed August 19, 2010).

McCabe, M. T., J. C. Brandes, and P. M. Vertino. 2009. Cancer DNA methylation: molecular mechanisms and clinical implications. *Clinical Cancer Research* 15:3927-3937.

McCarty, M., and K. Young. 2007. FDA to push ahead with assay guidance despite opposition. In *Advances in Diagnostics & Imaging* 2:15-19. http://www.medicaldevicedaily.com/img/S07414SamplePages.pdf (accessed August 5, 2010).

Medline Plus. 2008. *Beriberi*. July 12. http://www.nlm.nih.gov/medlineplus/ency/article/000339.htm (accessed August 5, 2010).

MedPAC (Medicare Payment Advisory Commission). 2007. *Report to the Congress: Impact of Changes in Medicare Payments for Part B Drugs*. http://www.medpac.gov/documents/Jan07_PartB_mandated_report.pdf (accessed August 5, 2010).

MedPAC. 2008. *Outpatient Hospital Services Payment System*. http://www.medpac.gov/documents/MedPAC_Payment_Basics_08_OPD.pdf (accessed August 5, 2010).

MedPAC. 2009. Medicare payment systems and follow-on biologics. *Report to the Congress: Improving Incentives in the Medicare Program*. http://www.medpac.gov/chapters/Jun09_Ch05.pdf (accessed August 5, 2010).

MedPAC. 2010a. Chapter 5: Status report on Part D. In *Report to the Congress: Medicare Payment Policy*. http://www.medpac.gov/chapters/Mar10_Ch05.pdf (accessed August 5, 2010).

MedPAC. 2010b. Chapter 2: Improving traditional Medicare's benefit design. In *Report to the Congress: Aligning Incentives in Medicare*. http://www.medpac.gov/chapters/Jun10_Ch02.pdf (accessed August 5, 2010).

Medtronic, Inc. 2009. *Melody® Transcatheter Pulmonary Valve Ensemble® Transcatheter Valve Delivery System.* http://wwwp.medtronic.com/Newsroom/LinkedItemDetails. do?itemId=1260978939170&itemType=fact_sheet&lang=en_US (accessed August 5, 2010).

Medtronic, Inc. 2010. First Publication of Data from Pivotal Clinical Trial for Medtronic Deep Brain Stimulation Therapy for Epilepsy Published Today in Epilepsia. http://wwwp. medtronic.com/Newsroom/NewsReleaseDetails.do?itemId=1268914059828 (accessed August 5, 2010).

Mehta, S., T. G. Myers, J. H. Lonner, G. R. Huffman, and B. J. Sennett. 2007. The ethics of sham surgery in clinical orthopaedic research. *Journal of Bone and Joint Surgery* 89(7):1650-1653.

Melese, T., S. M. Lin, J. L. Chang, and N. H. Cohen. 2009. Open innovation networks between academia and industry: an imperative for breakthrough therapies. *Nature Medicine* 15:502-507.

Merkens, L. S., C. Wassif, K. Healy, A. S. Pappu, A. E. DeBarber, J. A. Penfield, R. A. Lindsay, et al. 2009. Smith-Lemli-Opitz syndrome and inborn errors of cholesterol synthesis: summary of the 2007 SLOS/RSH foundation scientific conference sponsored by the National Institutes of Health. *Genetic Medicine* 11(5):359-364.

Meyers, A., and M. L. Di Paola. 2003. The orphan medicinal products: an international challenge. *Minerva Biotechnologica.* http://www.rarediseases.org/news/images/minerva_ biotech_orphmed_article_11504.jpg (accessed August 5, 2010).

Mikhail, I. S. 2005. Design issues in the study of rare cancers. Presented at the 2nd NCI Epidemiology Leadership Workshop: Understudied Rare Cancers, Boston, MA. http:// epi.grants.cancer.gov/documents/Conference2/slides/Mikhail.pdf (accessed September 1, 2010).

Miller, F. G. 2003. Sham surgery: an ethical analysis. *American Journal of Bioethics* 3(4): 41-48.

Milne, C. P. 2002. Orphan products—pain relief for clinical development headaches. *Nature Biotechnology* 20(8):780-784.

Mingozzi, F., and K. A. High. 2009. Gateway to the diseased brain. *Nature Medicine* 15:1123-1124. http://www.nature.com/nm/journal/v15/n10/abs/nm1009-1123.html (accessed August 12, 2010).

Mitka, M. 2009. Off-label cancer drug compendia found outdated and incomplete. *Journal of the American Medical Association* 301(16):1645-1646.

Mitsumoto, J., E. R. Dorsey, C. A. Beck, K. Kieburtz, and R. C. Griggs. 2009. Pivotal studies of orphan drugs approved for neurological diseases. *Annals of Neurology* 66(2):184-190.

Mizrachi, I. 2007. GenBank: The Nucleotide Sequence Database. In *The NCBI Handbook*, edited by J. McEntyre and J. Ostell. http://www.ncbi.nlm.nih.gov/bookshelf/br.fcgi? book=handbook&part=ch1 (accessed August 22, 2010).

MMF (Minnesota Medical Foundation). 2007. *Setting the Pace: What Do You Get When You Combine a Heart Surgeon and an Electrical Engineer?* http://www.mmf.umn.edu/bulletin/2007/fall/lookback/index.cfm (accessed August 5, 2010).

MMV (Medicines for Malaria Venture). 2002. *Annual Report.* http://www.mmv.org/news room/publications/annual-report-2002 (accessed August 5, 2010).

MMV. 2003. *Annual Report.* http://www.mmv.org/newsroom/publications/annual-report-2003 (accessed August 5, 2010).

Monroe, C. D., L. Potter, M. Millares, A. Barrueta, and R. Wagner. 2006. Kaiser Permanente's evaluation and management of biotech drugs: assessing, measuring, and affecting use. *Health Affairs* 25(5):1340-1346.

Moore, J. H., and M. D. Ritchie. 2004. The challenges of whole-genome approaches to common diseases. *Journal of the American Medical Association* 291(13):1642-1643.

Moran, M. 2005. A breakthrough in R&D for neglected diseases: new ways to get the drugs we need. *PLoS Medicine* 2(9):e302. http://www.ncbi.nlm.nih.gov/pmc/articles/PMC1198042/ (accessed December 1, 2010).

Moran, M., Ropars A-L., Guzman J., Diaz J., and Garrison C. 2004. *The New Landscape of Neglected Disease Drug Development*. The Wellcome Trust and London School of Economics and Political Sciences. London: The Wellcome Trust Publications Department.

Morel, C. M. 2000. Reaching maturity—25 years of the TDR. *Parasitology Today* 16(12):522-528.

Moseley, J. B., K. O'Malley, N. J. Petersen, T. J. Menke, B. A. Brody, D. H. Kuykendall, J. C. Hollingsworth, et al. 2002. A controlled trial of arthroscopic surgery for osteoarthritis of the knee. *New England Journal of Medicine* 347(2):81-88.

Moser, A. B., S. J. Steinberg, and G. V. Raymond. 2009. X-linked adrenoleukodystrophy. *Gene Reviews*. http://www.ncbi.nlm.nih.gov/bookshelf/br.fcgi?book=gene&part=x-ald (accessed August 5, 2010).

Mossinghoff, G. J. 1999. Overview of the Hatch-Waxman Act and its impact on the drug development process. *Food and Drug Law Journal* 54(2):187-194.

Moyer, V. A., N. Calonge, S. M. Teutsch, and J. R. Botkin. 2008. Expanding newborn screening: process, policy, and priorities. *Hastings Center Report* 38(3):32-39.

MRF (Myelin Research Foundation). 2010. *Comparisons Between ARC vs. Traditional Research*. http://www.myelinrepair.org/research_model/arc_vs_traditional_research.shtml (accessed August 5, 2010).

Munos, B. 2009. Lessons from 60 years of pharmaceutical innovation. *Nature Reviews Drug Discovery* 8(12):959-968.

Munos, B. 2010. Can open-source drug R&D repower pharmaceutical innovation? *Clinical Pharmacology and Therapeutics* 87:534-536.

Nathan, D. 2009. Musings on genome medicine: enzyme-replacement therapy of the lysosomal storage diseases. *Genome Medicine* 1(114).

Nathan, D. G., and S. H. Orkin. 2009. Musings on genome medicine: gene therapy. *Genome Medicine* 1(38).

NAS (National Academy of Sciences). 2003. *Materials and Society: From Research to Manufacturing—Report of a Workshop*. Washington, DC: The National Academies Press.

NCCAM (National Center for Complementary and Alternative Medicine). 2008. *Milk Thistle*. http://nccam.nih.gov/health/milkthistle/ataglance.htm (accessed August 5, 2010).

NCBI (National Center for Biotechnology Information). 2009. *GENETests: Growth of Laboratory Directory*. http://www.ncbi.nlm.nih.gov/projects/GeneTests/static/whatsnew/labdirgrowth.shtml (accessed August 4, 2010).

NCBI. 2010. *Questions and Answers: Genetic Testing Registry*. http://www.ncbi.nlm.nih.gov/gtr/qa/ (accessed August 4, 2010).

NCI (National Cancer Institute). 2009a. *Adult Brain Tumors Treatment (PDQ®)*. http://www.cancer.gov/cancertopics/pdq/treatment/adultbrain/HealthProfessional/page10 (accessed August 5, 2010).

NCI. 2009b. *States That Require Health Plans to Cover Patient Care Costs in Clinical Trials*. http://www.cancer.gov/clinicaltrials/developments/laws-about-clinical-trial-costs (accessed August 5, 2010).

NCI. 2009c. *Table 1.4: Age-Adjusted SEER Incidence and U.S. Death Rates and 5-Year Relative Survival Rates by Primary Cancer Site, Sex and Time Period*. http://www.seer.cancer.gov/csr/1975_2006/results_merged/topic_survival.pdf (accessed August 5, 2010).

NCOD (National Commission on Orphan Diseases). 1989. *Report of the National Commission on Orphan Diseases*. Rockville, MD: Public Health Service, U.S. Department of Health and Human Services.

NDRI (National Disease Research Interchange). 2003. *The Genetics of Rare Disease: Window to Common Disorders* (conference). Washington, DC. March 23.

NDRI. 2010. *NDRI Initiatives: Rare Diseases.* http://www.ndriresource.org/NDRI_Initiatives/Rare_Disease/30/ (accessed August 4, 2010).

Neschadim, A., J. A. McCart, A. Keating, and J. A. Medin. 2007. A roadmap to safe, efficient, and stable lentivirus-medicated gene therapy with hematopoietic cell transplantation. *Biology of Blood and Marrow Transplantation* 13(12):1407-1416.

Newhouse, J. P., and the Insurance Experiment Group. 1993. *Free for All? Lessons from the RAND Health Insurance Experiment.* Cambridge, MA: Harvard University Press.

Ng, S. B., K. J. Buckingham, C. Lee, A. W. Bigham, H. K. Tabor, K. M. Dent, C. D. Huff, et al. 2009. Exome sequencing identifies the cause of a Mendelian disorder. *Nature Genetics* 42(1):30-35.

NHGRI (National Human Genome Research Institute). 2009. *Learning About Gaucher Disease.* http://www.genome.gov/25521505 (accessed August 4, 2010).

NHLBI (National Heart, Lung, and Blood Institute). 2000. *Expert Panel Review of the NHLBI Total Artificial Heart (TAH) Program June 1998-November 1999.* http://www.nhlbi.nih.gov/resources/docs/tahrpt.pdf (accessed August 4, 2010).

NHLBI. 2008a. *NHLBI Working Group Report: Computational Models for Analyzing Genotype-Phenotype Associations in Rare Diseases.* http://www.nhlbi.nih.gov/meetings/workshops/gpa_rarediseases.htm (accessed August 4, 2010).

NHLBI. 2008b. *What Is LAM?* http://www.nhlbi.nih.gov/health/dci/Diseases/lam/lam_all.html (accessed August 4, 2010).

NHLBI. 2009. *What Is Aplastic Anemia?* http://www.nhlbi.nih.gov/health/dci/Diseases/aplastic/aplastic_whatis.html (accessed August 4, 2010).

NHLBI. 2010. *Sickle Cell Disease Awareness and Education Strategy Development Workshop Report.* http://www.nhlbi.nih.gov/meetings/workshops/Sickle_Cell_Disease_Workshop.pdf (accessed August 20, 2010).

NIAMS (National Institute of Arthritis and Musculoskeletal and Skin Diseases). 2010. *Polymyalgia Rheumatica and Giant Cell Arteritis.* http://www.niams.nih.gov/Health_Info/Polymyalgia/default.asp (accessed August 4, 2010).

NIBIB (National Institute of Biomedical Imaging and Bioengineering). 2009. *About NIBIB: Mission & History.* http://www.nibib.nih.gov/About/MissionHistory (accessed August 4, 2010).

NICHD (National Institute of Child Health and Human Development). 2009. *NIH Newborn Screening Research Program Named in Memory of Hunter Kelly.* http://www.nichd.nih.gov/news/releases/101909-Hunter-Kelly.cfm (accessed August 4, 2010).

NIH (National Institutes of Health). 2002. *Report on Steps to Coordinate Rare Diseases Research Programs.* http://rarediseases.info.nih.gov/Wrapper.aspx?src=asp/html/reports/fy1999/SEP.html (accessed October 11, 2010).

NIH. 2003. *Final NIH statement on sharing research data. Notice NOT-OD-03-032.* February 26. http://grants.nih.gov/grants/guide/notice-files/NOT-OD-03-032.html (accessed August 24, 2010).

NIH. 2007. *NIH Policy Manual: 1167—Public-Private Partnerships.* September 25. http://oma.od.nih.gov/manualchapters/management/1167/ (accessed August 20, 2010).

NIH. 2008. *Nocardia Infection.* http://www.nlm.nih.gov/medlineplus/ency/article/000679.htm (accessed August 4, 2010).

NIH. 2009a. *NIH Announces Expansion of Rare Diseases Clinical Research Network.* http://www.nih.gov/news/health/oct2009/od-05.htm (accessed August 4, 2010).

NIH. 2009b. *NIH Announces New Program to Develop Therapeutics for Rare and Neglected Diseases.* http://rarediseases.info.nih.gov/files/TRND%20Press%20Release.pdf (accessed August 4, 2010).

NIH. 2010a. *The Cancer Genome Atlas Identifies Distinct Subtypes of Deadly Brain Cancer That May Lead to New Treatment Strategies* (news release). http://cancergenome.nih.gov/media/glioblastoma4subtypes.asp (accessed August 4, 2010).

NIH. 2010b. *Advancing Regulatory Science Through Novel Research and Science-Based Technologies (U01). Request for Applications Number: RFA-RM-10-006.* http://grants.nih.gov/grants/guide/rfa-files/RFA-RM-10-006.html (accessed August 4, 2010).

Nijsten, T., and P. R. Bergstresser. 2010. Patient advocacy groups: let's stick together. *Journal of Investigative Dermatology* 130(7):1757-1759. http://www.nature.com/jid/journal/v130/n7/pdf/jid2010131a.pdf (accessed September 8, 2010).

NNSGRC (National Newborn Screening and Genetics Resource Center). 2010. *National Newborn Screening Status Report.* http://genes-r-us.uthscsa.edu/nbsdisorders.pdf (accessed August 4, 2010).

NORD (National Organization for Rare Disorders). 2003. *NORD Guide to Rare Disorders.* Philadelphia, PA: Lippincott Williams & Wilkins.

NORD. 2007. *Testimony Before the Social Security Administration Public Hearing on Compassionate Allowances. Washington, DC. December 4.* http://www.ssa.gov/compassionateallowances/NORDTestimonyCompassionateAllowances120407.pdf (accessed August 4, 2010).

NORD. 2010. *NORD Reports Progress in Appropriations Bill.* http://www.rarediseases.org/news/Appropriations_Progress (accessed August 4, 2010).

NRC (National Research Council). 2000. *Bioinformatics: Converting Data to Knowledge: Workshop Summary.* Washington, DC: National Academy Press.

NRC. 2006. *Reaping the Benefits of Genomic and Proteomic Research: Intellectual Property Rights, Innovation and Public Health.* Washington, DC: The National Academies Press.

NRC. 2007. *The New Science of Metagenomics: Revealing the Secrets of Our Microbial Planet.* Washington, DC: The National Academies Press.

NRC. 2009. *A New Biology for the 21st Century: Ensuring the United States Leads the Coming Biology Revolution.* Washington, DC: The National Academies Press.

NTP (National Toxicology Program). 2004. *Technical Report on the Toxicology and Carcinogenesis Studies of Elmiron.* http://ntp.niehs.nih.gov/ntp/htdocs/LT_rpts/tr512.pdf (accessed August 13, 2010).

Nussbaum, R. L., R. R. McInnes, and H. F. Willard. 2004. *Thompson & Thompson Genetics in Medicine, 7th Edition.* Philadelphia, PA: W.B. Saunders Company.

Nutt, B. 2007. *From the Other Side of the Stethoscope.* http://www.thelamfoundation.org/patients/living-with-lam/patient-storiesAll.html/#Nutt (accessed August 4, 2010).

Nwaka, S., and R. G. Ridley. 2003. Virtual drug discovery and development for neglected diseases through public-private partnerships. *Nature Reviews Drug Discovery* 2:919-928.

Öfverholm, A., E. Arkblad, S. Skrtic, P. Albertsson, E. Shubbar, and C. Enerbäck. 2010. Two cases of 5-fluorouracil toxicity linked with gene variants in the DPYD gene. *Clinical Biochemistry* 43(3):331-334.

OHRP (Office of Human Research Protections). 2008. *OHRP Research Involving Children Frequently Asked Questions.* http://www.hhs.gov/ohrp/researchfaq.html (accessed August 4, 2010).

OIG (Office of the Inspector General, DHHS). 2001a. *Medicare Hospital Prospective Payment System: How DRG Rates Are Calculated and Updated.* http://oig.hhs.gov/oei/reports/oei-09-00-00200.pdf (accessed August 4, 2010).

OIG. 2001b. *The Orphan Drug Act Implementation and Impact.* http://oig.hhs.gov/oei/reports/oei-09-00-00380.pdf (accessed August 4, 2010).

OIG. Undated. *Rare Diseases and Related Terms.* http://rarediseases.info.nih.gov/RareDiseaseList.aspx (accessed August 4, 2010).

OOPD (Office of Orphan Product Development, FDA). 2009. *Recipients of the FY09 Pediatric Device Consortia Grant Program Awards.* http://www.fda.gov/ForIndustry/Developing ProductsforRareDiseasesConditions/WhomtoContactaboutOrphanProductDevelopment/ ucm184125.htm (accessed August 4, 2010).

OOPD. 2010. *New Resource for Drug Developers: The Rare Disease Repurposing Database (RDRD).* http://www.fda.gov/ForIndustry/DevelopingProductsforRareDiseasesCondi tions/HowtoapplyforOrphanProductDesignation/ucm216147.htm (accessed September 24, 2010).

ORDR (Office of Rare Diseases Research, NIH). 2009. *Office of Rare Diseases Research (ORDR) Brochure.* http://rarediseases.info.nih.gov/Wrapper.aspx?src=asp/resources/ord_ brochure.html (accessed August 4, 2010).

Orphanet. 2009. *Prevalence of Rare Diseases.* Orphanet Report Series, No. 1, November. http://www.orpha.net/orphacom/cahiers/docs/GB/Prevalence_of_rare_diseases_by_alpha betical_list.pdf (this link is to a more recent version of the report than was used by the committee).

Orphanet. Undated a. *About Orphanet: Mission.* http://www.orpha.net/consor/cgi-bin/ Education_AboutOrphanet.php?lng=EN (accessed August 4, 2010).

Orphanet. Undated b. *About Rare Diseases.* http://www.orpha.net/consor/cgi-bin/Education_ AboutRareDiseases.php?lng=EN (accessed August 4, 2010).

Outterson, K., and A. S. Kesselheim. 2009. How Medicare could get better prices on prescrip- tion drugs. *Health Affairs* 28(5):w832-841.

Pannicke, U., M. Honig, I. Hess, C. Friesen, K. Holzmann, E. M. Rump, T. F. Barth, et al. 2009. Reticular dysgenesis (aleukocytosis) is caused by mutations in the gene encoding mitochondrial adenylate kinase 2. *Nature Genetics* 41(1):101-105.

Pariser, A. 2010. FDA regulation and review of small clinical trials. Presentation to IOM Committee on Accelerating Rare Diseases Research and Orphan Product Development, Washington, DC. February 4.

Patel, C. J., J. Bhattacharya, and A. J. Butte. 2010. An environment-wide association study (EWAS) on type 2 diabetes mellitus. *Public Library of Science ONE* 5(5):e10746.

Patterson, M. 2008. *Niemann-Pick Disease Type C.* http://www.ncbi.nlm.nih.gov/bookshelf/ br.fcgi?book=gene&part=npc (accessed August 3, 2010).

Pfizer. 2010. *Pfizer Prepares for Voluntary Withdrawal of U.S. New Drug Application and for Discontinuation of Commercial Availability of Mylotarg®* (press release). http:// media.pfizer.com/files/news/press_releases/2010/mylotarg_discontinuation_062110.pdf (accessed August 3, 2010).

Pharmaceutical Forum, E.C. 2008. Improving access to orphan medicines for all affected EU citizens. *Reference Document 3 in High Level Pharmaceutical Forum 2005-2008 Final Report.* http://ec.europa.eu/pharmaforum/docs/pricing_orphans_en.pdf (accessed August 3, 2010).

PhRMA (Pharmaceutical Research and Manufacturers of America). 2007. *Drug Discovery and Development: Understanding the R & D Process.* Washington, DC. http://www.phrma. org/files/attachments/RD%20Brochure%20022307.pdf (accessed August 27, 2010).

Pietzsch, J. B., L. A. Shluzas, M. E. Paté-Cornell, P. G. Yock, and J. H. Linehan. 2009. Stage- gate process for the development of medical devices. *Journal of Medical Devices* 3(2).

Pion, G., and M. Ionescu-Pioggia. 2003. Bridging postdoctoral training and a faculty position: initial outcomes of the Burroughs Wellcome Fund Career Awards in the Biomedical Sci- ences. *Academic Medicine* 78(2):177-186.

PMC (Personalized Medicine Coalition). 2009. *Comments on Development of Companion Diagnostics and the April 2005 Food and Drug Administration ("FDA") Drug-Diagnostic Co-development Concept Paper.* December 9. http://www.personalizedmedicinecoalition.org/sites/default/files/files/FDA%20CoDevelopment%20FINAL%20Version%20PDF.pdf (accessed August 4, 2010)

Pober, B. R. 2010. Williams-Beuren syndrome. *New England Journal of Medicine* 362(3): 239-252.

Pollack, A. 2008. Cutting dosage of costly drug spurs a debate. *New York Times*, March 16.

Pollack, A. 2009. Pfizer deal signals a move into treating rare diseases. *New York Times*, December 2. http://query.nytimes.com/gst/fullpage.html?res=9C0DE5D8153BF931A35751C1A96F9C8B63&sec=&spon=&pagewanted=print (accessed August 3, 2010).

Pollack, A. 2010. After gene patent is invalidated, taking stock. *New York Times*, March 30. http://www.nytimes.com/2010/03/31/business/31gene.html (accessed August 20, 2010).

PRF (Progeria Research Foundation). 2008. *The Progeria Research Foundation Timeline.* http://progeriaresearch.org/assets/files/pdf/Timeline%20Nov%202007.pdf (accessed August 3, 2010).

Prosser, L. A., C. Y. Kong, D. Rusinak, and S. L. Waisbren. 2010. Projected costs, risks, and benefits of expanded newborn screening for MCADD. *Pediatrics* 125:e286-e294.

Q1Medicare.com. 2009. *PDP—Facts: 2010 Medicare Part D Plan Statistics—Region (State) and National.* http://www.q1medicare.com/PartD-MedicarePartDPlanStatisticsState.php?crit=National (accessed August 3, 2010).

Radcliffe, S. 2009. BIO (Biotechnology Industry Organization). Statement to IOM Committee on Accelerating Rare Diseases Research and Orphan Product Development, Washington, DC. November 23. http://www.bio.org/reg/20091123.pdf (accessed August 2, 2010).

Radley, D. C., S. N. Finkelstein, and R. S. Stafford. 2006. Off-label prescribing among office-based physicians. *Archives of Internal Medicine* 166(9):1021-1026.

Rai, A. K., J. H. Reichman, P. F. Uhlir, and C. Crossman. 2008. Pathways across the valley of death: novel intellectual property strategies for accelerated drug discovery. *Yale Journal of Health Policy, Law, and Ethics* VIII(I):52-89. http://scholarship.law.duke.edu/cgi/viewcontent.cgi?article=2329&context=faculty_scholarship (accessed August 3, 2010).

Rappaport, B. 2010. Division director summary basis for recommendation of approval action. *Summary Review, Application Number 125338 [Xiaflex].* February 1. http://www.accessdata.fda.gov/drugsatfda_docs/nda/2010/125338s000SumR.pdf (accessed August 3, 2010).

Ray, T. 2010. *FDA Chief Commits to Completing Rx/Dx Codevelopment Guidance This Year, Improving Regulatory Science.* http://www.genomeweb.com/dxpgx/fda-chief-commits-completing-rxdx-codevelopment-guidance-year-improving-regulato (accessed August 3, 2010).

RegenceRx. 2010. *Off-Label Use of FDA-Approved Drugs.* http://blue.regence.com/trgmedpol/drugs/dru031.pdf (accessed August 3, 2010).

Reich, M. R. 2000. The global drug gap. *Science* 287(5460):1979-1981.

Reichert, J. M., C. J. Rosensweig, L. B. Faden, and M. C. Dewitz. 2005. Monoclonal antibody successes in the clinic. *Nature Biotechnology* 23:1073-1078.

Reiffen, D., and M. R. Ward. 2005. Generic drug industry dynamics. *Review of Economics and Statistics* 87(1):37-49.

Richey, E. A., E. A. Lyons, J. R. Nebeker, V. Shankaran, J. M. McKoy, T. H. Luu, N. Nonzee, et al. 2009. Accelerated approval of cancer drugs: improved access to therapeutic breakthroughs or early release of unsafe and ineffective drugs? *Journal of Clinical Oncology* 27(26):4398-4405.

Ridley, D. 2009. *Business of Drug Discovery.* http://gspp.berkeley.edu/iths/RDStrategies/lecture4.ppt#425,1,Business of Drug Discovery (accessed August 3, 2010).

Ridley, R. G. 2002. Medical need, scientific opportunity and the drive for antimalarial drugs. *Nature* 415(6872):686-693.

Ridley, R. G. 2003. Product R&D for neglected diseases. Twenty-seven years of WHO/TDR experiences with public-private partnerships. *EMBO Reports*. Spec No: S43-46. http://www.ncbi.nlm.nih.gov/pmc/articles/PMC1326445/pdf/4-embor858.pdf (accessed August 3, 2010).

Rinaldi, A. 2005. Adopting an orphan. *EMBO Reports* 6(6):507-510.

Riordan J. R., J. M. Rommens, B. Kerem, N. Alon, R. Rozmahel, Z. Grzelczak, J. Zielenski, et al. 1989. Identification of the cystic fibrosis gene: cloning and characterization of complementary DNA. *Science* 245(4922):1066-1073.

Roach, J. C., G. Glusman, A. F. Smit, C. D. Huff, R. Hubley, P. T. Shannon, L. Rowen, et al. 2010. Analysis of genetic inheritance in a family quartet by whole-genome sequencing. *Science*. http://www.sciencemag.org/cgi/rapidpdf/science.1186802v1.pdf (accessed August 3, 2010).

Roca, R. 2009. Summary review for regulatory action. *Summary Review, Application Number 22-352 [Colcrys / colchicine]*. July 30. http://www.accessdata.fda.gov/drugsatfda_docs/nda/2009/022352s000_SumR.pdf (accessed August 19, 2010).

Rockoff, R. D. 2010. An old gout drug gets new life and a new price, riling patients. *Wall Street Journal*, April 12. http://online.wsj.com/article/NA_WSJ_PUB:SB1000142405274 8703630404575053303739829726.html (accessed August 27, 2010).

Rosebraugh, C. 2010. *Approval Letter to Auxilium Pharmaceuticals, Inc. for BLA 125338/0 [Xiaflex]*. February 2. http://www.accessdata.fda.gov/drugsatfda_docs/appletter/2010/125338s000ltr.pdf (accessed August 20, 2010).

Rosecrans, H. 2010. Understanding the premarket notification (510(k)) process. Presentation at Public Health Effectiveness of the FDA 510(k) Clearance Process, Washington, DC. February 18.

Rosenberg, H., M. Davis, D. James, N. Pollock, and K. Stowell. 2007. Malignant hyperthermia. *Orphanet Journal of Rare Diseases* 2(1):21.

Rosenstein, B. J., and G. R. Cutting. 1998. The diagnosis of cystic fibrosis: a consensus statement. Cystic Fibrosis Foundation Consensus Panel. *Journal of Pediatrics* 132(4):589-595.

Rubinstein, Y. R., S. C. Groft, R. Barteck, K. Brown, R. A. Christensen, E. Collier, A. Farber, et al. 2010. Creating a global rare disease patient registry linked to a rare diseases biorepository database: Rare Disease-HUB (RD-HUB). *Contemporary Clinical Trials* 31(5):394-404.

SACGHS (Secretary's Advisory Committee on Genetics, Health, and Society). 2008. *U.S. System of Oversight of Genetic Testing*. http://oba.od.nih.gov/oba/SACGHS/reports/SACGHS_oversight_report.pdf (accessed August 3, 2010).

Sands, S. 2010. IFib. *Living with DMD*. May 19. http://dmdpioneers.org/home/living-with-dmd/ifib (accessed August 20, 2010).

Sardiello, M. P., A. di Ronza, D. L. Medina, M. Valenza, V. A. Gennarino, C. D. Malta, F. Donaudy, et al. 2009. A gene network regulating lysosomal biogenesis and function. *Science* 325(5939):473-477.

Sasinowski, F. 2010. Statement of the National Organization for Rare Disorders (NORD) at the U.S. Food and Drug Administration Part 15 Public Hearing: Considerations Regarding FDA Review and Regulation of Articles for the Treatment of Rare Disease. Silver Spring, MD, June 29. http://www.rarediseases.org/files/NORD-statement-FDA-hearing-06-29-10.pdf (accessed August 3, 2010).

Sauer M., S. Grewal, and C. Peters. 2004. Hematopoietic stem cell transplantation for mucopolysaccharidoses and leukodystrophies. *Klinische Pädiatrie* 216:163-168.

Sawyers, C. L. 2010. Even better kinase inhibitors for chronic myeloid leukemia. *New England Journal of Medicine* 362:2314-2315.

Schact, W. H. 2007. *The Bayh-Dole Act: Selected Issues in Patent Policy and the Commercialization of Technology*. Congressional Research Service Report RL32076. http://fpc.state.gov/documents/organization/96463.pdf (accessed September 2, 2010).

Schact, W. H., and J. R. Thomas. 2009. *Follow-on Biologics: Intellectual Property and Innovation Issues*. Congressional Research Service Report RL33901. http://assets.opencrs.com/rpts/RL33901_20090803.pdf (accessed August 3, 2010).

Schadt, E. E., A. Sachs, and S. Friend. 2005a. Embracing complexity, inching closer to reality. *Science Signaling* 295:pe40.

Schadt, E. E., J. Lamb, X. Yang, J. Zhu, S. Edwards, D. Guhathakurta, S. K. Sieberts, et al. 2005b. An integrative genomics approach to infer causal associations between gene expression and disease. *Nature Genetics* 37(7):710-717.

Scheinberg, I. H., and J. M. Walshe. 1986. *Orphan Diseases and Orphan Drugs*. Manchester, UK: Manchester University Press.

Schickedanz, A. D., and R. D. Herdman. 2009. Direct-to-consumer genetic testing: the need to get retail genomics right. *Clinical Pharmacology and Therapeutics* 86(1):17-20.

Schimke, R. N., D. L. Collins, and C. A. Stolle. 2009. *Von Hippel-Lindau Syndrome*. http://www.ncbi.nlm.nih.gov/bookshelf/br.fcgi?book=gene&part=vhl#vhl.grID1694 (accessed August 3, 2010).

Schmitz, J., L. W. Poll, and S. vom Dahl. 2007. Therapy of adult Gaucher disease. *Haematologica* 92(2):148-152.

Schofield, P. N., T. Bubela, T. Weaver, L. Portilla, S. D. Brown, J. M. Hancock, D. Einhorn, et al. 2009. Post-publication sharing of data and tools. *Nature* 461:171-173.

Schulte, F., and D. Donovan. 2007. Drug earning millions despite "orphan" label: Status granted before law increased use of "bupe." *Baltimore Sun*.

Schultz, D. 2008. FDA public health notification: life-threatening complications associated with recombinant human bone morphogenetic protein in cervical spine fusion. *FDA, Alerts and Notices (Medical Devices)*. July 1. http://www.fda.gov/MedicalDevices/Safety/AlertsandNotices/PublicHealthNotifications/UCM062000 (accessed August 12, 2010).

Scriver, C. R., and P. J. Lee. 2004. The last day of the past is the first day of the future: transitional care for genetic patients. *American Journal of Medicine* 117(8):615-617.

Scriver, C. R., and E. P. Treacy. 1999. Is there treatment for "genetic" disease? *Molecular Genetics and Metabolism* 68(2):93-102.

Segal, J. B., J. J. Strouse, M. C. Beach, C. Haywood, C. Witkop, H. Park, R. F. Wilson, et al. 2008. *Evidence Report/Technology Assessment: Hydroxyurea for the Treatment of Sickle Cell Disease*. AHRQ Publication No. 08-E007. http://www.ahrq.gov/downloads/pub/evidence/pdf/hydroxyurea/hydroxscd.pdf (accessed August 3, 2010).

Seoane-Vazquez, E., R. Rodriguez-Monguio, S. L. Szeinbach, and J. Visaria. 2008. Incentives for orphan drug research and development in the United States. *Orphanet Journal of Rare Diseases* 3(33). http://www.ojrd.com/content/pdf/1750-1172-3-33.pdf (accessed August 3, 2010).

Shah, R. R. 2006. Regulatory framework for the treatment of orphan diseases. In *Fabry Disease: Perspectives from 5 Years of FOS*, edited by A. Mehta, M. Beck, and G. Sunder-Plassmann. Oxford, UK: Oxford PharmaGenesis. http://www.ncbi.nlm.nih.gov/bookshelf/br.fcgi?book=fabry&part=A745 (accessed August 3, 2010).

Sing, C. F., J. H. Stengard, and S. L. R. Kardia. 2003. Genes, environment, and cardiovascular disease. *Arteriosclerosis, Thrombosis, and Vascular Biology* 23(7):1190-1196.

Smith, V. K., K. Gifford, E. Ellis, R. Rudowitz, M. O. M. Watts, and C. Marks. 2009. *The Crunch Continues: Medicaid Spending, Coverage and Policy in the Midst of a Recession*. http://www.kff.org/medicaid/upload/7985.pdf (accessed August 3, 2010).

Smits, P., A. D. Bolton, V. Funari, M. Hong, E. D. Boyden, L. Lu, D. K. Manning, et al. 2010. Lethal skeletal dysplasia in mice and humans lacking the golgin GMAP-210. *New England Journal of Medicine* 362(3):206-216.

So, A. D., and E. Stewart. 2009. Appendix F: Sharing knowledge for global health. In *The U.S. Commitment to Global Health: Recommendations for the Public and Private Sectors.* Institute of Medicine. Washington, DC: The National Academies Press. http://www.ncbi. nlm.nih.gov/bookshelf/br.fcgi?book=nap12642&part=a2001902dddd00191#a2001902d nnn00053 (accessed August 24, 2010).

Solomon, M. D., D. P. Goldman, G. F. Joyce, and J. J. Escarce. 2009. Cost sharing and the initiation of drug therapy for the chronically ill. *Archives of Internal Medicine* 169(8):740-748.

Sotos, J. G. 1989. *Zebra Cards: An Aid to Obscure Diagnoses.* Philadelphia, PA: American College of Physicians.

Sox, H. C. 2009. Evaluating off-label uses of anticancer drugs: time for a change. *Annals of Internal Medicine* 150(5):353-354.

Spiration, Inc. 2009. *CMS Approves New Technology Add-on Payment for Spiration® IBV Valve System (press release). August 3.* http://www.spiration.com/downloads/NTAPPress ReleaseFinal.pdf (accessed August 3, 2010).

SSA (Social Security Administration). 2010a. *Compassionate Allowances.* http://www.social security.gov/compassionateallowances/ (accessed August 3, 2010).

SSA. 2010b. *Medicare.* http://www.ssa.gov/pubs/10043.pdf (accessed August 3, 2010).

Statistics Bureau (Japan). 2008. *Statistical Handbook of Japan: Chapter 2 Population.* http:// www.stat.go.jp/english/data/handbook/c02cont.htm (accessed August 3, 2010).

Stein, R. 2010. FDA considers revoking approval of Avastin for advanced breast cancer. *Washington Post,* August 16. http://www.washingtonpost.com/wp-dyn/content/article/ 2010/08/15/AR2010081503466.html (accessed September 1, 2010).

Stein, S., M. G. Ott, S. Schultze-Strasser, A. Jauch, B. Burwinkel, A. Kinner, M. Schmidt, et al. 2010. Genomic instability and myelodysplasia with monosomy 7 consequent to EVI1 activation after gene therapy for chronic granulomatous disease. *Nature Medicine* 16(2):198-204. E-pub January 24.

Steinberg, K. K., M. E. Cogswell, J. C. Chang, S. P. Caudill, G. M. McQuillan, B. A. Bowman, L. M. Grummer-Strawn, et al. 2001. Prevalence of C282Y and H63D mutations in the hemochromatosis (*HFE*) gene in the United States. *Journal of the American Medical Association* 285:2216-2222.

Steiner, R. 2009. *Sitosterolemia. March 26.* http://emedicine.medscape.com/article/948892- overview (accessed August 3, 2010).

Steiner R. D., S. L. Huhn, T. Koch, A. Al-Uzri, G. Guillaume, T. Sutcliffe, H. Vogel, and N. Selden. 2009. CNS transplantation of purified human neural stem cells in infantile and late-infantile neuronal ceroid lipofuscinoses: summary of the Phase I trial. Abstracts for the 11th International Congress of Inborn Errors of Metabolism. *Molecular Genetics and Metabolism* 98(1-2):76 (A422).

Stoffels, P. 2009. Collaborative innovation for the post-crisis world. *Boston Globe,* February 2. http://www.boston.com/bostonglobe/editorial_opinion/oped/articles/2009/02/02/ collaborative_innovation_for_the_post_crisis_world?mode=PF (accessed August 3, 2010).

Stossel, T. P. 2008. The discovery of statins. *Cell* 134(6): 903-905. http://download.cell.com/ pdf/PIIS0092867408011276.pdf?intermediate=true (accessed August 11, 2010).

Stratman, R. C., J. D. Flynn, and K. W. Hatton. 2009. Malignant hyperthermia: a pharmaco-genetic disorder. *Orthopedics* 32:835.

Straube, B. M. 2009. Update: CMS and genetic applications in health care. Presentation to SACGHS Meeting, Washington, DC. March 12. http://oba.od.nih.gov/oba/SACGHS/ meetings/March2009/Straube_slides.pdf (accessed August 3, 2010).

Sung, N. S., W. F. Crowley, Jr., M. Genel, P. Salber, L. Sandy, L. M. Sherwood, S. B. Johnson, et al. 2003. Central challenges facing the national clinical research enterprise. *Journal of the American Medical Association* 289(10):1278-1287.

Suthram, S., J. T. Dudley, A. P. Chiang, R. Chen, T. J. Hastie, and A. J. Butte. 2010. Network-based elucidation of human disease similarities reveals common functional modules enriched for pluripotent drug targets. *PLoS Computational Biology* 6(2): e1000662. http://www.ploscompbiol.org/article/info%3Adoi%2F10.1371%2Fjournal. pcbi.1000662 (accessed August 3, 2010).

Suzuki, M., K. Wlers, E. B. Brooks, K. D. Grels, K. Halnes, M. S. Klein-Gittleman, J. Olson, et al. 2009. Initial validation of a novel protein biomarker for active pediatric lupus nephritis. *Pediatric Research* 65(5):530-536.

Swann, J. P. 2003. The history of the FDA. In *The Food and Drug Administration*, edited by M. A. Hickman. Hauppauge, NY: Nova Science Publishers.

Swanson, J. 2009. Companion diagnostics take off. *Genome Technology.* http://www.genome web.com/dxpgx/companion-diagnostics-take (accessed August 3, 2010).

Tabor, H. K., and M. Bamshad. 2010. Exome sequencing and rare diseases. Presentation to IOM Committee on Accelerating Rare Diseases Research and Orphan Product Development, Washington, DC. February 4.

TDR (Special Programme for Research and Training in Tropical Diseases). 2008. BL3—drug discovery on fast track says expert advisors. *TDRnews.* May. http://apps.who.int/tdr/svc/ publications/tdrnews/issue-80/drug-discovery-fast-track (accessed August 20, 2010).

Tejada, P. 2009. *Towards an International Standard of Coding and Classification of Rare Diseases.* http://archive.eurordis.org/imprimer.php3?id_article=2014 (accessed August 3, 2010).

Terry, S. F. 2009. Written statement for Subcommittee on Agriculture, Rural Development, Food and Drug Administration, and Related Agencies, U.S. House of Representatives, March 18. http://www.geneticalliance.org/statements.terry (accessed August 3, 2010).

Terry, S. F. 2010. Accelerate medical breakthroughs by ending disease earmarks. *Nature Reviews Genetics* 11:310-311.

Thaul, S. 2008. *FDA Fast Track and Priority Review Programs.* Congressional Research Service RS22814 (http://nationalaglawcenter.org/assets/crs/RS22814.pdf) (accessed August 27, 2010).

Therrell, B., F. Lorey, R. Eaton, D. Frazier, G. Hoffman, C. Boyle, D. Green, et al. 2008. Impact of expanded newborn screening. *Morbidity and Mortality Weekly Report* 57(37):1012-1015. http://www.cdc.gov/mmwr/preview/mmwrhtml/mm5737a2.htm (accessed August 3, 2010).

Thomson, G., N. Marthandan, J. A. Hollenbach, S. J. Mack, H. A. Erlich, R. M. Single, M. J. Waller, et al. 2010. Sequence feature variant type (sfvt) analysis of the *hla* genetic association in juvenile idiopathic arthritis. *Pacific Symposium on Biocomputing* 15:359-370.

Tillman, D. B. 2010. Approval letter for Medtronic Melody® Transcatheter Pulmonary Valve and Medtronic Ensemble® Transcatheter Valve Delivery System (H080002). January 25. http://www.accessdata.fda.gov/cdrh_docs/pdf8/H080002a.pdf (accessed August 19, 2010).

Tillman, D. B., and S. Gardner. 2004. Letter to Institute of Medicine committee on postmarket surveillance of pediatric medical devices, September 27. As cited in *Safe Medical Devices for Children.* 2006. Washington, DC: The National Academies Press.

Tollefson, L. 2008. *Letter to Donald M. Poretz, President, Infectious Diseases Society of America Concerning the Orphan Drug Act,* October 15. http://www.hivma.org/ WorkArea/DownloadAsset.aspx?id=16139 (accessed August 24, 2010).

Torreele, E., M. Usdin, and P. Chirac. 2004. A needs-based pharmaceutical R&D agenda for neglected diseases. Paper prepared for the *WHO Commission on Intellectual Property Rights, Innovation and Public Health*. Version 31. July. http://www.who.int/intellectual property/topics/research/Needs%20based%20R&D%20for%20neglected%20diseases%20Els%20Pierre%20Martine.pdf (accessed September 7, 2010).

Trafton, A. 2010. Revolutionizing medicine one chip at a time. *MIT News*, March 9.

Travis, J. 2008. Science by the masses. *Science* 319(5871):1750-1752.

Trikalinos, T. A., M. Chung, J. Lau, and S. Ip. 2009. Systematic review of screening for bilirubin encephalopathy in neonates. *Pediatrics* 124(4):1162-1171.

Tse, T., R. J. Williams, and D. A. Zarin. 2009. Reporting "basic results" in ClinicalTrials.gov. *Chest* 136(1):295-303.

Tufts Center for the Study of Drug Development. 2010. U.S. orphan product designations more than doubled from 2000-02 to 2006-08. *Impact Report* 12(1).

Ulatowski, T. 2009. *Warning Letter to William Birdsall, Chief Executive Officer, MicroMed Technology, Inc. RE: DeBakey VAD Child.* http://www.fda.gov/ICECI/Enforcement Actions/WarningLetters/ucm195995.htm (accessed August 19, 2010).

Unger, E. F., A. M. Thompson, M. J. Blank, and R. Temple. 2010. Erythropoiesis-stimulating agents—time for a reevaluation. *New England Journal of Medicine* 362(3):189-192.

UNOS (United Network for Organ Sharing). 2010. *Financing a Transplant*. http://www.transplantliving.org/beforethetransplant/finance/costs.aspx (accessed August 3, 2010).

U.S. Census Bureau. 2001. *Monthly Estimates of the United States Population: April 1, 1980 to July 1, 1999, with Short-Term Projections to November 1, 2000.* http://www.census.gov/population/estimates/nation/intfile1-1.txt (accessed August 3, 2010).

U.S. Census Bureau. 2009. *Annual Estimates of the Resident Population for the United States, Regions, States, and Puerto Rico: April 1, 2000 to July 1, 2009 (NST-EST2009-01). Washington, DC.* http://www.census.gov/popest/states/tables/NST-EST2009-01.xls (accessed August 3, 2010).

U.S. Congress, Senate Committee on Appropriations. 2008. *Report on S. 1710 Departments of Labor, Health and Human Services, and Education, and Related Agencies Appropriation Bill.* Washington, DC.

UTHSCSA (University of Texas Health Science Center San Antonio). 2004. *Titanium Rib Becomes 1st New FDA-Approved Spine Deformity Treatment in 40 Years (press release).* http://www.uthscsa.edu/hscnews/singleformat2.asp?newID=1148 (accessed August 3, 2010).

Valeo, T. 2010. New molecule found to cross the blood-brain barrier: reported safe for patients with progressive glioma. *Neurology Today* 10(1):12-13. http://journals.lww.com/neurotodayonline/Fulltext/2010/01070/New_Molecule_Found_to_Cross_the_Blood_Brain.8.aspx (accessed August 3, 2010).

Van Eyk, J. E. 2010. Development of biomarkers. Presentation to IOM Committee on Accelerating Rare Diseases Research and Orphan Product Development, Washington, DC. February 4.

VCRC (Vasculitis Clinical Research Consortium). 2010. *What Is the VCRC?* http://rarediseases network.epi.usf.edu/vcrc/about/index.htm (accessed August 3, 2010).

Villa, S., A. Compagni, and M. R. Reich. 2008. Orphan drug legislation: lessons for neglected tropical diseases. *International Journal of Health Planning and Management.* http://www.wcfia.harvard.edu/sites/default/files/Reich_Orphan.pdf (accessed August 3, 2010).

Villarreal, M. A. 2001. *Orphan Drug Act: Background and Proposed Legislation in the 107th Congress.* Congressional Research Service Report RS20971. http://www.policyarchive.org/handle/10207/bitstreams/3490.pdf (accessed August 3, 2010).

Vodovotz, Y., M. Csete, J. Bartels, S. Chang, and G. An. 2008. Translational systems biology of inflammation. *Public Library of Science Journal Computational Biology* 4(4).

Wade, N. 2010. Disease cause is pinpointed with genome. *New York Times.* http://www.nytimes.com/2010/03/11/health/research/11gene.html (accessed August 3, 2010).

Wagner, J. A., M. Prince, E. C. Wright, M. M. Ennis, J. Kochan, D. J. R. Nunez, B. Schneider, et al. 2010. The biomarkers consortium: practice and pitfalls of open-source precompetitive collaboration. *Clinical Pharmacology and Therapeutics* 87:539-542.

Walpoth, B. H., and G. L. Bowlin. 2005. The daunting quest for a small diameter vascular graft. *Expert Review of Medical Devices* 2(6):647-651.

Wang, D., T. Wood, M. Sadilek, C. R. Scott, F. Turecek, and M. H. Gelb. 2007. Tandem mass spectrometry for the direct assay of enzymes in dried blood spots: application to newborn screening for mucopolysaccharidosis II (Hunter disease). *Clinical Chemistry* 53:137-140.

Wang, S. S. 2010. Drug makers will share data from failed Alzheimer's trials. *Wall Street Journal,* June 11. http://online.wsj.com/article/SB1000142405274870362770457529878
83153884208.html (accessed August 3, 2010).

Wasserstein, J. N., and K. R. Karst. 2007. *Orphan Drug Designation Not Sacrosanct—FDA Revokes Orphan Designation for TheraCLEC for EPI, but Other Exclusivity Issues Remain. July 11.* http://www.fdalawblog.net/fda_law_blog_hyman_phelps/2007/07/fda-revokes-alt.html (accessed August 3, 2010).

Watson, M. S., Marie Y. Mann, M. A. Lloyd-Puryear, P. Rinaldo, and R. R. Howell. 2006. Newborn screening: toward a uniform screening panel and system. *Genetics in Medicine* 8(5).

Waxman, H. J. Undated. *Orphan Drugs.* http://waxman.house.gov/IssueList/Internal/orphan drugs.htm (accessed August 3, 2010)

Wechsler, J. 2008. Orphan drug R&D challenges sponsors. *Applied Clinical Trials.* http://appliedclinicaltrialsonline.findpharma.com/appliedclinicaltrials/Articles/Orphan-Drug-RampD-Challenges-Sponsors/ArticleStandard/Article/detail/527733 (accessed August 3, 2010).

Weiss, K. D. 2005. *Approval Letter to BioMarin Pharmaceutical, Incorporated for BLA* 125117 [Galsulfase / Naglazyme]. May 31. http://www.accessdata.fda.gov/drugsatfda_docs/appletter/2005/125117_0000_ltr.pdf (accessed August 23, 2010).

Wellman-Labadie, O., and Y. Zhou. 2009. The U.S. Orphan Drug Act: rare disease research stimulator or commercial opportunity? *Health Policy* 95(2-3):216-228.

Wellmark Blue Cross Blue Shield. 2009. *Humanitarian Use Devices: Medical Policy 10.01.14.* http://www.wellmark.com/Provider/MedPoliciesAndAuthorizations/MedicalPolicies/Policies/Humanitarian_Use_Devices.aspx (accessed August 3, 2010).

Wellmark Blue Cross Blue Shield. 2010. *Off-label Drug Use (Medical Policy).* http://wwwprep.wellmark.com/Provider/MedPoliciesAndAuthorizations/MedicalPolicies/policies/_Off-label_Drug_UsePrinterFriendly.aspx (accessed August 3, 2010).

Whalen, J. 2009. Novartis shifts focus to rare diseases. *Wall Street Journal,* December 21.

WHO (World Health Organization). 2009a. *Global Tuberculosis Control, Epidemiology.* http://www.who.int/tb/publications/global_report/2009/pdf/chapter1.pdf (accessed August 3, 2010).

WHO. 2009b. *Leishmaniasis: Burden of Disease.* http://www.who.int/leishmaniasis/burden/en/ (accessed August 3, 2010).

Wolf, B. 2008. *Biotinidase Deficiency [Late-Onset Biotin-Responsive Multiple Carboxylase Deficiency, Late-Onset Multiple Carboxylase Deficiency].* http://www.ncbi.nlm.nih.gov/bookshelf/br.fcgi?book=gene&part=biotin (accessed August 3, 2010).

Wolfe, J. H. 2009. Gene therapy in large animal models of human genetic diseases. *Institute for Laboratory Animal Research Journal* 50(2):107-111.

Wolfe, L. C. 2010. Chronic granulomatous disease: treatment and medication. *eMedicine* April 16. http://emedicine.medscape.com/article/956936-treatment (accessed August 11, 2010).

Wolff, A. C. 2009. The controversy: perspectives on HER2 testing for breast cancer. *ASCO News & Forum.* http://www.ascoconnection.org/LinkClick.aspx?fileticket= gN-fxKFh0xA%3d&tabid=78 (accessed August 3, 2010).

Wong, H. R., N. Cvijanovich, G. L. Allen, R. Lin, N. Anas, K. Meyer, R. J. Freishtat, et al. 2009. Genomic expression profiling across the pediatric systemic inflammatory response syndrome, sepsis, and septic shock spectrum. *Critical Care Medicine* 37(5):1558-1566.

Wong, H. S., and H. Q. Wang. 2008. Constructing the gene regulation-level representation of microarray data for cancer classification. *Journal of Biomedical Informatics* 41(1):95-105. E-pub April 11, 2007.

Wood, A. J. J. 2006. A proposal for radical changes in the drug-approval process. *New England Journal of Medicine* 355(6):618-623.

Woodward, E. R., and E. R. Maher. 2006. Von Hippel-Lindau disease and endocrine tumor susceptibility. *Endocrine-Related Cancer* 13(2):415-425. http://www.ncbi.nlm.nih.gov/pubmed/16728571?dopt=Abstract (accessed August 20, 2010).

Woolf, S. H. 2008. The meaning of translational research and why it matters. *Journal of the American Medical Association* 299(2):211-213.

Yaplito-Lee, J., J. Pitt, J. Meijer, L. Zoetekouw, R. Meinsma, and A. B. van Kuilenburg. 2008. beta-Ureidopropionase deficiency presenting with congenital anomalies of the urogenital and colorectal systems. *Molecular Genetics and Metabolism* 93(2):190-194.

Yong, G., M. H. Salinger, and T. E. Feldman. 2007. Device closure for PFO: the data and devices associated with percutaneous PFO closure. *Cardiac Interventions Today* June:32-40.

Zacks, R. 2008. Artificial heart finally ready for market? Abiomed's potential "billion-dollar monopoly." *xconomy,* January 23. http://www.xconomy.com/2008/01/23/artificial-heart-finally-ready-for-market-abiomeds-potential-billion-dollar-monopoly/ (accessed August 3, 2010)

Zenios, S., J. Makower, P. Yock, T. J. Brinton, U. N. Kumar, L. Denend, and T. M. Krummel. 2010. *Biodesign: The Process of Innovating Medical Technologies.* New York: Cambridge University Press.

Zhang, F. R., W. Huang, S. M. Chen, L. D. Sun, H. Liu, Y. Li, Y. Cui, et al. 2009. Genomewide association study of leprosy. *New England Journal of Medicine* 361(27):2609-2618.

Zielinska, E. 2009. Team of rivals. *TheScientist.com* 23(11):62.

Zipes, D. P., P. Libby, R. O. Bonow, and E. Braunwald, eds. 2007. *Braunwald's Heart Disease: A Textbook of Cardiovascular Medicine,* 8 ed. St. Louis, MO: W.B. Saunders.

Zlotogora, J. 2009. Population programs for the detection of couples at risk for severe monogenic genetic diseases. *Human Genetics* 126(2):247-253.

A

Study Activities

During the summer of 2008, officials from the National Institutes of Health (NIH) and the Food and Drug Administration (FDA) approached the Institute of Medicine (IOM) about an examination of strategies for rare diseases research and orphan product development. Workshops organized by the IOM Forum on Drug Discovery, Development, and Translation in 2007 and 2008 had helped to sharpen ideas for an IOM study. As discussions progressed, the focus expanded beyond drugs and devices to include medical devices, including certain aspects of genetic tests. The charge to the IOM committee appointed to oversee the study was

To prepare a report that will assess existing strategies to promote research discoveries and development of orphan products to improve the health of people with rare diseases. To that end, the report will:

1. Describe the epidemiology and societal impact of rare diseases and provide an overview of current methods for their prevention, diagnosis, and treatment.

2. Describe the strengths and limitations of the current development pathways for new drugs, medical devices, and biologics for rare diseases (taking into account developments in genetic testing) and discuss the special challenges that rare diseases create for research and product regulation.

3. Examine current public policies relevant to product development for rare diseases, including the Orphan Drug Act, the Humanitarian Use Device exemption, the approaches of the National Institutes of Health and the Food and Drug Administration, reimbursement policies, and other legislative and regulatory initiatives.

4. Consider, as part of a national policy framework, a wide range of public and private strategies and innovations, such as:

- enhancing multidisciplinary collaboration and government-university-industry partnerships in basic and translational research;
- expanding public engagement and enhancing the roles of patient organizations;
- facilitating research data and biomaterials collection and dissemination, including the use of bio-repositories and registries;
- strengthening training of investigators;
- disseminating information to clinicians, patients, and families;
- revising policies and regulations;
- encouraging alternative research financing mechanisms; and
- developing research agendas and coordinating resources and development efforts throughout the product development pathways.

5. Make recommendations for an integrated national rare disease policy on research and development, including responding to the proposals included in a white paper that will be prepared by the sponsors and provided to the committee approximately six months after the contract begins.

NIH and FDA concluded after further consideration that it was not feasible to present the white paper with proposals for the committee, but NIH and FDA staff made presentations to the committee and answered numerous committee questions. The committee reviewed a broad range of government, industry, and academic resources. It commissioned two background papers that appear as Appendixes B and C.

The study committee met five times between August 2009 and May 2010. Three of these meetings included public sessions during which the committee heard from a range of interested parties, including government officials, basic and clinical researchers, representatives of advocacy groups that are engaged in supporting research and product development, and representatives of industry trade associations and individual companies involved in developing drugs and devices. (The agendas for the public sessions follow this overview of study activities.) The committee also worked with the National Organization for Rare Disorders and the Genetic Alliance to solicit views from member organizations that are involved in research. (A list of organizations that submitted written statements follows the November meeting agenda below.)

INSTITUTE OF MEDICINE
COMMITTEE ON ACCELERATING RARE DISEASES
RESEARCH AND ORPHAN PRODUCT DEVELOPMENT

Room 204, Keck Center of the National Academies
500 Fifth Street, N.W., Washington, DC
August 12, 2009—Open Session

2:00   **Welcome and introductions**
        Thomas Boat, M.D., Committee Chair

        Sponsor objectives for study
        Stephen Groft, Pharm.D, Director, NIH Office of Rare Diseases
            Research
        Timothy R. Coté, M.D., M.P.H., Director, FDA Office of Orphan
            Products Development

3:00   **Break**

3:15   **Discussion of background paper prepared by NIH and FDA**
        Stephen Groft, Pharm.D., Director, NIH Office of Rare Diseases
            Research
        Timothy R. Coté, M.D., M.P.H., Director, FDA Office of Orphan
            Products Development

4:30   **Adjourn open session**

INSTITUTE OF MEDICINE
COMMITTEE ON ACCELERATING RARE DISEASES
RESEARCH AND ORPHAN PRODUCT DEVELOPMENT

Lecture Room, National Academy of Sciences Building
2101 C Street, N.W., Washington, DC
November 23, 2009—Open Session

8:20   **Welcome and introductions**
        Thomas Boat, M.D., Committee Chair

8:30   **Panel 1**
        National Organization for Rare Disorders
        Wayne Pines, Consultant

Genetic Alliance
Sharon F. Terry, President and Chief Executive Officer
Discussion

9:10   **Panel 2**
Cystic Fibrosis Foundation Therapeutics, Inc.
Diana R. Wetmore, Ph.D., Vice President of Alliance
      Management

Multiple Myeloma Research Foundation and Multiple Myeloma
      Research Consortium
Susan Kelley, M.D., Chief Medical Officer

Friedreich's Ataxia Research Alliance
Jennifer Farmer, M.S., Executive Director

Fanconi Anemia Research Fund (by phone)
Dave Frohnmayer, J.D., Co-founder and Board Vice President;
Lynn Frohnmayer, M.S.W., Co-founder and Advisor to the Board

10:10   **Break**

10:30   **Discussion before and after break**

11:00   **Panel 3**
Pharmaceutical Research and Manufacturers Association (PhRMA)
Alan Goldhammer, Ph.D., Vice President Scientific and
      Regulatory Affairs

Advanced Medical Technology Association (AdvaMed)
Susan Alpert, Ph.D., M.D., Senior Vice President, Global
      Regulatory Affairs, Medtronic, Inc.

Biotechnology Industry Organization (BIO)
Sara Radcliffe, M.P.H., Acting Executive Vice President, Health,
      and Vice President for Science and Regulatory Affairs

Discussion

Noon   **Working lunch for committee and speakers and other invited guests**

1:00   **Panel 4**
Mark L. Batshaw, M.D.

Principal Investigator, Urea Cycle Disorders Consortium (NIH Rare Diseases Clinical Research Network); Chief Academic Officer, Children's National Medical Center; Chairman of Pediatrics and Associate Dean for Academic Affairs, George Washington University School of Medicine and Health Sciences

Frederick Kaplan, M.D.
Isaac & Rose Nassau Professor of Orthopaedic Molecular Medicine; Director, Center for Research in FOP (Fibrodysplasia Ossificans Progressiva) & Related Disorders, University of Pennsylvania School of Medicine

Alan K. Percy, M.D.
Principal Investigator, Angelman, Rett, and Prader-Willi Syndromes Consortium (NIH Rare Diseases Clinical Research Network); Medical Director, Civitan International Research Center; Professor of Pediatric Neurology, University of Alabama at Birmingham

Discussion

2:20   **Open discussion**

2:45   **Adjourn open session**

Organizations submitting written statements to the committee

In addition to the organizations presenting statements during the November meeting, the committee worked with the Genetic Alliance and the National Organization for Rare Disorders to solicit views from their members on issues before the committee. The following organizations responded:

American Partnership for Eosinophilic Disorders
Brown-Vialetto-Van Laere International
Children's Tumor Foundation
FRAXA Research Foundation (Fragile X)
Genetic Alliance BioBank
International Rett Syndrome Foundation
NBIA Disorder Association (Neurodegeneration with Brain Iron Accumulation)
Pancreatic Cancer Action Network

INSTITUTE OF MEDICINE
COMMITTEE ON ACCELERATING RARE DISEASES
RESEARCH AND ORPHAN PRODUCT DEVELOPMENT

Lecture Room, National Academy of Sciences Building
2101 C Street, N.W., Washington, DC
February 4, 2010—Open Session

8:30   **Welcome and introductions**
Thomas F. Boat, M.D., Chair

Melissa Ashlock, M.D.
Senior Consultant, Therapeutics for Rare and Neglected Diseases
    Program, National Institutes of Health

Discussion

9:00   **Update from FDA**
Debra Lewis, O.D., M.B.A.
Associate Director, Office of Orphan Products Development, FDA

Introduction to Humanitarian Device Exemption (HDE) Process
Debra Lewis, O.D., M.B.A.

One Company's Experiences and Perspectives with the HDE Process
Nancy Hill
Vice President, Marketing and Business Development, Spirations,
    Inc.

Discussion

10:10 **Break**

10:30 **Environment for Orphan Drug Development**
Bernard Munos, M.B.A., Ph.D.
Advisor, Corporate Strategy, Eli Lilly and Company

Emil D. Kakkis, M.D., Ph.D.
President, Kakkis EveryLife Foundation

Discussion

11:30 **Advances in Biomedicine: Exome Sequencing and Rare Diseases**
Holly K. Tabor, Ph.D.
Assistant Professor, Treuman Katz Center for Pediatric Bioethics
and Department of Pediatrics, University of Washington School
of Medicine

Discussion

Noon **Working lunch for committee and speakers and other invited
guests**
Update from NIH
Stephen Groft, Pharm.D.
Director, Office of Rare Diseases Research, NIH

1:00 **Translational and Clinical Research for Rare Diseases and
Orphan Products**
Christopher P. Austin, M.D.
Director, Chemical Genomics Center; Senior Advisor to the
Director for Translational Research, National Human Genome
Research Institute

Anne Pariser, M.D.
Medical Team Leader, Division of Gastroenterology Products and
Inborn Errors of Metabolism, Center for Drug Evaluation and
Research, U.S. Food and Drug Administration

Discussion

2:00 **Trial Design, Biomarkers, and Other Issues in Clinical Research for
Rare Diseases and Orphan Products**
William A. Gahl, M.D., Ph.D.
Clinical Director, National Human Genome Research Institute;
Director, NIH Undiagnosed Diseases Program

Jennifer Van Eyk, Ph.D.
Professor of Medicine, Biological Chemistry, and Biomedical
Engineering; Director, Johns Hopkins Bayview Proteomics
Center, Johns Hopkins School of Medicine

Discussion

3:15 **Open discussion**

3:45 **Adjourn open session**

B

Innovation and the Orphan Drug Act, 1983-2009: Regulatory and Clinical Characteristics of Approved Orphan Drugs

Aaron S. Kesselheim[1]

INTRODUCTION

Pharmaceutical research in the United States relies on both government funding for the basic science behind drug development and private investment, which finances the majority of clinical research and manufacturing process.[2] The revenue potential of a drug in treating a particular disease can influence for-profit manufacturers' willingness to devote necessary resources to its development. If a disease affects a limited number of patients and does not allow recovery of private research investment, then therapeutic products for that condition may be developed slowly or not at all. In the United

[1] Aaron S. Kesselheim, M.D., J.D., M.P.H., is Instructor in Medicine, Harvard Medical School; Division of Pharmacoepidemiology and Pharmacoeconomics, Brigham and Women's Hospital. This work was conducted under a contract from the Institute of Medicine (IOM). The author would like to thank Uzaib Saya for his research assistance. The author would like to acknowledge the helpful comments from Kui Xu and Anne Pariser at the FDA Office for Orphan Products Development and from members of the IOM committee. This work was also conducted with support from Harvard Catalyst | The Harvard Clinical and Translational Science Center (NIH Award #UL1 RR 025758 and financial contributions from Harvard University and its affiliated academic health care centers). Dr. Kesselheim is currently supported by a grant from the Agency for Healthcare Research and Quality and a Robert Wood Johnson Foundation Investigator Award in Health Policy Research. The content is solely the responsibility of the author and does not necessarily represent the official views of Harvard Catalyst, Harvard University and its affiliated academic health care centers, the National Center for Research Resources, the FDA, the National Institutes of Health, or the Institute of Medicine or its committees and convening bodies.

[2] Moses H III, Dorsey ER, Matheson DH, Thier SO. Financial anatomy of biomedical research. JAMA 2005;294(11):1333-1342.

States, Congress passed the Orphan Drug Act in 1983 to provide incentives for industry investment in treatments for such rare conditions.[3]

The Orphan Drug Act provided manufacturers with three primary incentives: (1) federal funding of grants and contracts to perform clinical trials of orphan products; (2) a tax credit of 50 percent of clinical testing costs; and (3) an exclusive right to market the orphan drug for 7 years from the date of marketing approval. The market exclusivity incentive protects orphan drug manufacturers from competition for 7 years, which allows greater discretion in pricing.[4] Additional benefits available to sponsors of orphan-designated products include close coordination with the Food and Drug Administration (FDA) throughout the drug's development, priority FDA review, and a waiver of drug application fees. (The first two benefits may also be available to sponsors of nonorphan drugs for serious or life-threatening conditions and unmet needs.) The legislation initially targeted drugs for which there was "no reasonable expectation" that sales in the United States could support development of the drug. Because that criterion was difficult to assess and manufacturers were wary of showing the government their internal financial projections,[5] an amendment in 1984 defined a rare disease as a condition affecting fewer than 200,000 people in the United States.

The act empowered the FDA to review and approve requests for orphan drug status, coordinate drug development, and award research grants. The FDA created the Office of Orphan Product Development (OOPD) to help manage this regulatory function. Although the initial legislation permitted manufacturers to apply for orphan product designation at any time, a 1988 amendment required sponsors to apply for orphan designation before submitting applications for marketing approval.

From 1983 through 2009, a total of 2,112 orphan designations were assigned by the OOPD. Of those designations, 347 (16 percent) had been approved by the FDA as of the end of 2009. In contrast, 34 drugs that were approved from 1967 to 1983 would have qualified under the Orphan Drug Act based on their approval for a rare condition. Some authors have regarded the act as crucial in the development of certain important products. For example, an effective treatment for infant botulism, a rare neurological disease affecting about 100 U.S. children per year, was described as being developed due to concerted efforts of the California Department of Health

---

[3] 21 USC 360bb(a)(2) (2008).

[4] Prices for orphan drugs can reach more than $400,000 per year. Health plans may cover these drugs, but many require substantial patient cost sharing. See Appendix C. See also Walsh B. The tier IV phenomenon—shifting the high cost of drugs to consumers. March 9, 2009. Available at http://assets.aarp.org/rgcenter/health/tierfour.pdf.

[5] Asbury CH. The Orphan Drug Act: the first 7 years. JAMA 1991;265(7):893-897.

Services, supported by OOPD grants and close coordination with the FDA.[6] As pharmaceutical manufacturers are cited as focusing more attention on developing orphan products,[7] policy makers are considering whether to offer orphan-like incentives to basic and translational research aimed at other conditions.[8] Congress recently passed a law that directs the Commissioner of the FDA to "convene a public meeting regarding which serious and life threatening infectious diseases potentially qualify for available grants and contracts under the Orphan Drug Act or other incentives for development," thereby opening the door to providing orphan drug-like incentives for new antibiotics to treat multidrug-resistant infections in the United States.[9]

This appendix was developed to provide some background data on the implementation of the Orphan Drug Act. Data from publicly available FDA files were collected to provide a comprehensive overview of drugs approved with orphan designations, with attention paid to the drugs' innovativeness as well as their scientific and regulatory characteristics. In addition, characteristics of the clinical trial development process of orphan-designated drugs were analyzed.

PRIOR ORPHAN DRUG ACT RESEARCH

Prior research has been done on various aspects of the Orphan Drug Act. A few studies provided perspectives on the early implementation of the incentive. One analysis by Asbury of the first 42 orphan-designated products approved from 1983 to 1989 found that among the 33 nonbiologic drugs, 21 (64 percent) were New Molecular Entities (NMEs). The FDA ranked 38 percent of these NMEs as "important" therapeutic gains and 48 percent as "moderate" therapeutic gains.[10] Asbury reported that annual sales of 25 of 40 orphan drugs were less than $1 million, while annual sales of 3 were for greater than $100 million. A study by Shulman and Manocchia analyzed 121 orphan drug approvals from 1983 to 1995 (involving 102 different drugs).[11] Fifteen drugs were approved for more than one orphan indication. They found that the drugs averaged about 8 years in clinical development

---

[6] Arnon SS. Creation and development of the public service orphan drug human botulism immune globulin. Pediatrics 2007;119(4):785-789.

[7] Business Wire. "Big pharma" and biotechnology companies boost US pulmonary arterial hypertension markets. Jan. 24, 2007.

[8] Villa S, Compagni A, Reich MR. Orphan drug legislation: lessons for neglected tropical diseases. Int J Health Planning and Management 2009;24(1):27-42.

[9] Food and Drug Administration Amendments Act of 2007 § 1112 (codified at 21 USC § 524) (2007).

[10] Asbury CH. The Orphan Drug Act: the first 7 years. JAMA 1991;265(7):893-897.

[11] Shulman SR, Manocchia M. The US orphan drug programme 1983-1995. Pharmacoeconomics 1997;12(3):312-326.

(from Investigational New Drug [IND] to New Drug Application [NDA]) and approximately 1.8 years in FDA review.

Both Asbury and Shulman and Manocchia provide some data on the types of manufacturers sponsoring orphan-designated drugs. Asbury notes that 39 of the 42 drugs she analyzed were sponsored by members of the biopharmaceutical industry, from a total of 30 different firms. Shulman and Manocchia report that small-sized firms (categorized by annual worldwide sales) made up more than half of all drug sponsors, and small- and mid-sized firms together made up approximately three-quarters of the sample.

Three more recent studies have examined trends in orphan drug approvals. For the period 1983-2007, Seoane-Vazquez and colleagues studied 322 orphan-designated drug approvals, including 72 biologicals (22.4 percent) and 250 nonbiological drugs (77.6 percent).[12] The most common group of diseases targeted was cancer (25.5 percent). The approved drugs emerged from 155 different sponsors but were concentrated in 83 companies (54 percent of the total) that accounted for 67.7 percent of the total number of orphan approvals. During 1983-2007, the FDA approved 635 NMEs, and the authors reported that the first NDAs for 115 (18.1 percent) of these NMEs were approved by the FDA for an orphan indication. Seoane-Vazquez and colleagues also examined the market exclusivity period for orphan drugs. Orphan-designated drugs had a shorter FDA review time on average than nonorphan NMEs (1.6 years versus 2.2 years). The authors found that the minimum effective market exclusivity life (including orphan drug market exclusivity) was 9.9 ± 3.7 years for orphan NMEs and 10.5 ± 4.1 years for other NMEs (no statistically significant difference), while the maximum effective patent and market exclusivity life (including orphan drug market exclusivity) was 11.7 ± 5.0 years for orphan NMEs and 13.9 ± 5.5 years for other NMEs ($p < 0.001$). They concluded that the orphan drug market exclusivity incentive had a positive yet relatively modest overall effect on the market exclusivity life.

Another review of orphan drugs conducted by Wellman-Labadie and Zhou included drugs approved from 1983 through May 2009.[13] Charting the number of orphan approvals as a function of time, the authors found that an average of about eight orphan-designated drugs per year were approved, although the annual approval rates included a number of peaks (in the mid-1990s and mid-2000s) and valleys (early 1990s and early 2000s). Wellman-Labadie and Zhou concluded that the highest rate of orphan drug

---

[12] Seoane-Vazquez E, Rodriguez-Monguio R, Szeinbach SL, Visaria J. Incentives for orphan drug research and development in the United States. Orphanet Journal of Rare Diseases 2008;3:33.

[13] Wellman-Labadie O, Zhou Y. The US Orphan Drug Act: rare disease research stimulator or commercial opportunity? Health Policy 2010;95(2-3):216-228.

approvals overall was in the field of oncology (27 percent), followed by endocrine-metabolic, hematology, infectious diseases, and neurological disorders. They found that the "top 10" pharmaceutical and biological companies (by U.S. revenue) accounted for about 75 percent of the approvals.

Finally, Coté and colleagues compared trends in orphan drug approval from 1983 through July 2009 with trends for all drug approvals during the same time.[14] They found that while there has been a peak and more recent decline in the number of new drugs approved overall, the number of new orphan drugs remained relatively constant from 1984 through 2008. As a result, the number of orphan drug approvals as a percentage of all drug approvals increased from 17 percent (1984-1988) to 31 percent (2004-2008) and was 35 percent in 2008. They concluded that orphan products now represent about one-third of FDA-approved drugs and biologics. In 2009, they reported that 11 of the 29 new molecular entities approved were orphan-designated products.

These studies report trends in absolute numbers of approvals, as well as of other characteristics of orphan drugs, including the characteristics of their sponsors, lengths of market exclusivity, and fields of use. This appendix provides further data about additional regulatory and clinical features of U.S. orphan drug approvals through a comprehensive review of orphan drugs (1983-2009), as well as a detailed analysis of smaller subsets of more recently approved orphan drugs.

METHODS

The primary source for this analysis was a public domain master list of orphan product designations and approvals published by the FDA OOPD.[15] From this source, a list of all drugs with orphan product designations between January 1, 1983, and December 31, 2009, was extracted. The OOPD database records all brand or generic names, date of orphan designation, date of approval, proposed indication, specific indication, and sponsoring company. To avoid double counting specific products, the list was manually searched for drugs with multiple orphan designations, which were then combined into single entries if they had the same generic name and were marketed by the same manufacturer. This process allowed identification of the number of total orphan designations attached to each approved product, as well as the number of those designations that were approved by the FDA.

---

[14] Coté T, Kelkar A, Xu k, Braun MM, Phillips MI. Orphan products: an emerging trend in drug approvals. Nature Rev: Drug Discovery 2010;9(1):84-85.
[15] http://www.accessdata.fda.gov/scripts/opdlisting/oopd/index.cfm.

Once a full list of separate products was completed, it was supplemented with additional data obtained from a variety of sources. First, the FDA website was employed for individual product searches.[16] From this source, a number of regulatory characteristics with respect to each drug were identified:

- whether it was approved under a New Drug Application or a Biologics Licensing Application;
- the original FDA approval date for a drug that was already on the market at the time of its orphan designation;
- the review classification as priority (P), defined by the FDA as a drug that appears to represent an advance over available therapy; standard (S), defined as a drug that appears to have therapeutic qualities similar to those of an already-marketed drug; and/or orphan (O), defined as a product that treats a rare disease affecting fewer than 200,000;
- the route of administration of the drug;
- whether generic versions of the product are available and the date these generics were first made available; and
- whether the drug product has been discontinued or removed from the market.

Further information was sought from the current product label for each orphan drug identified in the initial search. The product label is a formal, FDA-approved document describing the product, its approved indications, and pertinent safety and efficacy information. From the orphan-designated drug product labels, the following items were identified:

- the chemical description of the product;
- whether the product was intended to be a drug or a diagnostic tool;
- the existence of nonorphan indications for the product; and
- the existence of any "black box warnings" (the most severe product safety warning recommended by the FDA).

Finally, more in-depth information was obtained about a subset of drugs with orphan designations. For some approved drugs, individual product searches on the FDA website can also provide links to digital copies of the full FDA review packets. The review packets typically include the regulatory reviews by different FDA officers (medical, statistical, pharmacologic, etc.) and other formal regulatory documents associated with the agency evaluation of the drug. The medical officer review contains the

---

[16] See http://www.accessdata.fda.gov/scripts/cder/drugsatfda/index.cfm.

final statement from the medical officer, including a detailed description of the regulatory history, product development, and trials performed to prove efficacy and safety. Through this search process, copies of the full medical officer review were obtained for 81 approved orphan drugs from 2000 to 2009. From these data, the following items were identified:

- the innovativeness of each drug, including whether it was (1) completely new, defined as a drug with a unique molecular structure that was unrelated to any drug previously approved by the FDA (i.e., "first in class"); (2) a variation of a prior drug, defined as a drugs with similar chemical structure that differed either by method of administration or peripheral chemical components;[17] or (3) an old drug, defined as a drug that had already been available in U.S. and/or overseas markets;
- comparative regulatory information about whether the drug was previously approved for its orphan indication in another similar market or whether the drug had been approved for any nonorphan indications; and
- whether other treatments had been approved for the indication being sought.

For medical officer reviews obtained in the past 3 years ($N = 30$), further details about the clinical trial development process were extracted for the drug leading to its orphan designation and FDA approval. The goal was to describe the length and rigor of the clinical trial development process. During development, drugs undergo a number of trials intended to measure their effect on a certain disease. FDA medical officers designate the particular trials used to support a drug's efficacy for a particular condition as either pivotal efficacy trials or supportive efficacy trials.

Apart from efficacy trials, drugs may also undergo a number of other human trials that impact knowledge about the safety of the drug; such trials could include early-stage Phase I trials on healthy volunteers, as well as open-label continuations of efficacy trials for drugs intended to treat chronic diseases. Efficacy trials, whether pivotal or supportive, also provide evidence of safety. The FDA judges the safety of a product for a particular indication based on all studies done on that product at the time of its review.

In this part of the analysis, the following items were identified:

- the dates of IND application, orphan drug designation, NDA or Biologics License Application (BLA) submission, and approval;

---

[17] Two drugs that differ by peripheral chemical components could be defined as members of the same general "class" as a previously approved product.

- the number of pivotal and supportive efficacy trials conducted on which the approval was based, including the number of comparator arms in those trials;
- whether the efficacy trials were controlled and, if so, whether the drug was compared against an active comparator or a placebo;
- whether efficacy trials were blinded;
- whether the efficacy trials were classified as Phase I, II, III, or IV by the FDA medical officer;
- whether the efficacy trials were multicenter or single-center studies;
- the average time of exposure during the efficacy trials;
- whether the end points of the efficacy trials were surrogate (hematologic markers, interval response rate, etc.) or final (i.e., mortality, disease cure, etc.);
- the number of patients enrolled in efficacy trials;
- the existence of a data safety monitoring board or independent review committee organized by the manufacturer to assist in evaluation of the efficacy trials;
- the total number of human trials conducted by the manufacturer;
- the total number of human subjects in whom the drug was tested;
- whether the FDA identified methodological concerns about the clinical development trials;
- whether published data were used to support the application;
- whether the FDA convened an Advisory Committee to evaluate the drug prior to approval and, if so, whether the vote was unanimous; and
- whether the FDA imposed postmarketing commitments on the manufacturer, and the nature of those requirements (i.e., additional trials, a patient registry, a Risk Evaluation and Mitigation Strategy [REMS]).

RESULTS

All Approved Drugs

From 1983 through 2009, the FDA approved 347 total drugs with orphan designations. However, a single drug can be approved for multiple orphan indications. For example, while somatropin (human growth hormone) accounted for 16 approvals overall, these approvals involved 9 brand-name drugs (some with multiple orphan approvals); the criteria used in this study—drugs having the same active ingredients and manufacturers—identified 6 "separate" products for further study (see Table B-1). Novartis' imatinib (Gleevec) was approved for the treatment of chronic myelogenous leukemia (2001), gastrointestinal stromal tumors (2002), eosinophilic leukemia (2006), mastocytosis (2006), myeloproliferative disease

(2006), acute lymphoblastic leukemia (2006), and dermatofibrosarcoma (2006). Imatinib is therefore a single orphan drug with seven different disease-based approvals. To cite a different situation, the combination product benzoate-phenylacetate was initially approved in 1987 as Ucephan (Immunex Corp.), an oral formulation for management of hyperammonemia, but the manufacturer later withdrew it from the market. Another company then sought new approval as an orphan product for the same indication (but in an intravenous formulation) under the name Ammonul (Ucyclyd, a subsidiary of Medicis Pharmaceutical Corp.) in 2005. For the purposes of analyzing the impact of the Orphan Drug Act in this study, benzoate-phenylacetate counted as two separate products because it appears to have originated from two separate manufacturers and also to differ in formulation.

This process identified a subset of 279 separate orphan products among the original sample that were approved for 347 designations or indications. Within this subset, 233 products had a single approved orphan designation, 36 products had two designations, 5 products had three designations, 3 drugs had four designations, and 2 products had seven designations each

TABLE B-1 Orphan Approvals for Somatropin Products (human growth hormone, hGH)

Brand Name	Year Approved	Manufacturer(s)	Comments	Separate Product?
Nutropin	1985	Genentech		Y
Protropin	1985	Genentech	Identical to Nutropin, except for single amino acid on the N-terminus of the molecule	N
Humatrope	1987	Lilly		Y
Serostim	1996	Serono		Y
Saizen	1996	Serono	Designated as an orphan but not granted market exclusivity. Structurally equivalent to Serostim, but given a different brand name for a different indication	N
Genotropin	1997	Pharmacia and Upjohn		Y
Nutropin Depot	1999	Genentech	New delivery system and slightly different formulation	Y
Zorbtive	2003	Serono	Same structure as Serostim and same manufacturer, although given different brand name for different orphan indication	N
Norditropin	2007	Novo Nordisk	Originally approved in 1995	Y

(including imatinib). The sample included 275 therapeutic products and 4 drugs used as diagnostic agents. The FDA-defined regulatory classification of orphan-designated products could be identified for 208 products. Among that group, there were 133 products (64 percent) classified as NMEs.[18] Information about review status was assessed for drugs approved after 1992, when the priority review classification was created; among orphan products, 144 (70 percent) were listed as Priority drugs, whereas 61 (30 percent) were classified as Standard.

Among the 279 products, small molecules (183, 65 percent) outnumbered biologic-based orphan products (96, 35 percent), although the ratio has changed in recent years as the number of new biologic products overall has increased. From 1990 to 1999, 27 orphan products were approved under a BLA (21 percent) and 101 were approved under an NDA (79 percent), while from 2000 to 2009, 32 products were approved under a BLA (29 percent) and 78 were approved under an NDA (71 percent). In the full product group, there were 214 (77 percent) products approved under an NDA and 65 (23 percent) approved under a BLA.[19] Among the biologic-based drugs were 24 hormones, 18 clotting factors, 12 enzymes, 11 monoclonal antibodies, 9 antibodies, 9 protein conjugates, 7 cytokines, 4 proteins, and 2 biological mixtures.

The greatest number of the 279 orphan products was approved primarily for use in oncology-related conditions (79, 28 percent), predominantly chemotherapy, but also management of cancer-related conditions such as electrolyte disturbances and adverse effects of drug management. In the second-largest group, 43 products (15 percent) were approved for various infectious diseases, including HIV/AIDS-related conditions. The next largest clinical indications were neurological or psychiatric conditions (31, 11 percent) and enzyme deficiencies (28, 10 percent).[20] Renal, cardiovascular, rheumatologic, dermatological, gastroenterological, and pulmonary conditions each made up less than 10 percent of the approvals. Thirty-six (13 percent) different products had indications specifically for pediatric

---

[18] By way of comparison, FDA officials report that the overall number of NMEs and significant new BLAs for the period 1983 to 2009 was 178 or 64 percent of the total NDAs and BLAs.

[19] These numbers differ somewhat from the numbers of small molecules and biologic-based orphan products because not all biologic-based drugs are reviewed via a BLA. For historical reasons, some biologic-based products, including monoclonal antibodies and hormones, have been regulated under the NDA process.

[20] Enzyme deficiencies include all replacement products (clotting factors, etc.) as well as other therapies aimed at treating patients with congenital enzyme deficiencies through exogenous administration of the enzyme itself (e.g., pegademase bovine [Adagen] for ADA [adenosine deaminase] deficiency in patients with severe combined immunodeficiency). By contrast, hormone replacement therapies such as somatropin were defined as being endocrine products.

patients. Of the approved products, 83 were intended to be taken orally (33 percent); 136 through intramuscular, subcutaneous, or intravenous injection (54 percent); 6 directly applied to the eye (2 percent); 5 topical preparations (2 percent); 4 inhalants (2 percent); and 16 other miscellaneous preparations (6 percent).[21]

The data show that compared to nonorphan drugs, relatively few drugs approved with orphan designations are exposed to generic competition. Focusing on just those drugs approved before the year 2000 provides a fair assessment of the rate of generic competition, because the 7-year market exclusivity period is now over for that entire group. This analysis excluded

- a number of orphan drugs because they were approved as biologic drugs under a BLA, for which no generic approval pathway existed;[22]
- some of the more complex hormones approved under NDAs (e.g., somatropin) that the FDA has determined are not appropriate to approve as generics based on bioequivalence data under the current guidelines; and
- 25 drugs that have been removed from the market—no further explanation was provided on the FDA website for these removals, except in the case of two products, where the removal was listed as being "unrelated to safety issues." Additional details about withdrawals could not be identified from the FDA website or online archives.

Among 108 qualifying products with orphan designation approved under an NDA from 1984 to 1999 that are still available, 49 (45 percent) had A-rated generic alternatives that were manufactured by a competitor.

Regulatory and Scientific Characteristics of Orphan Drugs

In the entire group of approved orphan drugs, among the 248 orphan products for which data could be found on the FDA website, there were 164 (66 percent) products for which the original FDA approval date coincided with the initiation of their orphan drug market exclusivity, meaning that their original approval in the United States was for an orphan indication. The remaining 84 (34 percent) had all been approved by the FDA for another indication prior to their orphan drug designation. To cull more information about the inventiveness, regulatory histories, and other clinical uses of drugs approved with orphan designations, full medical reviews from the NDA were available from the FDA website for 81 of the 101 drugs ap-

---

[21] Based on 250 products for which information was listed.
[22] Such a pathway was recently enacted by the 2010 health reform legislation but remains far from implementation.

proved with orphan designations from 2000 to 2009.[23] Additional information, including the current drug label, was available from the FDA website for all products, except nine clotting factors, approved during this time.

Among the drugs in this subset, 34 met the study definition of "new" (34 percent). Such drugs included those approved as a New Molecular Entity that had not previously been available in any other form anywhere in the world before the current regulatory submission.[24]

Another 36 (36 percent) were adaptations of or related to prior-approved drugs. Seventeen (47 percent) of these drugs involved changes in method of administration. For example, the intravenous orphan drug So-Aqueous (sotalol IV), approved in 2009 for ventricular tachyarrhythmias, was a variation based on method of administration of the oral orphan drug Betapace (sotalol) approved in 1992 for the same indication. The remaining 19 (53 percent) drugs were members of the same class as previously approved products. For example, ambrisentan (Letairis), approved in 2007 for pulmonary artery hypertension, is in the same drug class as the orphan drug bosentan (Tracleer), approved in 2001 for the same indication.[25]

Finally, there were 31 drugs (31 percent) that had previously been approved in the United States or elsewhere.[26] Thirteen of the 31 old drugs (42 percent) were available in the United States at the time of their orphan drug approval.[27] For example, raloxifene (Evista), approved in 2007 to reduce the risk of invasive breast cancer in certain high-risk post-menopausal women, was approved in 1997 for the prevention of osteoporosis in post-menopausal women. Twenty-seven of the 31 drugs (87 percent) were previously available overseas or in Canada. For example, Tindamax (tinidazole), approved by the FDA in 2004 for treatment of intestinal giardiasis, had

---

[23] The FDA now posts reviews for all new molecular entities and prioritizes posting for other NDAs (including supplemental New Drug Applications [sNDAs, which are for supplemental indications related to already-approved drugs]) and historical materials based on inquiries. The FDA does not post all reviews in a timely manner due to lack of resources, including a backlog of Freedom of Information Act requests and the burden of reviewing all posted material for redaction.

[24] A drug approved in Europe or Canada within the past 2 years for a similar indication was considered fully new.

[25] Ambrisentan may have different receptor selectivity. It is administered on a daily basis, compared to bosentan, which was recommended to be used twice a day. Monitoring recommendations are virtually the same. See, e.g., Cada DJ, Levien T, Baker DE. Ambrisentan. Hosp Pharm 2007;42:1145-1154.

[26] This result is consistent with the results from the overall sample that about a third of the drugs (84 out of 238 or 34 percent) had previously been approved in the United States.

[27] This number does not include three products (colchicine, quinine, and capsaicin) that were available in the United States despite not ever being officially approved by the FDA because they had been introduced prior to the passage of the Food, Drug, and Cosmetic Act.

been approved for such use since 1975 in Australia and 1982 in the United Kingdom.

As seen in Figure B-1, numbers of approvals for these different categories show considerable variability from year to year. In 2000, three new drugs, two variations, and one old drug were approved as orphans. In 2009, one new drug, six variations, and seven old drugs were approved as orphans.

The data also show that a number of drugs from this sample were approved for orphan indications where approved therapy already existed for some aspect of the disease. Fifty-seven (56 percent) orphan drugs approved during this period were approved for diseases or conditions that had other approved therapeutic alternatives. For example, two antiepileptic drugs—topiramate (Topamax) and rufinamide (Banzel)—were approved during the period to manage Lennox-Gastaut syndrome, an extremely rare childhood form of epilepsy that occurs in about 0.2-2.8 per 10,000 live births. At the time that rufinamide was approved, felbamate (Felbatol) and lamotrigine (Lamictal) had also already been approved as orphan drugs for the condition.[28] Similarly, five orphan products have been approved to treat pulmonary artery hypertension.[29] This measure does not address whether different drugs were more or less effective for the particular condition, but in nearly all cases, head-to-head studies comparing two drugs approved for the same indication have not been conducted.

Orphan Drug Clinical Trials Development Process

The FDA lists 47 unique drugs approved for orphan designations between 2007 and 2009.[30] In the final step of the analysis, the clinical trial development of these drugs was investigated in depth. For these drugs, the full medical officer reviews for 30 (64 percent) were located. The 17 drugs

---

[28] A cost-effectiveness analysis organized by the manufacturer of rufinamide suggest that this drug could be cost-effective compared to a brand-name version of topiramate, and even cost-effective when compared to an inexpensive generic treatment (lamotrigine) "due to the importance of patient choice." See Verdian L, Yi Y. Cost-utility analysis of rufinamide versus topiramate and lamotrigine for the treatment of children with Lennox-Gastaut syndrome in the United Kingdom. Seizure 2010;19(1):1-11.

[29] They are bosentan (Tracleer) for "treatment of pulmonary arterial hypertension," treprostinil (Remodulin) for "treatment of pulmonary arterial hypertension," iloprost (Ventavis) for "treatment of pulmonary arterial hypertension (World Health Organization [WHO] Group I) in patients with New York Heart Association [NYHA] Class III or IV symptoms," ambrisentan (Letairis) for "treatment of pulmonary arterial hypertension," and tadalafil (Adcirca) for "treatment of pulmonary arterial hypertension (WHO Group I) to improve exercise ability."

[30] Treprostinil inhalational (Tyvaso) for the treatment of pulmonary arterial hypertension was excluded because it was approved in 2010, although its market exclusivity start date was subsequently revised to July 2009.

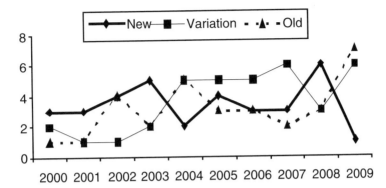

FIGURE B-1 Annual orphan drug approvals by "newness." The thick line represents number of orphan drugs approved each year where the molecular structure is completely new. The dotted line represents the number of orphan approvals each year for drugs previously available on the market in the United States or elsewhere. The thin line represents the number of orphan drugs approved each year that were variations or members of the same class of previously approved drugs.

for which the details were not located included 9 clotting factors or immune globulins, 7 already-marketed drugs,[31] and 1 other product.[32]

Of the 30 drugs for which the full medical officer reviews were analyzed, the NDA and IND dates were obtained for 17 of the products. An average of 3.8 years lapsed from the date of the IND to the date of the orphan drug designation, while an average of 5.9 years lapsed from the date of the IND to the date of the NDA. Approximately 0.7 years passed from NDA submission to approval.

The 30 drugs collectively underwent a total of 71 trials evaluating their efficacy. These efficacy trials enrolled a median of 75 participants (inter-

---

[31] They are raloxifene (Evista) for reduction in the risk of breast cancer in postmenopausal women with osteoporosis, adalimumab (Humira) for the treatment of juvenile rheumatoid arthritis, bevacizumab (Avastin) for renal cell carcinoma and glioblastoma with progressive disease following prior therapy, sorafenib (Nexavar) for treatment of unresectable hepatocellular carcinoma, doxorubicin liposomal injection (Doxil) for use in combination with bortezomib for the treatment of patients with multiple myeloma who have not previously received bortezomib and have at least one prior therapy, thyrotropin alfa (Thyrogen) for use as an adjunctive treatment for radioiodine ablation of thyroid tissue remnants in patients who have undergone thyroidectomy for well-differentiated thyroid cancer and who do not have evidence of metastatic thyroid cancer, and somatropin (Norditropin) for short stature associated with Noonan's syndrome. This information theoretically could be obtained via a Freedom of Information Act (FOIA) request, although the long duration required for such requests to be filled made the FOIA pathway impractical for this study.

[32] Capsaicin (Qutenza) for management of neuropathic pain associated with postherpetic neuralgia.

quartile range [IQR]: 34-157) and took a median of 8.5 weeks (IQR: 2-20 weeks). Fifty-five of those trials were considered "pivotal" efficacy trials for the approval of the product, while the remaining 16 were considered supportive. In total, 13 orphan drugs in this sample were approved based on a single efficacy trial, including 8 based on a single Phase III trial, 4 based on a single Phase II trial, and 1 based on a single Phase I trial. The sample as a whole was approved on the basis of a median of two efficacy trials (IQR: 1-2) per drug.[33]

Among the 55 pivotal trials, 27 were conducted in a double-blind fashion (49 percent), 5 were single-blinded (9 percent), and 23 were not blinded at all (42 percent). Thirteen of the trials were single-arm (24 percent). Thirty-eight of the trials were randomized (69 percent). Twenty-six of the pivotal trials were placebo-controlled (47 percent), while 11 used active comparators (20 percent) (these do not include historical controls or different doses of the drug itself). There were 30 pivotal Phase III studies (55 percent), 17 pivotal Phase II studies (31 percent), 1 pivotal Phase I study (2 percent), and 4 pivotal Phase IV studies (7 percent).[34] There were 39 (71 percent) multicenter trials and 16 (29 percent) single-center trials.

Thirty-two of the pivotal trials (58 percent) used final end points, while 23 used surrogate end points (42 percent). For example, nilotinib (Tasigna), a drug approved in 2007 for "chronic phase (CP) and accelerated phase (AP) Philadelphia chromosome positive chronic myelogenous leukemia (CML) in adult patients resistant to or intolerant to prior therapy that included Gleevec (imatinib)," was approved on the basis of one pivotal efficacy trial measuring cytogenetic and hematologic response rates, not overall survival. FDA medical officers pointed out methodological concerns with efficacy trials relating to 7 of the 30 drugs in the sample (23 percent), although all drugs were approved. Notably, for four of the pivotal trials, the primary efficacy end point was not achieved or the improvement was not statistically significant (7 percent).

For the safety analysis, which included all efficacy trials as well as Phase I and Phase II trials and open-label extension studies, the sample of drugs approved for orphan designations underwent a median of 11.5 trials (IQR: 4.5-15), involving a median of 502 participants (IQR: 263-980). Among all 389 safety trials, 28 percent were Phase I trials (individuals without the disease in question), 45 percent were Phase II trials, and 13 percent

---

[33] Notably, some products such as colchicine (Colcrys) were approved based only on a literature review of prior studies. See Kesselheim AS, Solomon DH. Incentives for drug development—the curious case of colchicine. NEJM 2010; 362:2045-2047. In addition, sotalol-IV (So-Aqueous) was approved on the basis of a single Phase I pharmacokinetic study intending to show its bioequivalence to the oral formulation.

[34] For the remaining 3 studies, their classification was not provided by the FDA.

were Phase III trials.[35] Fifteen drugs (50 percent) supplemented their safety records with references to already-published data, including experiences with the drug in other settings such as Europe and Canada. For 6 of the 30 drugs (20 percent), an independent data safety monitoring board or review committee was used during the clinical development process.

FDA medical officers identified life-threatening adverse events with 8 of the 30 drugs in the sample (27 percent). Formal expert FDA Advisory Committees were organized to provide opinions regarding the approval of 9 drugs (30 percent), voting their approval each time (although they were unanimous only 3 times). Postmarketing commitments were required for 12 products (40 percent), 5 (17 percent) manufacturers were required to conduct specific trials, 8 (27 percent) were required to set up an official REMS program, and 3 (10 percent) were required to initiate a formal data safety registry of patients.

ANALYSIS

This review of the regulatory and scientific characteristics of drugs developed under the Orphan Drug Act involved three different subsets of orphan drugs. The first subset was the full list of orphan drugs approved from 1983 to 2009. While there were a total of 347 approvals, those approvals included 279 separate drugs. Among that sample, the vast majority of drugs were approved only for a single orphan condition (most likely in the field of oncology).

The second subset was the 101 orphan drugs approved from 2000 to 2009; in this sample, more details of the drugs' regulatory history and scientific context of their approval were assessed. The sample was roughly evenly divided among "new" drugs, drugs already available in the United States or abroad, and variations of previous drugs, although the numbers of old drugs and drug variations approved as orphan drugs increased over the time period.

The final subset consisted of the 30 products approved from 2007 to 2009 where full FDA medical officer reviews were available; in this sample, the clinical trial development process was analyzed. The results showed that clinical trial development took about 5.9 years, with official orphan drug designation occurring toward the end of the development process. Orphan drugs were generally approved on the basis of efficacy studies conducted in small numbers of participants. The efficacy studies varied in their complexity. Some pivotal studies were large, multicenter randomized trials where the product was tested against an active comparator. Others

---

[35] Based on data from 28 drugs where this information was available in the FDA medical review.

lacked randomization and blindedness.[36] Use of surrogate end points was common, although we do not know how the extent of use compares to trials of nonorphan drugs. A substantial minority of approved orphan drugs demonstrated important adverse events in their premarketing trials, and nearly half included postmarketing commitments intended to better assess their safety.

The study has a number of limitations. The data were obtained from freely available material on the FDA website, so to the extent that errors were made in posting that information, they may be reflected in these data as well. The medical officer reviews used for the in-depth analysis of trials followed a standard pattern but were composed by different authors. Though these reviews were often more than a hundred pages long, there may have been some details about the trials that were not mentioned in the final posted review. In addition, 14 medical officer reviews could not be obtained through the publicly accessible FDA website, a sample that included many replacement clotting factors and orphan drugs approved via a supplemental NDA pathway. Inclusion of these cases may have affected the proportions of efficacy and/or safety trials reported in this study.

The results from the clinical trial process suggest that the length of drug development for orphan drugs, on average, approximates similar estimates for nonorphan drugs and may even be slightly less. Orphan designation can be granted at any time during the development of a drug, even before IND designation. Although this analysis only included the IND and NDA dates for 17 products approved from 2007 to 2009, for these drugs, on average, orphan drug designation did not occur until well into the clinical testing phase. If a product was initially designed solely for a particular orphan disease, one might predict that orphan product designation would occur more frequently in close temporal proximity to the filing of the IND application that initiates manufacturers' clinical trials. On the other hand, it may be that a new drug demonstrates a potential application to an orphan disease once it reaches Phase I or II trials. These results show that orphan product designation can occur closer to the final step in drug development (the NDA).

A substantial number of pivotal efficacy trials for orphan drugs were open label, non-randomized, and placebo-controlled. Surrogate end points were also common. Surrogate end points, which must be considered "reasonably likely . . . to predict clinical benefit,"[37] can be well-suited to studies

---

[36] For a published analysis that tabulates these characteristics among a larger sample of orphan drugs approved for neurological indications, see Mitsumoto J, Dorsey ER, Beck CA, Kieburtz K, Griggs RC. Pivotal studies of orphan drugs approved for neurological diseases. Ann Neurol 2009;66(2):184-190.

[37] 21 CFR 314.510, subpart H.

of orphan drugs in cases where trials evaluating long-term clinical outcomes is not feasible and in cases where premarketing trials can be completed with fewer patients and with less cost. Mortality and other clinical outcomes can be rare and hard to measure, particularly in trials with a limited population of patients. However, because of their small numbers and shortened time frames, trials that assess surrogate end points may provide a limited view into a drug's safety. Drugs approved on the basis of surrogate end points must be followed up with Phase IV verification studies, although the GAO has pointed out that for a substantial number of drugs approved on the basis of surrogate end points, including midodrine (ProAmantine), approved as an orphan drug in 1996,[38] the required Phase IV studies have not been completed even after years of experience.[39]

From a safety standpoint, new orphan drugs were generally studied in fewer than 1,000 participant prior to approval, and nearly a third of those patients were young and healthy volunteers in Phase I trials. Therefore, the safety record for these products, as with all new drugs, is incomplete at the time of FDA approval. Monitoring the postapproval use of orphan drugs to evaluate potential safety concerns is important, especially for drugs approved despite serious methodological concerns expressed by FDA medical officer reviews. In the past, there have been cases where methodological concerns raised at the FDA level have not been translated adequately onto the label or in communications about an approved drug.[40]

---

[38] Harris G. F.D.A. backtracks and returns drug to market. NY Times. 3 Sept 2010, at A11.

[39] General Accounting Office. FDA needs to enhance its oversight of drugs approved on the basis of surrogate endpoints (GAO-09-866). 23 Sept 2009. Available at: http://www.gao.gov/new.items/d09866.pdf.

[40] Schwartz LM, Woloshin S. Lost in transmission—FDA drug information that never reaches clinicians. N Engl J Med 2009;361(18):1717-1720.

C

Medicare Part D Coverage and Reimbursement of Orphan Drugs

*Laura Faden and Haiden Huskamp**

INTRODUCTION

Given the small potential market for medications that treat rare conditions, pharmaceutical manufacturers may have reduced incentives to develop new medications for rare diseases. To increase incentives for manufacturers, the Orphan Drug Act (P.L. 97-414) provides the following provisions for drugs that receive an orphan drug indication[1] from the U.S. Food and Drug Administration (FDA): a 7-year period of market exclusivity, a tax credit of 50 percent of the cost of conducting clinical trials, eligibility for federal research grants, and a waiver of user fees (21 USC 360bb, OIG, 2001). However, health plan coverage and reimbursement also influence a pharmaceutical firm's decisions to invest in the development of a drug or biologic for a rare disease.

The purpose of this report is to examine stand-alone Medicare Part D prescription drug plan (PDP) coverage of a set of drugs and biologics that

---

*Laura Faden., M.P.H., is a doctoral student in the Harvard University Program in Health Policy. Haiden Huskamp, Ph.D., is Professor of Health Care Policy in the Department of Health Care Policy at Harvard Medical School. Responsibility for the content of this paper rests with the author and does not necessarily represent the views of the Institute of Medicine or its committees and convening bodies.

[1] The Orphan Drug Act of 1983 defines an orphan indication as follows: "in the case of a drug, any disease or conditions which (A) affects less than 200,000 persons in the United States, or (B) affects more than 200,000 in the United States and for which there is no reasonable expectation that the cost of developing and making available in the United States a drug for such disease or condition will be recovered from sales in the United States of such drug" (21 USC 360bb).

treat rare diseases or conditions—which we will refer to collectively as "orphan drugs"—in the Medicare population. This report does not address Medicare coverage and reimbursement of medical devices.

We focus on the Medicare population because the program covers approximately 15 percent of the U.S. population, including adults who have a disabling rare condition and who have Medicare coverage based on their qualification for Social Security Disability Insurance (SSDI). Furthermore, data on Medicare prescription drug coverage and reimbursement are more readily available than similar data from Medicaid and private plans—because Medicare is a public, federal program, the data are public and centrally collected.

There have been no comprehensive studies of Medicare PDP coverage and reimbursement of orphan drugs. In 2005, the National Organization for Rare Disorders (NORD) conducted a similar study that examined coverage of orphan drugs in 10 national Medicare Part D plans (NORD, 2006). This report extends the NORD report by including drugs approved since 2005 and by analyzing coverage of all Medicare prescription drug plans. Furthermore, this report goes beyond the NORD analysis, which only analyzed plan coverage, by also analyzing factors that may reduce access to covered drugs (i.e., formulary tier placement, utilization management).[2]

Medicare Beneficiaries

Medicare, which was created by the Social Security Act of 1965, is a federally administered health insurance program for people who are 65 years of age or older or who qualify for SSDI. There is typically a two-year waiting period before people who qualify for SSDI can receive Medicare benefits. Congress has waived that requirement for people with end-stage renal disease or Lou Gehrig's disease.

As of January 2010, Medicare covers 46 million Americans, 17 percent of whom are under 65 years and are permanently disabled (KFF, 2010c). Almost half (47 percent) of Medicare beneficiaries have low income (below 200 percent poverty), and 7 million beneficiaries meet income and asset criteria to quality for Medicaid—these beneficiaries are known as "dual-eligibles." Among the Medicare population, there is a high prevalence of comorbid conditions (44 percent suffer from three or more chronic conditions), and 29 percent have a cognitive or mental impairment (KFF, 2010c).

It is not known how many Medicare beneficiaries have a rare disease or, conversely, what proportion of people with a rare disease is covered by Medicare. However, the Social Security Compassionate Allowances program—

---

[2] Although the NORD report notes the tier placement and utilization management tools used for each drug, the authors do not provide any analysis of these aspects of drug coverage.

which guarantees immediate SSDI benefits for people who suffer from certain conditions—covers many rare diseases (Social Security Online, 2010).

Currently, more than 27 million Medicare beneficiaries are enrolled in a Medicare prescription drug plan, two-thirds of whom are enrolled in a stand-alone PDP (KFF, 2009d, 2010b).[3] In 2009, 36 percent of these beneficiaries received low-income subsidies (LIS) that cover their premiums and deductibles; LIS beneficiaries are responsible only for a small copayment that is determined by their income level (KFF, 2009a). Dual-eligibles and those eligible for Supplemental Security Income cash assistance are automatically eligible for LIS, and other low-income beneficiaries can apply for the subsidies. All LIS beneficiaries are enrolled in plans that have monthly premiums below the benchmark premium amount established for each region (hereafter referred to as "benchmark plans").

Medicare Prescription Drug Plans

Until 2006, Medicare did not cover outpatient prescription drugs. It covered hospital and physician services (Part A and B), which included coverage of inpatient drugs and drugs administered by a physician (e.g., infusions). The Balanced Budget Act of 1997 created an option for Medicare beneficiaries to receive insurance coverage from private health plans that contract with Medicare (Part C)—these plans are currently referred to as "Medicare Advantage Plans." The Medicare Prescription Drug Improvement and Modernization Act of 2003 created the Medicare Part D program, a voluntary drug benefit that is administered through private health plans or pharmaceutical benefit managers. As of January 1, 2006, Medicare beneficiaries could voluntarily enroll in either a stand-alone PDP or a Medicare Advantage plan with prescription drug coverage (MA-PD). Dual-eligibles are automatically enrolled in a benchmark plan.

The legislation does not require PDPs to have uniform cost sharing requirements or formulary design. However, PDPs are required to offer a plan that is at least actuarially equivalent to a standard benefit package as determined by the Centers for Medicare and Medicaid Services (CMS) (CMS, 2010). In 2010, the standard benefit package is

- $310 deductible;
- 25 percent coinsurance up to $2,830 of total drug costs;

---

[3] Of the remaining Medicare beneficiaries not covered by a Part D plan—approximately 19 million—most have drug coverage, either through a retiree drug plan (through an employer or union) or another form of drug coverage (e.g., Veterans Affairs, Indian Health Services, state pharmacy assistance programs, employer benefits for active workers, etc.). Approximately 10 percent of beneficiaries have no prescription drug coverage (KFF, 2009d, 2010b).

- no coverage from $2,830 to $6,330 of total drug costs—a coverage gap that is commonly referred to as the "doughnut hole," which, starting in 2010, will be partially subsidized (beneficiaries will receive a $250 rebate);[4] and
- 5 percent coinsurance, or a flat copayment of $2.50 for a generic drug and $6.30 for a brand drug, above $4,550 out-of-pocket expenses (i.e., catastrophic out-of-pocket spending limit) with no maximum limit on out-of-pocket expenses.

In addition, CMS requires that PDP and MA-PD formularies include at least two drugs in every drug class[5] and all, or substantially all, drugs in the following six "protected" therapeutic categories: antidepressants; antipsychotics; anticonvulsants; immunosuppressants (to prevent rejection of organ transplants); antiretrovirals (for the treatment of infection by retroviruses, primarily HIV); and antineoplastics (only those chemotherapy drugs that are generally are not covered under Medicare Part B) (CMS, 2010).

Even with these requirements, PDPs and MA-PDs have a considerable amount of flexibility in formulary design. First, plans decide whether or not to cover a drug. Second, plans can use a tiered formulary structure to create financial incentives for beneficiaries to choose lower-cost or preferred drugs. In 2010, approximately three-fifths of plans have the following four-tier structure (KFF, 2009c).

- Tier 1: generic drugs
- Tier 2: preferred brand-name drugs
- Tier 3: nonpreferred brand-name drugs
- Tier 4 ("specialty tier"): specialty drugs[6]

Each tier has a different cost sharing requirement—most plans assign a flat copayment to the first three tiers and a coinsurance to the specialty tiers (although a growing number of plans are requiring a coinsurance for the first three tiers) (KFF, 2009c). Almost all (94 percent) of plans have a

---

[4] The Patient Protection and Affordable Care Act of 2010 (P.L. 111-148) included provisions to reduce cost sharing in the doughnut hole. Starting in 2011, Medicare and manufacturers will phase in subsidies for generic and brand drugs with the goal of reducing out-of-pocket expenditure in the doughnut hole in 2010 to the same 25 percent coinsurance that applies to costs below the lower threshold of the coverage gap.

[5] The U.S. Pharmacopeia has developed a therapeutic classification system that serves as a guideline for Part D formularies. Model guidelines are publicly available: see http://www.usp.org/pdf/EN/mmg/modelGuidelinesV4.0WithFKDTs.pdf.

[6] CMS guidelines stipulate that drugs placed on the specialty tier must cost at least $600 per month and prohibit enrollees from requesting cost sharing exceptions for specialty drugs (CMS, 2009b).

specialty tier (KFF, 2009c).[7] In 2010, the specialty tier coinsurance ranges from 25 to 33 percent of the full cost of the drug (KFF, 2009c).

In addition to coverage decisions and tiered formularies, a third way in which plans influence prescription drug utilization is by employing utilization management tools such as prior authorization (PA) requirements, step therapy (ST) requirements, and quantity limits (QL). PA requirements create an administrative barrier to accessing a drug—a patient or provider must follow a certain procedure, created by the plan, to request coverage of the drug and then await the plan's approval of coverage. ST requirements establish a chronological course of recommended treatments for a condition that must be tried before coverage of the drug is approved. QL requirements set explicit criteria for the quantity of a drug that will be covered during a given period of time.

METHODS

Medicare Part D Plans Characteristics and Orphan Drug Coverage

We used the CMS Formulary and Pharmacy Network Information File (January 2010 quarterly release) to determine the coverage, tier placement, and utilization management requirements for each orphan drug. We classified drug plans as stand-alone drug plans (PDPs) and MA-PD plans.[8] Within PDPs, we identified national plans (i.e., plans offered in every region of the country) and benchmark plans. National plans were identified by contract number (CMS, 2009b), and benchmark plans were identified using the regional premium limits (CMS, 2009a).

We calculated the "plan coverage rate" for a particular drug as the percentage of plans that cover the drug. Similar to the NORD report (NORD, 2006), we categorized each drug by level of coverage rate, which we classified as the following:

- No or low coverage: <25 percent plan coverage rate
- Low coverage: 25-49 percent plan coverage rate
- Medium coverage: 50-74 percent plan coverage rate
- High coverage: 75-99 percent plan coverage rate
- Complete coverage: 100 percent plan coverage rate

We also examined tier placement and utilization management among drugs covered by PDPs. For each drug we calculated the "tier placement

---

[7] This excludes plans that offer the standard benefit package (i.e., plans that have no tiering).

[8] MA-PDs include both regional and local plans. However, for the analyses we removed duplicate MA-PDs by including each unique contract and plan combination only once.

rate" as the percentage of plans that cover that drug on a given tier. For example, if 20 percent of the plans that cover a drug have placed that drug on tier 4, the drug has a tier 4 placement rate of 20 percent. The tiers range from one to four. A few plans have more than four tiers—for these plans we included all tiers greater than four in the tier 4 category.[9]

Similarly, we examined rates of step therapy requirements, quantity limits, and prior authorization requirements ("utilization management rate").[10] We categorized each covered drug by the rate of tier placement and use of utilization management, which we classified into the following categories:

- No or low placement (or use): <25 percent of plans
- Low placement (or use): 25-49 percent of plans
- Medium placement (or use): 50-74 percent of plans
- High placement (or use): 75-99 percent of plans
- Complete placement (or use): 100 percent of plans

In terms of beneficiary access to drugs, a higher plan coverage rate will likely improve access, whereas a higher utilization management or tier 4 placement rate may pose barriers to access. These categories are subjective and were created only to simplify the interpretation of the results for all drugs along the three dimensions of access (i.e., plan coverage, tier placement, and utilization management). Therefore we also report the raw rates.

---

[9] For the purposes of this report, we refer to tiers 4-6 as "tier 4" and assume that tier 4 is equivalent to a specialty tier. However, given the heterogeneity of the PDPs' formulary structures, this assumption does not hold for all plans. As previously noted, three-fifths of the plans have a four tier structure—for these plans tier 4 is the specialty tier (CMS, 2009b). Some plans have no tiers (11 percent) or fewer than four tiers (7 percent)—for the latter, the specialty tier may actually be tier 3. Also, 21 percent of the plans have more than four tiers—for these plans, tier 4 may not be a specialty tier but rather a nonpreferred brand tier (CMS, 2009b) or a tier for injectible drugs (KFF, 2010a). Therefore, by collapsing tiers 4-6 and labeling this as a specialty tier, we may be misclassifying up to 28 percent of the plans. However, this misclassification may have a negligible effect in terms of concerns about beneficiary cost sharing because a large share (34 percent) of PDPs now use coinsurance rates for nonpreferred brand tiers (CMS, 2009b) and these coinsurance rates may actually be higher than specialty-tier coinsurance rates. Likewise, cost sharing for drugs placed in an injectible tier is also likely to be high because these drugs are quite expensive.

[10] Note that for these analyses, the rates are based on only the number of plans that cover each drug (i.e., the denominator is different for each drug). Since each drug is associated with multiple entries in the National Drug Code (NDC) directory, a drug may appear on multiple tiers of a plan's formulary (e.g., both the brand and generic version are covered, but the generic is on lower tier). For the purposes of our analyses, we assign drugs to the lowest tier on which they appear. A plan is counted as having a utilization management tool for a drug if the tool is applied to at least one of the covered NDCs associated with the drug.

To determine if coverage policies differed by type of plan, we repeated these analyses for several subgroups of plans: all PDPs, benchmark PDPs, national PDPs and MA-PDs. Although we present data on all analyses, we focus on the analyses of all PDPs in the results and discussion sections.

List of Orphan Drugs

We created a list of drugs that were approved by the FDA with an orphan indication between 1983 and December 2008. We included only drugs approved prior to 2009 in order to provide adequate time for marketing and plan coverage decisions. We included only outpatient drugs (i.e., not covered by Medicare Part B as of July 2010) that have an approved orphan indication relevant to the Medicare population (i.e., not for a pediatric indication[11]) and that have not been discontinued or withdrawn.

Our list excludes drugs that are covered by Medicare Part A or B and blood products. We also excluded drugs that are available on the market (for other FDA-approved indications) and that have been granted an orphan designation but have not yet received FDA approval for an orphan indication. Lastly, we excluded drugs for the treatment of rare diseases or conditions that appear in Medicare compendia unless the FDA has approved the drugs for the same orphan indication (see Chapter 6 of this report).

The National Drug Codes (NDCs) for each drug were obtained from First Data Bank (FDB), which was up-to-date as of January 2010. We noted which drugs are available in generic form and which are biologics versus new chemical entities.

RESULTS

List of Orphan Drugs

Ninety-nine orphan drugs met our inclusion criteria (see Addendum Table C-A1). Drugs are listed in chronological order of the date of approval of the first orphan indication relevant to the Medicare population (some drugs have multiple relevant orphan indications). Twenty-nine (29 percent) of the drugs are available in generic form and eleven (11 percent) are biologics.

Medicare Plan Characteristics—Part D and Medicare Advantage Plans

In 2010, there are 1,620 stand-alone PDPs and 2,418 MA-PDs. Of the PDPs, 1,295 (77 percent) are national plans and 398 (23 percent) are

---

[11] We performed a separate analysis of Medicare Part D coverage of orphan drugs with only a pediatric indication orphan approval. See Addendum Tables C-A3 and C-A4.

benchmark plans. The 1,295 national plans represent 12 plan sponsor organizations, 26 unique contracts, and 88 unique formularies (a sponsor may use the same formulary for multiple plans).

The average monthly premium is $46.39 (range: $1.50 to $120.20; standard deviation: $19.75) (see Table C-1). More than half (60 percent) of the plans have deductibles. The median deductible for all plan types is $310.00 (range: $10.00 to $310.00). Benchmark plans and nonnational plans are more likely to have a deductible and to have a higher deductible than nonbenchmark and national plans. Compared to stand-alone PDPs, MA-PDs have a lower average premium and are less likely to have a deductible.

Medicare Plans' Coverage of Orphan Drugs— Stand-Alone PDPs and MA-PDs

The coverage rate (percentage of plans covering a drug) for orphan drugs among Medicare prescription drug plans is high. On average, an orphan drug is covered by 84 percent (standard deviation: 24 percent) of stand-alone PDPs. Table C-2 shows a breakdown of coverage rate category by plan type. Of the 99 drugs, 44 (44 percent) are covered by all 1,620 PDPs (i.e., complete coverage category). An additional 29 drugs (29 percent) are covered by at least 75 percent of the plans (i.e., high-coverage category).

Table C-2 shows that 19 (19 percent) of the drugs fall into the medium-coverage category (i.e., only covered by 50-75 percent of plans) and that 7 (7 percent) are covered by less than half of the plans (i.e., no or very low coverage and low-coverage categories). As of January 2010 4 drugs are not covered by any PDP: citric acid, glucono-delta-lactone, and magnesium car-

TABLE C-1 Average Premium and Use of Deductible for Different Types of Medicare Prescription Drug Plans (99 drugs)

	N	Average Premium (std. dev.)	% with Deductible[a]
All stand-alone PDPs	1,620	46.39 (19.75)	60
Benchmark PDPs	398	28.70 (5.69)	94
Nonbenchmark PDPs	1,222	52.15 (19.27)	49
National PDPs	1,295	46.70 (20.14)	57
Nonnational PDPs	325	45.15 (18.07)	72
MA-PDs	2,418	20.12 (18.81)	23

[a] The median deductible across all plan types is $310.
NOTE: 2010 Data.

TABLE C-2 Orphan Drug Coverage by Type of Medicare Prescription Drug Plan (99 drugs)

	All Stand-alone PDPs (N)	MA-PDPs (N)	Stand-alone National PDPs (N)	Stand-alone Non-national PDPs (N)	Stand-alone Bench-mark PDPs (N)	Stand-alone Non-bench-mark PDPs (N)
No or very low coverage (<25% plan coverage rate)	4	4	4	10	4	4
Low coverage (25-49% plan coverage rate)	3	0	0	13	7	2
Medium coverage (50-74% plan coverage rate)	19	17	19	8	15	19
High coverage (75-99% plan coverage rate)	29	36	19	25	24	29
Complete coverage (100% plan coverage rate)	44	42	57	43	49	45

NOTE: Number of drugs that fall into each coverage rate category. Because the number of drugs in the analysis is 99, the numbers and percentages of drugs are identical; the percentages have therefore not been included in the table.

bonate (Renacidin Irrigation); clofazimine (Lamprene); glutamine (Nutrestore); zinc acetate (Galzin). Three other drugs—lodoxamide tromethamine (Alomide Ophthalmic Solution), tinidazole (Tindamax), and metronidazole topical (Metrogel)—are covered by 45 to 50 percent of PDPs (see Table C-3). As explained in the note for the table, a search of formularies conducted in late spring 2010 found a few plans had initiated coverage of Galzin and Renacidin Irrigation.

Overall, MA-PD plans have slightly better coverage of orphan drugs than stand-alone PDPs. Compared to PDPs, the percentage of drugs falling into the no-very low and low-coverage categories is slightly lower among MA-PDs (4 percent in MA-PDPs versus 7 percent in PDPs). On average, an orphan drug is covered by 87 percent (standard deviation: 22 percent) of MA-PDPs, compared to 84 percent of stand-alone PDPs.

Within PDPs, there is some variation in coverage rates between benchmark and nonbenchmark plans, with nonbenchmark plans having slightly higher coverage rates. On average, an orphan drug is covered by 83 percent (standard deviation: 26 percent) of benchmark plans and 85 percent (standard deviation: 24 percent) of nonbenchmark plans. The benchmark plans have a higher percentage of drugs that fall within the no-very low

TABLE C-3 Orphan Drugs with No, Very Low, or Low Plan Coverage (less than 50% coverage among all stand-alone PDPs) (7 drugs)

Generic Name	Trade Name	Stand-alone PDP Coverage (% plans that cover drug)	Route of Administration	Orphan Designation(s) (year of orphan approval)
Citric acid, glucono-delta-lactone, and magnesium carbonate	Renacidin Irrigation	0[a]	Irrigation	Treatment of renal and bladder calculi of the apatite or struvite variety (1990)
Clofazimine	Lamprene	0	Oral	Treatment of lepromatous leprosy, including dapsone-resistant lepromatous leprosy and lepromatous leprosy complicated by erythema nodosum leprosum (1986)
Glutamine	Nutrestore	0	Oral	For use with human growth hormone in the treatment of short bowel syndrome (nutrient malabsorption from the gastrointestinal tract resulting from an inadequate absorptive surface) (2004)
Zinc acetate	Galzin	0[a]	Oral	Treatment of Wilson's disease (1997)
Lodoxamide tromethamine	Alomide Ophthalmic Solution	46	Ophthalmic	Treatment of vernal keratoconjunctivitis (1993)
Tinidazole	Tindamax	47	Oral	(1) Treatment of giardiasis; (2) treatment of amebiasis (2004)
Metronidazole (topical)	Metrogel	49	Topical	Treatment of acne rosacea (1988)

[a] These drugs had 0% coverage according to our analysis, which was limited to coverage of the drugs' NDCs (listed in the FDB) in the January 2010 CMS data release. Through a systematic search of all national PDP formularies and an unsystematic Internet search of all Medicare PDPs, we determined that Renacidin and Galzin are in fact covered by some PDPs as of June 2010. Galzin, which was a "high priority access problem drug" in the NORD analysis, is not on any national PDP formularies but appears on at least two nonnational formularies. Renacidin also appears on two national formularies and a few nonnational PDP formularies.

and low-coverage categories (11 percent in benchmark versus 6 percent in nonbenchmark plans).

There is considerably more variation in coverage rates between national and nonnational plans, with national plans having higher coverage rates. On average, an orphan drug is covered by only 77 percent (standard deviation: 32 percent) of nonnational plans, compared to 86 percent (standard deviation: 24 percent) of national plans. Within nonnational plans, almost a quarter (23 percent) of the drugs are classified as having a no-very low or low-coverage rate, compared to only 4 percent of drugs within national plans. Aside from the four drugs covered by no PDPs, no other drug is covered by less than 50 percent of the national plans. Conversely, 19 of the 95 covered drugs are covered by less than 50 percent of the nonnational plans.

Formulary Tier Placement by Stand-Alone PDPs

The orphan drugs are commonly placed on high cost sharing tiers. Table C-4 shows the tier 4 placement rate by plan type. For these analyses, and the utilization management analyses below, we excluded the four drugs not covered by any plan. Of the 95 remaining drugs, 84 (88 percent) are placed on tier 4 or higher by at least one PDP. Twenty-eight (29 percent) are placed on tier 4 by at least 75 percent of the plans (i.e., high tier 4 placement), and another 15 (16 percent) are placed on tier 4 by at least 50 percent of the plans (i.e., medium tier 4 placement).

Utilization Management Tools Used by Stand-Alone PDPs

PDPs rarely use step therapy to manage orphan drugs. ST is used by at least one plan only for 18 (19 percent) of the covered orphan drugs. Of these 18 drugs, half (9) have a ST use rate of less than 10 percent. The drug with the highest use of ST—interferon beta-1b—is given ST requirements by almost one-quarter (23 percent) of PDPs. The use of quantity limits to manage utilization of orphan drugs is more common among PDPs than the use of ST, although most plans do not use quantity limits for these drugs. QLs are used by at least one plan for 57 (60 percent) of the covered drugs. Twenty-seven (28 percent) of these drugs have QL use rates greater than 20 percent, and an additional 4 drugs (4 percent) have QL use rates greater than 50 percent (interferon beta-1a, lidocaine patch, raloxifene, and modafinil).

Prior authorization is the most widely used form of utilization management employed by PDPs. Table C-5 shows PA rates by plan type. PA is used by at least one plan for 80 (84 percent) of the covered orphan drugs. Thirty-three (35 percent) of the drugs are given a PA requirement by at least

TABLE C-4 Orphan Drugs by Rate of Tier 4 Placement and Type of Medicare Prescription Drug Plan (95 drugs)

	Stand-alone PDPs N (%)	MA-PDPs N (%)	Stand-alone National PDPs N (%)	Stand-alone Non-national DPs N (%)	Stand-alone Bench-mark PDPs N (%)	Stand-alone Non-benchmark PDPs N (%)
No or very low tier 4 placement (<25% plans)	47 (49)	52 (55)	47 (49)	43 (45)	49 (52)	47 (49)
Low tier 4 placement (25-49% plans)	5 (5)	2 (2)	5 (5)	12 (13)	4 (4)	5 (5)
Medium tier 4 placement (50-74% plans)	15 (16)	8 (8)	12 (13)	29 (31)	35 (37)	12 (13)
High tier 4 placement (75-99% plans)	28 (29)	33 (35)	31 (33)	11 (12)	7 (7)	31 (33)
Complete tier 4 placement (100% plans)	0 (0)	0 (0)	0 (0)	0 (0)	0 (0)	0 (0)

NOTE: Number (percentage) of drugs that fall into each coverage rate category; excludes 4 drugs not covered by any plan.

TABLE C-5 Orphan Drugs by Rate of Prior Authorization Use and Type of Medicare Prescription Drug Plan (95 drugs)

	Stand-alone PDPs N (%)	MA-PDPs N (%)	Stand-alone National PDPs N (%)	Stand-alone Non-national PDPs N (%)	Stand-alone Bench-mark PDPs N (%)	Stand-alone Non-benchmark PDPs N (%)
No or very low use of PA (<25% plans)	47 (49)	52 (55)	46 (48)	56 (59)	45 (47)	48 (51)
Low tier use of PA (25-49% plans)	15 (16)	13 (14)	15 (16)	19 (20)	14 (15)	17 (18)
Medium use of PA (50-74% plans)	19 (20)	17 (18)	15 (16)	14 (15)	18 (19)	16 (17)
High use of PA (75-99% plans)	14 (15)	13 (14)	9 (9)	6 (6)	13 (14)	14 (15)
Complete use of PA (100% plans)	0 (0)	0 (0)	10 (11)	0 (0)	5 (5)	0 (0)

NOTE: Number (percentage) of drugs that fall into each coverage rate category; excludes 4 drugs not covered by any plan.

half of the PDPs (i.e., medium and high use of PA). Ten drugs are given a PA requirement by at least 90 percent of the PDPs, and 5 of these are given a PA requirement by 99 percent of the plans (somatropin (R-DNA), somatropin for injection, somatropin, immune globulin (human), and tacrolimus).

The PA use rate and tier 4 placement rate are highly correlated (correlation coefficient = .75). That is, drugs that are more likely to be placed on tier 4 are also more likely to have PA requirements.

Table C-A2 shows coverage rate, tier placement, and utilization management rates by drug. See Tables C-A3 and C-A4 for a list of orphan drugs with only a pediatric orphan indication (N = 27) and the coverage rate, tier placement, and utilization management rates by drug.

DISCUSSION

Medicare beneficiaries' access to orphan drugs is jointly determined by the following three factors: whether or not the plan covers the drug, the formulary tier the drug is placed on (and the cost sharing requirements associated with each tier), and whether there are any utilization management requirements for the drug.

In terms of the percentage of plans that cover the drugs, Medicare prescription drug plan coverage of orphan drugs is relatively extensive. The majority of drugs have complete coverage (100 percent) or high rates of coverage (>75 percent) among PDPs. The fact that many of these drugs are in protected classes (for either the orphan indication or another approved indication) may explain the high coverage rates of these drugs.

Nonetheless, it is important to emphasize that 26 orphan drugs are covered by less than 75 percent of PDPs, and 4 of these are not covered by any PDP. Also, only 4 of these 26 drugs are available in generic form. If a drug is not covered by a PDP, beneficiaries in that PDP must pay out-of-pocket for the full cost of a brand-name drug unless a lower-cost generic alternative is available.

There is also variation in orphan coverage between types of PDPs—notably, there is much higher coverage in national than nonnational plans. There is also slightly higher coverage among nonbenchmark than benchmark plans.

However, plan coverage alone does not guarantee access—tier placement and utilization management requirements may limit access of covered drugs by imposing financial barriers (e.g., high cost sharing on specialty tiers) or administrative barriers (e.g., paperwork required for PA). We found that PDPs often place covered orphan drugs on a high cost sharing tier and/or require prior authorization. However, we found minimal use of quantity limits or step therapy, the latter of which was expected since there are often few, if any, therapeutic substitutes for these orphan drugs.

Our findings are similar to a recent analysis of tier placement and use of utilization management by national PDPs for 10 common specialty drugs (KFF, 2009b). The authors found that almost all of the PDPs covered the 10 drugs and that 7 of the drugs were placed on a specialty tier by more than 75 percent of the plans. The authors also found high rates of utilization management for these drugs. Four of the 10 drugs analyzed are on our list of orphan drugs—Sensipar, Copaxone, Thalomid, and Tracleer; the last 3 are placed on tier 4 or above by approximately four out of five PDPs in 2010.

Non-low-income subsidy PDP enrollees typically face high levels of out-of-pocket spending for drugs on a specialty tier. In 2009, the national PDP average *monthly* specialty tier cost sharing amount for these three orphan drugs was $602, $1,512, and $1,916 (for Copaxone, Tracleer, and Thalomid, respectively) (KFF, 2009b). Patients taking these drugs typically reached the catastrophic out-of-pocket payment limit, which was $4,350 in 2009, in less than 3 months for both Thalomid and Tracleer and in 7 months for Copaxone—this is assuming no deductible and no doughnut hole, the latter of which will be partially eliminated with the recent health care reform (KFF, 2010a). After reaching the limit, these patients were then responsible for paying 5 percent of the full cost of the drug—these monthly out-of-pocket payments were an average of $99, $247, and $314 (for Copaxone, Tracleer, and Thalomid, respectively), calculated using data in reference (KFF, 2009b). For beneficiaries in the majority of PDPs, these financial barriers to access were compounded by utilization management requirements, predominantly PA.

When used appropriately, formulary management techniques such as tier placement and PA can improve the appropriate use of drugs and save costs. However, orphan diseases, by definition, have limited treatment options and there may not be a lower-cost therapy available to patients. Although most orphan drugs are covered by PDPs, patients who require drugs that are placed on high cost sharing tiers are forced to either pay large out-of-pocket costs or forgo treatment. The cost-related and utilization management-related nonadherence for orphan drugs among the Medicare population is not known. Also, although the financial barriers are largely removed for those receiving low-income subsidies, it is not known how utilization management requirements affect these beneficiaries' access to orphan drugs.

ADDENDUM

TABLE C-A1 Orphan Drugs Relevant to Medicare Population (1983-2008 approvals) (99 drugs)

Exclusivity Start Date	Generic Name	Trade Name	Indication for Original Approval[a]
10/3/84	Cromolyn sodium 4% ophthalmic solution[b]	Opticrom 4% ophthalmic solution	Treatment of vernal keratoconjunctivitis
11/30/84	Naltrexone HCl[b]	Revia	For blockade of the pharmacological effects of exogenously administered opioids as an adjunct to the maintenance of the opioid-free state in detoxified formerly opioid-dependent individuals
8/30/85	Potassium citrate[b]	Urocit-K	(1) Prevention of calcium renal stones in patients with hypocitraturia. (2) Prevention of uric acid nephrolithiasis. (3) For avoidance of the complication of calcium stone formation in patients with uric lithiasis.
11/8/85	Trientine HCl	Syprine	Treatment of patients with Wilson's disease who are intolerant of, or inadequately responsive to, penicillamine
4/10/86	Levocarnitine[b]	Carnitor	Treatment of genetic carnitine deficiency
12/15/86	Clofazimine	Lamprene	Treatment of lepromatous leprosy, including dapsone-resistant lepromatous leprosy and lepromatous leprosy complicated by erythema nodosum leprosum
12/30/86	Tranexamic acid[c]	Cyklokapron	Treatment of patients with congenital coagulopathies who are undergoing surgical procedures (e.g., dental extractions)
3/19/87	Zidovudine[b]	Retrovir	(1) Treatment of AIDS-related complex. (2) Treatment of AIDS.
8/11/88	Tiopronin	Thiola	Prevention of cystine nephrolithiasis in patients with homozygous cystinuria
11/22/88	Metronidazole (topical)[b]	Metrogel	Treatment of acne rosacea
5/2/89	Mefloquine HCl[b]	Lariam	(1) Prophylaxis for *Plasmodium falciparum* malaria that is resistant to other available drugs. (2) Treatment of acute malaria due to *Plasmodium falciparum* and *Plasmodium vivax*.

continued

TABLE C-A1 Continued

Exclusivity Start Date	Generic Name	Trade Name	Indication for Original Approval[a]
5/25/89	Rifampin[b,c]	Rifadin I.V.	For antituberculosis treatment where use of the oral form of the drug is not feasible
6/5/89	Selegiline HCl[b]	Eldepryl	As an adjuvant to levodopa and carbidopa treatment of idiopathic Parkinson's disease (paralysis agitans), postencephalitic Parkinsonism, and symptomatic Parkinsonism
12/22/89	Cromolyn sodium	Gastrocrom	Treatment of mastocytosis
10/2/90	Citric acid, glucono-delta-lactone and magnesium carbonate[c]	Renacidin irrigation	Treatment of renal and bladder calculi of the apatite or struvite variety
12/10/90	Calcium acetate[b]	Phos-lo	Treatment of hyperphosphatemia in end-stage renal failure
12/26/90	Altretamine	Hexalen	Palliative treatment of patients with persistent or recurrent ovarian cancer following first-line therapy
10/30/92	Sotalol HCl[b]	Betapace	Treatment of life-threatening ventricular tachyarrhythmias
11/25/92	Atovaquone	Mepron	For the acute oral treatment of mild to moderate *Pneumocystis carinii* pneumonia in patients who are intolerant to trimethoprim-sulfamethoxazole
12/23/92	Rifabutin	Mycobutin	Prevention of disseminated *Mycobacterium avium* complex disease in patients with advanced HIV infection
7/23/93	Interferon beta-1b[c,d]	Betaseron	In ambulatory patients with relapsing-remitting multiple sclerosis to reduce the frequency of clinical exacerbations
9/10/93	Megestrol acetate[b]	Megace	Treatment of anorexia, cachexia, or an unexplained significant weight loss in patients with a diagnosis of acquired immune deficiency syndrome
9/23/93	Lodoxamide tromethamine	Alomide ophthalmic solution	Treatment of ocular disorders referred to by the terms vernal keratoconjunctivitis, vernal conjunctivitis, vernal keratitis
3/7/94	Desmopressin acetate[b]	N/A	Treatment of patients with hemophilia A or von Willebrand's disease (type I) whose factor VIII coagulant activity level is greater than 5%

TABLE C-A1 Continued

Exclusivity Start Date	Generic Name	Trade Name	Indication for Original Approval[a]
3/22/94	Pilocarpine[b,d]	Salagen	Treatment of symptoms of xerostomia from salivary gland hypofunction caused by radiotherapy for cancer of the head and neck
5/31/94	Rifampin, isoniazid, pyrazinamide	Rifater	For the short-course treatment of tuberculosis
6/30/94	Aminosalicylic acid	Paser granules	Treatment of tuberculosis infections
7/29/94	Sulfadiazine[b]	N/A	Toxoplasmosis, as adjunctive with pyrimethamine
8/15/94	Cysteamine	Cystagon	Treatment of nephropathic cystinosis in adults and children
8/3/95	Amiodarone HCl[b]	Cordarone	For initiation of treatment and prophylaxis of frequently recurring ventricular fibrillation and hemodynamically unstable ventricular tachycardia in patients refractory to other therapy
11/22/95	Tretinoin[b,d]	Vesanoid	Induction of remission in patients with acute promyelocytic leukemia who are refractory to or unable to tolerate anthracycline-based cytotoxic chemotherapeutic regimens
12/12/95	Riluzole[b,d]	Rilutek	Treatment of patients with amyotrophic lateral sclerosis
4/30/96	Sodium phenylbutyrate[d]	Buphenyl	Adjunctive therapy in the chronic management of patients with urea cycle disorders involving deficiencies of carbamylphosphate synthetase, ornithine transcarbamylase, or argininosuccinic acid synthetase
5/17/96	Interferon beta-1a[c,e]	Avonex	Treatment of relapsing forms of multiple sclerosis to slow the accumulation of physical disability and decrease the frequency of clinical exacerbations
5/17/96	Allopurinol sodium[b,c]	Aloprim for injection	Management of patients with leukemia, lymphoma, and solid tumor malignancies who are receiving cancer therapy that causes elevations of serum and urinary uric acid levels and who cannot tolerate oral therapy
5/22/96	Ofloxacin[b]	Ocuflox ophthalmic solution	Treatment of bacterial corneal ulcers

continued

TABLE C-A1 Continued

Exclusivity Start Date	Generic Name	Trade Name	Indication for Original Approval[a]
6/11/96	Albendazole	Albenza	(1) Treatment of cystic hydatid disease of the liver, lung, and peritoneum, caused by the larval form of the dog tapeworm, *Echinococcus granulosus*. (2) Treatment of parenchymal neurocysticercosis due to active lesions caused by larval forms of the pork tapeworm, *Taenia solium*.
8/23/96	Somatropin for injection[c,e]	Serostim	Treatment of AIDS wasting or cachexia
9/6/96	Midodrine HCl[b]	Amatine	Treatment of symptomatic orthostatic hypotension
9/26/96	Pentosan polysulfate sodium	Elmiron	Relief of bladder pain or discomfort associated with interstitial cystitis
10/25/96	Betaine	Cystadane	Treatment of homocystinuria
11/27/96	Tizanidine HCl[b]	Zanaflex	Treatment of spasticity associated with multiple sclerosis and spinal cord injury
12/20/96	Glatiramer acetate[c]	Copaxone	For reduction of the frequency of relapses in patients with relapsing-remitting multiple sclerosis
1/28/97	Zinc acetate	Galzin	For maintenance treatment of patients with Wilson's disease who have been initially treated with a chelating agent
3/14/97	Anagrelide[b]	Agrylin	Treatment of patients with essential thrombocythemia
5/29/97	Toremifene[d]	Fareston	Treatment of metastatic breast cancer in postmenopausal women with estrogen positive or receptor unknown tumors
12/10/97	Ursodiol[b]	Urso	Treatment of patients with primary biliary cirrhosis
2/25/98	Hydroxyurea[b]	Droxia	To reduce the frequency of painful crises and to reduce the need for blood transfusions in adult patients with sickle cell anemia with recurrent moderate to severe painful crises
4/9/98	Sacrosidase	Sucraid	Oral replacement therapy of the genetically determined sucrase deficiency
6/5/98	Mafenide acetate solution	Sulfamylon solution	For use as an adjunctive topical antimicrobial agent to control bacterial infection when used under moist dressings over meshed autografts on excised burn wounds

TABLE C-A1 Continued

Exclusivity Start Date	Generic Name	Trade Name	Indication for Original Approval[a]
6/22/98	Rifapentine	Priftin	Treatment of pulmonary tuberculosis
7/16/98	Thalidomide	Thalomid	Acute treatment of the cutaneous manifestations of moderate to severe erythema nodosum leprosum (ENL) and as maintenance therapy for prevention and suppression of the cutaneous manifestations of ENL recurrences
8/24/98	Lamotrigine[b]	Lamictal	Adjunctive treatment of Lennox-Gastaut syndrome in pediatric and adult patients
8/24/98	Infliximab[c,e]	Remicade	Treatment of moderately to severely active Crohn's disease for the reduction of signs and symptoms, in patients who have an inadequate response to conventional therapy; and treatment of patients with fistulizing Crohn's disease for reduction in the number of draining enterocutaneous fistula(s)
12/24/98	Modafinil	Provigil	Improve wakefulness in patients with excessive daytime sleepiness associated with narcolepsy
2/2/99	Alitretinoin	Panretin	Topical treatment of cutaneous lesions in patients with AIDS-related Kaposi's sarcoma
3/19/99	Lidocaine patch 5%	Lidoderm patch	For relief of allodynia (painful hypersensitivity) and chronic pain in postherpetic neuralgia
6/28/99	Doxorubicin liposome[c,d]	Doxil	Treatment of metastatic carcinoma of the ovary in patients with disease that is refractory to both paclitaxel- and platinium-based chemotherapy regimens
10/21/99	Exemestane[d]	Aromasin	Treatment of advanced breast cancer in postmenopausal women whose disease has progressed following tamoxifen therapy
12/29/99	Bexarotene	Targretin	Treatment of cutaneous manifestations of cutaneous T-cell lymphoma in patients who are refractory to at least one prior systemic therapy
5/10/01	Imatinib mesylate[d]	Gleevec	Treatment of patients with chronic myeloid leukemia (CML) in blast crisis, accelerated phase, or in chronic phase after failure of interferon-alpha therapy

continued

TABLE C-A1 Continued

Exclusivity Start Date	Generic Name	Trade Name	Indication for Original Approval[a]
8/28/01	Topiramate[d]	Topamax	As adjunctive therapy in patients 2 years and older with seizures associated with Lennox-Gastaut syndrome
11/20/01	Bosentan	Tracleer	Treatment of pulmonary arterial hypertension
1/18/02	Nitisinone	Orfadin	Adjunctive therapy to dietary restriction of tyrosine and phenylalanine in treatment of hereditary tyrosinemia type 1
7/17/02	Oxybate	Xyrem	Treatment of cataplexy associated with narcolepsy
10/8/02	Buprenorphine in combination with naloxone	Suboxone	Treatment of opioid dependence in patients 16 years of age or older
10/8/02	Buprenorphine hydrochloride[d]	Subutex	Treatment of opioid dependence in patients 16 years of age or older
11/22/02	Nitazoxanide	Alinia	Treatment of diarrhea caused by *Cryptosporidium parvum* and *Giardia lamblia*
3/25/03	Pegvisomant[c]	Somavert	Treatment of acromegaly in patients who have had an inadequate response to surgery and/or radiation therapy and/or other medical therapies, or for whom these therapies are not appropriate
7/31/03	Miglustat[d]	Zavesca	Treatment of mild to moderate Type I Gaucher disease in adults for whom enzyme replacement therapy is not a therapeutic option
12/1/03	Somatropin (r-DNA)[c,e]	Zorbtive	Treatment of short bowel syndrome in patients receiving specialized nutritional support
3/8/04	Cinacalcet[d]	Sensipar	Treatment of hypercalcemia in patients with parathyroid carcinoma
4/20/04	Apomorphine HCl[c]	Apokyn	For the acute, intermittent treatment of hypomobility, "off" episodes, associated with advanced Parkinson's disease
5/17/04	Tinidazole	Tindamax	(1) Treatment of giardiasis caused by *G. duodenalis* (also termed *G. lamblia*). (2) Treatment of intestinal amebiasis and amebic liver abcess caused by *E. histolytica*.

TABLE C-A1 Continued

Exclusivity Start Date	Generic Name	Trade Name	Indication for Original Approval[a]
6/10/04	Glutamine	Nutrestore	Treatment of short bowel syndrome in patients receiving specialized nutritional support when used in conjunction with a recombinant human growth hormone that is approved for this indication
8/12/05	Quinine sulfate	Qualaquin	Treatment of uncomplicated *Plasmodium falciparum* malaria
10/28/05	Nelarabine[c,d]	Arranon	Treatment of patients with T-cell acute lymphoblastic leukemia and T-cell lymphoblastic lymphoma whose disease has not responded to or has relapsed following treatment with at least two chemotherapy regimens
11/2/05	Deferasirox	Exjade	Treatment of chronic iron overload due to blood transfusions (transfusional hemosiderosis) in patients 2 years of age or older
12/20/05	Sorafenib	Nexavar	Treatment of patients with advanced renal cell carcinoma
12/27/05	Lenalidomide	Revlimid	Treatment of patients with transfusion dependant anemia due to low or intermediate-1 risk myelodysplastic syndromes associated with a deletion 5 q cytogenetic abnormality with or without additional cytogenetic abnormalities
3/1/06	Cetuximab[c,d,e]	Erbitux	For use in combination with radiation therapy, for the treatment of locally or regionally advanced squamous cell carcinoma of the head and neck (SCCHN) and for use as a single agent for the treatment of patients with recurrent or metastatic SCCHN for whom prior platinum-based therapy has failed
3/29/06	Tacrolimus[b,c]	Prograf	Prophylaxis of organ rejection in patients receiving allogenic heart transplants
4/28/06	Recombinant human acid alpha-glucosidase[c,e]	Myozyme	For use in patients with Pompe disease (GAA deficiency)
5/2/06	Decitabine[c]	Dacogen	For treatment of patients with myelodysplastic syndromes

continued

TABLE C-A1 Continued

Exclusivity Start Date	Generic Name	Trade Name	Indication for Original Approval[a]
6/28/06	Dasatinib[d]	Sprycel	(1) Treatment of adults with Philadelphia chromosome-positive acute lymphoblastic leukemia with resistance or intolerance to prior therapy. (2) Treatment of adults with CML with resistance or intolerance to prior therapy including imatinib.
7/24/06	Idursulfase[c,d,e]	Elaprase	Indicated for patients with Hunter syndrome (mucopolysaccharidosis II, MPS II)
10/6/06	Vorinostat	Zolinza	Treatment of cutaneous manifestations in patients with cutaneous T-cell lymphoma (CTCL) who have progressive, persistent, or recurrent disease on or following two systemic therapies
5/30/07	Temsirolimus[c]	Torisel	Treatment of advanced renal cell carcinoma
5/31/07	Somatropin[c,e]	Norditropin	Treatment of short stature in patients with Noonan's syndrome
6/15/07	Ambrisentan	Letairis	Treatment of pulmonary arterial hypertension (WHO group I) in patients with WHO class II or III symptoms to improve exercise capacity and delay clinical worsening
8/30/07	Lanreotide[c]	Somatuline depot	Long-term treatment of acromegalic patients who have had an inadequate response to or cannot be treated with surgery and/or radiotherapy
9/13/07	Raloxifene	Evista	Reduction in risk of invasive breast cancer in postmenopausal women with osteoporosis and reduction in risk of invasive breast cancer in postmenopausal women at high risk for invasive breast cancer
10/29/07	Nilotinib[d]	Tasigna	For the use for chronic phase (CP) and accelerated phase (AP) Philadelphia chromosome positive chronic myelogenous leukemia (CML) in adult patients resistant to or intolerant to prior therapy that included imatinib

TABLE C-A1 Continued

Exclusivity Start Date	Generic Name	Trade Name	Indication for Original Approval[a]
12/13/07	Sapropterin	Kuvan	Indicated to reduce blood phenylalanine (Phe) levels in patients with hyperphenylalaninemia (HPA) due to tetrahydrobiopterin-(BH4-) responsive phenylketonuria (PKU)
2/27/08	Rilonacept[c,e]	Arcalyst	Treatment of cryopyrin-assisted periodic syndromes (CAPS)
8/15/08	Tetrabenazine	Xenazine	Treatment of chorea associated with Huntington's disease
9/12/08	Immune globulin (human)[c,e]	Gamunex	Treatment of chronic inflammatory demyelinating polyneuropathy
11/14/08	Rufinamide	Banzel	Adjunctive therapy of seizures associated with Lennox-Gastaut syndrome
11/20/08	Eltrombopag	Promacta	Treatment of thrombocytopenia in patients with chronic immune (idiopathic) thrombocytopenic purpura who have had an insufficient response to corticosteroids, immunoglobulins, or splenectomy

NOTE: CIAS1 = cold-induced autoinflammatory syndrome.

[a] We excluded drugs that are covered under Medicare Part B or that are not relevant for the Medicare population (i.e., removed orphan approvals for a pediatric indication). The drugs are sorted by the exclusivity date (i.e., date of approval of orphan indication) for first orphan approval with a relevant indication. Drugs with multiple orphan designations often have exclusivity different dates associated with each approved indication. The text for some indications has been abbreviated.

[b] These drugs are available in generic form.

[c] These drugs have one of the following routes of administration: injection, intravenous, intramuscular, irrigation, or subcutaneous.

[d] These drugs have one or more indications on the Social Security Compassionate Allowances List.

[e] These are biologics, as opposed to chemical entities.

TABLE C-A2 Medicare Stand-Alone PDP Coverage of Orphan Drugs: Inclusion on Formulary (i.e., Plan Coverage), Tier Placement, and Utilization Management (99 drugs)

Generic Name	Trade Name	% Plans That Cover Drug
Citric acid, glucono-delta-lactone, and magnesium carbonate	Renacidin irrigation	0.0
Clofazimine	Lamprene	0.0
Glutamine	Nutrestore	0.0
Zinc acetate	Galzin	0.0
Lodoxamide tromethamine	Alomide ophthalmic solution	45.6
Tinidazole	Tindamax	47.4
Metronidazole (topical)	Metrogel	49.3
Somatropin for injection	Serostim	50.4
Recombinant human acid alpha-glucosidase	Myozyme	51.8
Rifampin, isoniazid, pyrazinamide	Rifater	52.7
Doxorubicin liposome	Doxil	53.0
Nelarabine	Arranon	53.6
Cetuximab	Erbitux	53.6
Somatropin (r-DNA)	Zorbtive	53.6
Temsirolimus	Torisel	54.1
Allopurinol sodium	Aloprim for injection	56.6
Decitabine	Dacogen	57.8
Mafenide acetate solution	Sulfamylon solution	59.1
Rilonacept	Arcalyst	61.2
Lanreotide	Somatuline depot	64.1
Rifampin	Rifadin I.V.	65.9
Somatropin	Norditropin	69.1
Buprenorphine hydrochloride	Subutex	71.1
Pentosan polysulfate sodium	Elmiron	72.0
Buprenorphine in combination with naloxone	Suboxone	73.6
Immune globulin (human)	Gamunex	73.8
Albendazole	Albenza	75.9
Idursulfase	Elaprase	76.0
Nitazoxanide	Alinia	78.1
Quinine sulfate	Qualaquin	83.1
Cromolyn sodium	Gastrocrom	83.9
Sapropterin	Kuvan	84.0
Levocarnitine	Carnitor	84.4
Interferon beta-1a	Avonex	84.5
Apomorphine HCl	Apokyn	85.4
Tetrabenazine	Xenazine	86.4
Oxybate	Xyrem	87.1
Atovaquone	Mepron	88.8
Rifapentine	Priftin	89.0

% Plans That Place on Tier 3	% Plans That Place on Tier 4	% Plans That Have ST	% Plans That Have QL	% Plans That Have PA
—	—	—	—	—
—	—	—	—	—
—	—	—	—	—
—	—	—	—	—
65.2	32.8	0.0	0.5	0.0
46.4	30.7	0.0	0.3	0.0
39.5	4.6	0.0	0.0	0.1
12.5	82.9	0.0	21.1	99.6
13.5	81.8	0.0	0.0	37.8
45.8	20.2	0.0	0.0	0.0
17.4	74.3	0.0	0.0	56.7
30.8	65.0	0.0	0.0	28.1
26.0	69.6	0.0	0.0	74.6
14.0	81.8	0.0	19.8	99.5
9.3	86.0	0.0	0.0	69.5
8.4	24.2	0.0	0.0	1.1
9.2	82.1	0.0	0.0	71.7
38.5	14.3	0.0	7.1	0.0
7.9	91.7	0.0	18.2	63.2
7.3	92.2	9.8	33.4	80.4
14.2	16.0	0.0	0.0	7.4
15.6	80.9	0.0	15.4	99.7
45.9	15.3	0.0	28.2	51.9
46.2	12.3	0.0	14.7	0.0
39.1	22.7	0.0	11.5	34.5
18.4	80.9	0.0	0.0	99.8
34.7	16.3	0.0	0.0	0.0
9.4	84.6	0.0	0.0	45.9
49.3	18.7	0.0	33.9	1.3
41.0	18.1	0.0	30.7	52.1
32.0	17.0	0.0	0.0	0.0
13.8	83.5	0.0	0.3	44.7
5.0	0.0	0.0	0.0	7.9
12.8	82.0	0.1	51.9	91.1
11.6	70.5	0.0	8.6	56.5
14.8	82.0	0.0	22.7	69.8
12.4	58.5	0.0	27.6	37.9
17.7	74.5	12.0	19.7	13.6
45.6	28.7	0.0	0.0	0.0

continued

TABLE C-A2 Continued

Generic Name	Trade Name	% Plans That Cover Drug
Eltrombopag	Promacta	90.5
Cysteamine	Cystagon	91.9
Midodrine HCl	Amatine	92.3
Modafinil	Provigil	93.5
Trientine HCl	Syprine	94.0
Anagrelide	Agrylin	95.6
Riluzole	Rilutek	95.7
Mefloquine HCl	Lariam	95.8
Ambrisentan	Letairis	98.3
Tiopronin	Thiola	99.4
Betaine	Cystadane	99.8
Pegvisomant	Somavert	99.9
Tizanidine HCl	Zanaflex	99.9
Cromolyn sodium 4% ophthalmic solution	Opticrom 4% ophthalmic solution	99.9
Deferasirox	Exjade	99.9
Ofloxacin	Ocuflox ophthalmic solution	99.9
Alitretinoin	Panretin	100.0
Altretamine	Hexalen	100.0
Aminosalicylic acid	Paser granules	100.0
Amiodarone HCl	Cordarone	100.0
Bexarotene	Targretin	100.0
Bosentan	Tracleer	100.0
Calcium acetate	Phos-lo	100.0
Cinacalcet	Sensipar	100.0
Dasatinib	Sprycel	100.0
Desmopressin acetate	N/A	100.0
Exemestane	Aromasin	100.0
Glatiramer acetate	Copaxone	100.0
Hydroxyurea	Droxia	100.0
Imatinib mesylate	Gleevec	100.0
Infliximab	Remicade	100.0
Interferon beta-1b	Betaseron	100.0
Lamotrigine	Lamictal	100.0
Lenalidomide	Revlimid	100.0
Lidocaine patch 5	Lidoderm patch	100.0
Megestrol acetate	Megace	100.0
Miglustat	Zavesca	100.0
Naltrexone HCl	Revia	100.0
Nilotinib	Tasigna	100.0
Nitisinone	Orfadin	100.0
Pilocarpine	Salagen	100.0
Potassium citrate	Urocit-K	100.0
Raloxifene	Evista	100.0
Rifabutin	Mycobutin	100.0
Rufinamide	Banzel	100.0

% Plans That Place on Tier 3	% Plans That Place on Tier 4	% Plans That Have ST	% Plans That Have QL	% Plans That Have PA
19.3	78.0	0.0	46.0	88.7
51.0	12.0	0.0	0.0	16.1
3.5	0.0	0.0	11.5	0.2
48.8	6.9	0.2	74.3	98.5
49.2	11.5	0.0	0.0	0.0
0.1	0.0	0.0	0.1	11.5
11.5	65.9	0.0	11.1	29.1
0.0	0.0	0.0	11.2	0.2
15.5	79.8	10.8	33.6	50.7
48.2	12.5	0.0	0.0	0.0
52.0	11.0	0.0	0.0	15.0
13.7	68.9	6.3	30.2	85.9
4.3	0.0	0.0	0.1	0.1
0.0	0.0	0.0	0.9	0.2
15.3	79.3	0.0	0.0	51.2
2.1	0.0	0.0	5.3	0.2
16.2	57.6	0.0	4.2	10.8
19.3	74.6	0.0	0.0	28.6
45.5	25.6	0.0	0.0	4.4
0.0	0.0	0.0	0.0	5.1
14.0	68.0	0.0	21.5	55.2
15.0	80.0	10.6	29.8	62.4
4.3	2.2	0.0	0.0	0.2
27.9	2.2	10.5	39.8	28.6
15.2	79.7	10.7	40.9	55.4
6.3	0.0	1.4	9.3	0.1
40.4	16.9	10.7	21.1	0.0
13.0	82.4	0.0	43.8	91.7
0.0	0.0	0.0	0.0	0.2
15.2	82.3	0.0	28.8	69.0
12.6	82.5	1.1	0.0	94.4
15.3	82.4	22.6	43.0	92.1
4.2	0.0	13.8	30.6	33.5
15.0	80.2	0.0	34.6	69.9
33.6	8.4	6.3	56.4	45.7
2.1	0.0	0.0	21.3	7.4
15.9	62.4	0.0	6.7	31.1
0.0	0.0	0.0	0.0	0.2
15.2	80.0	10.7	38.7	53.2
15.6	75.3	0.0	0.0	26.4
3.1	0.0	0.0	0.0	0.2
0.0	0.0	0.0	0.0	0.2
21.1	2.2	0.0	63.8	0.0
38.5	12.4	0.0	0.0	0.0
45.7	25.6	0.0	48.3	40.9

continued

TABLE C-A2 Continued

Generic Name	Trade Name	% Plans That Cover Drug
Sacrosidase	Sucraid	100.0
Selegiline HCl	Eldepryl	100.0
Sodium phenylbutyrate	Buphenyl	100.0
Sorafenib	Nexavar	100.0
Sotalol HCl	Betapace	100.0
Sulfadiazine	N/A	100.0
Tacrolimus	Prograf	100.0
Thalidomide	Thalomid	100.0
Topiramate	Topamax	100.0
Toremifene	Fareston	100.0
Tranexamic acid	Cyklokapron	100.0
Tretinoin	Vesanoid	100.0
Ursodiol	Urso	100.0
Vorinostat	Zolinza	100.0
Zidovudine	Retrovir	100.0

% Plans That Place on Tier 3	% Plans That Place on Tier 4	% Plans That Have ST	% Plans That Have QL	% Plans That Have PA
20.5	66.6	0.0	0.0	21.9
0.0	0.0	0.3	0.1	0.2
16.1	61.7	0.0	0.0	19.3
12.9	79.9	0.0	41.2	83.1
0.0	0.0	0.0	0.0	0.2
1.4	4.3	0.0	0.0	0.0
39.9	18.6	0.0	7.6	99.8
10.2	79.8	0.0	33.5	71.4
11.6	2.1	0.1	38.8	13.7
48.3	16.6	0.0	16.9	4.1
17.0	11.8	0.0	0.0	24.0
8.2	50.5	0.0	0.0	31.9
2.1	0.0	0.0	0.0	0.2
15.3	80.0	0.0	34.5	64.1
2.1	0.0	0.0	0.2	0.0

TABLE C-A3 Drugs with a Pediatric Orphan Indication (1983-2008 Approvals) (27 drugs)

Exclusivity Start Date	Generic Name	Trade Name	Indication for Original Approval
10/17/85	Somatropin	Nutropin	For use in the long-term treatment of children who have growth failure due to a lack of adequate endogenous growth hormone secretion
10/17/85	Somatrem for injection	Protropin	For long-term treatment of children who have growth failure due to a lack of adequate endogenous growth hormone secretion
3/8/87	Somatropin for injection	Humatrope	For the long-term treatment of children who have growth failure due to inadequate secretion of normal endogenous growth hormone
8/2/90	Colfosceril palmitate, cetyl alcohol, tyloxapol	Exosurf neonatal for intratracheal suspension	Treatment of established hyaline membrane disease at all gestational ages
1/30/91	Succimer	Chemet capsules	Treatment of lead poisoning in children
7/1/91	Beractant	Survanta intratracheal suspension	(1) Prevention of RDS (hyaline membrane disease) in premature infants less than 1250 grams birth weight or with evidence of surfactant deficiency. (2) Treatment of ("rescue") premature infants with RDS confirmed by x-ray and requiring mechanical ventilation.
12/24/91	Histrelin acetate	Supprelin injection	Treatment of central precocious puberty
2/26/92	Nafarelin acetate	Synarel nasal solution	Treatment of central precocious puberty
7/14/92	Teniposide	Vumon for injection	Induction therapy in patients with refractory childhood acute lymphoblastic leukemia
4/16/93	Leuprolide acetate	Lupron injection	Treatment of children with central precocious puberty
7/29/93	Felbamate	Felbatol	As adjunctive therapy in the treatment of partial and generalized seizures associated with the Lennox-Gastaut syndrome in children
12/27/93	Immune globulin intravenous, human	Gamimune N	Infection prophylaxis in pediatric patients affected with the human immunodeficiency virus

TABLE C-A3 Continued

Exclusivity Start Date	Generic Name	Trade Name	Indication for Original Approval
1/18/96	Respiratory syncytial virus immune globulin (human)	Respigam	Prophylaxis of respiratory syncytial virus (RSV) lower respiratory tract infections in infants and young children at high risk of RSV disease
9/26/97	Sermorelin acetate	Geref	Treatment of idiopathic or organic growth hormone deficiency in children with growth failure
5/27/99	Etanercept	Enbrel	Reduction in signs and symptoms of moderately to severely active polyarticular-course juvenile rheumatoid arthritis in patients who have had an inadequate response to one or more disease-modifying antirheumatic drugs
9/21/99	Caffeine	Cafcit	Short-term treatment of apnea of prematurity in infants between 28 and less than 33 weeks gestational age
6/20/00	Somatropin (r-DNA)	Genotropin	Long-term treatment of pediatric patients who have growth failure due to Prader-Willi syndrome (PWS)
7/12/02	Rasburicase	Elitek	Treatment of malignancy-associated or chemotherapy-induced hyperuricemia
7/29/03	Ribavirin	Rebetol	Treatment of chronic hepatitis C among previously untreated pediatric patients at least 3 years of age or older
10/23/03	Botulism immune globulin	Babybig	Indicated for treatment of infant botulism caused by type A or type B *Clostridium botulinum*
12/28/04	Clofarabine	Clolar	Treatment of pediatric patients 1 to 21 years old with relapsed or refractory acute lymphoblastic leukemia after at least two prior regimens
8/11/05	Meloxicam	Mobic	For relief of the signs and symptoms of pauciarticular or polyarticular course juvenile rheumatoid arthritis in patients 2 years of age or older
8/30/05	Mecasermin	Increlex	Long-term treatment of growth failure in children with severe primary IGF-1 deficiency (Primary IGFD) or with growth hormone (GH) gene deletion who have developed neutralizing antibodies to GH
12/12/05	Mecasermin rinfabate	Iplex	Treatment of growth failure in children with severe primary IGF-1 deficiency (Primary IGFD) or with growth hormone (GH) gene deletion who have developed neutralizing antibodies to GH

continued

TABLE C-A3 Continued

Exclusivity Start Date	Generic Name	Trade Name	Indication for Original Approval
4/13/06	Ibuprofen lysine	Neoprofen	For closure of a clinically significant patent ductus arteriosus in premature infants weighing between 500 and 1500 g, who are no more than 32 weeks gestational age when usual medical management (e.g., fluid restriction, diuretics, respiratory support) is ineffective
12/20/06	Balsalazide disodium	Colazal	Treatment of mildly to moderately active ulcerative colitis in patients 5 years of age and older
2/21/08	Adalimumab	Humira	Treatment of juvenile rheumatoid arthritis

NOTE: This list includes drugs that received approval only for a pediatric orphan indication. Remicade, which received a pediatric orphan approval for the treatment of pediatric Crohn's disease, is also approved for an adult orphan indication and was therefore included in a previous list of drugs. The drugs are sorted by the exclusivity date (i.e., date of approval of orphan indication) for first orphan approval with a relevant indication. Drugs with multiple orphan designations often have different exclusivity dates associated with each approved indication. The text for some indications has been abbreviated.

TABLE C-A4 Medicare Stand-Alone PDP Coverage for Drugs with a Pediatric Orphan Indication: Inclusion on Formulary (i.e., Plan Coverage), Tier Placement, and Utilization Management (27 drugs)

Generic Name	Trade Name	No. of Plans That Cover Drug	% Plans That Cover Drug	%- Plans That Place on Tier 3	% Plans That Place on Tier 4	% Plans That Have ST	% Plans That Have QL	% Plans That Have PA
Beractant	Survanta intratracheal suspension	0	0.0	—	—	—	—	—
Botulism immune globulin	Babybig	0	0.0	—	—	—	—	—
Caffeine	Cafcit	0	0.0	—	—	—	—	—
Colfosceril palmitate, cetyl alcohol, tyloxapol	Exosurf neonatal for intratracheal suspension	0	0.0	—	—	—	—	—
Histrelin acetate	Supprelin injection	0	0.0	—	—	—	—	—
Ibuprofen lysine	Neoprofen	0	0.0	—	—	—	—	—
Immune globulin intravenous, human	Gamimune n	0	0.0	—	—	—	—	—
Mecasermin rinfabate	Iplex	0	0.0	—	—	—	—	—
Respiratory syncytial virus immune globulin (human)	Respigam	0	0.0	—	—	—	—	—
Sermorelin acetate	Geref	0	0.0	—	—	—	—	—
Somatrem for injection	Protropin	0	0.0	—	—	—	—	—
Succimer	Chemet capsules	0	0.0	—	—	—	—	—
Teniposide	Vumon for injection	0	0.0	—	—	—	—	—
Somatropin [r-DNA]	Genotropin	622	38.4	57.6	25.6	0.0	27.8	99.5
Somatropin	Nutropin	625	38.6	16.6	77.6	0.0	28.0	99.5
Somatropin for injection	Humatrope	693	42.8	15.0	79.4	0.0	25.3	99.6

continued

TABLE C-A4 Continued

Generic Name	Trade Name	No. of Plans That Cover Drug	% Plans That Cover Drug	% Plans That Place on Tier 3	% Plans That Place on Tier 4	% Plans That Have ST	% Plans That Have QL	% Plans That Have PA
Clofarabine	Clolar	899	55.5	25.0	66.6	0.0	0.0	19.4
Mecasermin	Increlex	1,347	83.1	21.4	73.1	0.0	0.0	92.0
Nafarelin acetate	Synarel nasal solution	1,445	89.2	30.0	61.7	0.0	0.0	31.4
Etanercept	Enbrel	1,450	89.5	11.5	83.3	1.4	45.2	93.7
Balsalazide disodium	Colazal	1,536	94.8	4.4	0.0	0.0	0.0	0.2
Meloxicam	Mobic	1,546	95.4	0.0	0.0	0.1		0.2
Leuprolide acetate	Lupron injection	1,554	95.9	11.1	9.8	0.0	18.1	71.1
Adalimumab	Humira	1,618	99.9	13.0	82.4	1.2	46.8	94.3
Felbamate	Felbatol	1,620	100.0	38.1	18.9	0.0	0.0	0.0
Rasburicase	Elitek	1,620	100.0	17.7	77.3	0.0	0.0	49.0
Ribavirin	Rebetol	1,620	100.0	6.9	6.4	0.0	17.4	73.6

REFERENCES

CMS (Centers for Medicare and Medicaid Services). 2009a. *2010 Medicare Advantage Rate-book and Prescription Drug Rate Information: 2010 Low-Income Premium Subsidy Amounts.* http://www.cms.hhs.gov/MedicareAdvtgSpecRateStats/Downloads/Regional RatesBenchmarks2010.pdf (accessed September 2, 2010).

CMS. 2009b. *2010 Medicare Part D National Stand-Alone Prescription Drug Plans.* http://www.cms.hhs.gov/PrescriptionDrugCovGenIn/Downloads/NationalPDPs.pdf (accessed September 2, 2010).

CMS. 2010. *CMS Announces Course of Action to Identify Protected Class of Prescription Drugs.* http://www.cms.hhs.gov/apps/media/press/release.asp?Counter=3409 (accessed September 2, 2010).

KFF (Kaiser Family Foundation). 2009a. *Medicare: Low-Income Assistance Under the Medicare Drug Benefit.* http://www.kff.org/medicare/upload/7327-05.pdf (accessed September 2, 2010).

KFF. 2009b. *Medicare Part D 2009 Data Spotlight: Specialty Tiers.* http://www.kff.org/medicare/upload/7919.pdf (accessed September 2, 2010).

KFF. 2009c. *Medicare Part D 2010 Spotlight: Benefit Design and Cost-Sharing. December.* http://www.kff.org/medicare/upload/8033.pdf (accessed September 2, 2010).

KFF. 2009d. *Medicare Part D Spotlight: Part D Plan Availability in 2010 and Key Changes since 2006.* http://www.kff.org/medicare/upload/7986.pdf (accessed September 2, 2010).

KFF. 2010a. *Explaining Health Care Reform: Key Changes to the Medicare Part D Drug Benefit Coverage Gap.* http://www.kff.org/healthreform/upload/8059.pdf (accessed September 2, 2010).

KFF. 2010b. *Medicare: A Primer.* http://www.kff.org/medicare/upload/7615-03.pdf (accessed September 2, 2010).

KFF. 2010c. *Medicare at a Glance.* http://www.kff.org/medicare/upload/1066-12.pdf (accessed September 2, 2010).

NORD (National Organization for Rare Disorders). 2006. Letter to Mark B. McClellan, M.D., Ph.D., Administrator of CMS: Orphan Drug Coverage in Medicare Part D Formularies January. http://www.rarediseases.org/news/pdf/Final_ltr_CMS_011006_V2.pdf (accessed September 2, 2010).

OIG (Office of Inspector General, U.S. Department of Health and Human Services). 2001. *The Orphan Drug Act: Implementation and Impact.* http://oig.hhs.gov/oei/reports/oei-09-00-00380.pdf (accessed September 2, 2010).

Social Security Online. 2010. *Compassionate Allowances.* http://www.socialsecurity.gov/compassionateallowances/ (accessed September 2, 2010).

D

Glossary, Abbreviations, and Public Laws

GLOSSARY[*]

Acetylation. Attachment of an acetyl group, a chemical moiety, to a newly translated protein molecule (see also *Posttranslational modification*). (http://themedicalbiochemistrypage.org/protein-modifications.html)

Active treatment concurrent control. In a clinical trial, "the test drug is compared with known effective therapy." (21 CFR 314.126)

Adaptive design. A clinical study that "includes a prospectively planned opportunity for modification of one or more specified aspects of the study design and hypotheses based on analysis of data (usually interim data) from subjects in the study. Analyses of the accumulating study data are performed at prospectively planned timepoints." (http://www.fda.gov/downloads/Drugs/guidancecomplianceregulatoryinformation/guidances/ucm201790.pdf)

Allele. One of two or more versions of the genetic sequence that comprises a gene, found at a particular location on a chromosome. (Feero et al., 2010). (http://www.ncbi.nlm.nih.gov/bookshelf/br.fcgi?book=gene&part=glossary#IX-T)

Animal model. A laboratory animal possessing physical and/or genetic characteristics of a human disease or disorder used for medical research on that condition (see *Mouse model*). (http://www.genome.gov/glossary.cfm?key=mouse%20model)

---

[*]Consultant Alison Mack assisted with the preparation of the glossary.

Antibody. A protein produced by the immune system that circulates in the blood, where it recognizes foreign substances such as bacteria or viruses, binds to them, and destroys them. (http://www.genome.gov/glossary/index.cfm?id=7)

Approval. Authorization by the Food and Drug Administration (FDA) for the marketing of a drug (under a New Drug Application), medical device (under a Premarket Approval Application), or biological product (under a Biologics Licensing Agreement) (see also *Clearance*; *Humanitarian Device Exemption*; *New Drug Application*; *Premarket Approval application*).

Autosomal dominant. A pattern of inheritance that involves a gene located on one of the numbered pairs of autosomal chromosomes (i.e., not the sex chromosomes X or Y) in human cells. Dominant refers to the effect of the specific genetic sequence present at this location (see *Allele*). An allele is dominant if only one of the paired autosomal chromosomes needs to contain it in order for the person to exhibit the associated trait (see also *Autosomal recessive*). (http://www.genome.gov/glossary/index.cfm?id=12)

Autosomal recessive. A pattern of inheritance that involves a gene located on one of the numbered pairs of autosomal chromosomes (i.e., not the sex chromosomes X or Y) in human cells. Recessive refers to the effect of the specific genetic sequence present at this location (see *Allele*). An allele is recessive if both of the paired autosomal chromosomes must contain it in order for the person to exhibit the associated trait (see also *Autosomal dominant*). (http://www.genome.gov/glossary/index.cfm?id=12)

Benefit. A positive or valued outcome of an action or event.

Biobanking. See *Biorepository.*

Bioengineering. Integration of the physical, chemical, mathematical, and computational sciences with engineering principles for the study of biology, medicine, and behavior. (http://www.nibib.nih.gov/HealthEdu/ScienceEdu/BioengDef)

Bioinformatics. "The application of computers to the collection, organization, analysis, manipulation, presentation, and sharing of biological data" (see also *Translational bioinformatics*). (NRC, 2000, p. 4)

Biologic or biological product. A "virus, therapeutic serum, toxin, antitoxin, vaccine, blood, blood component or derivative, allergenic product, or analogous product, or arsphenamine or derivative of arsphenamine (or any other trivalent organic arsenic compound), applicable to the prevention, treatment, or cure of a disease or condition of human beings." (42 USC 262(1)) "Biologics can be composed of sugars, proteins, or nucleic acids or complex combinations of these substances, or may be living entities such as cells and tissues. Biologics are isolated from a variety of natural sources—human, animal, or microorganism." (http://www.fda.gov/AboutFDA/CentersOffices/CBER/ucm133077.htm)

Biologics Licensing Application. Form used by sponsors to request FDA approval to market a new biologic product in the United States based on information about its safety and effectiveness and other requirements.

Biomarker. A "characteristic that is objectively measured and evaluated as an indicator of normal biological processes, pathogenic processes, or pharmacologic responses to a[n] . . . intervention" (Biomarkers Definitions Working Group, 2001).

Biorepository. A "facility that collects, catalogs, and stores samples of biological material, such as urine, blood, tissue, cells, DNA, RNA, and protein, from humans, animals, or plants for laboratory research. If the samples are from people, medical information may also be stored along with a written consent to use the samples in laboratory studies." (http://www.cancer.gov/dictionary/?CdrID=561323)

Blood-brain barrier. A"network of blood vessels with closely spaced cells that makes it difficult for potentially toxic substances (such as anticancer drugs) to penetrate the blood vessel walls and enter the brain." (http://www.cancer.gov/dictionary/?CdrID=46504)

Cell therapy. Providing patients with cells (often from the immune system) that function in the treatment of disease or the support of other therapy. (http://www.celltherapysociety.org/index.php/glossarynv/40/160) (http://www.cancer.gov/dictionary/?CdrID=44024)

Chemical library. See *Compound library.*

Clearance. Action taken by FDA under section 510(k) of the Food, Drug, and Cosmetic Act to authorize the marketing of a medical device based on a review of evidence of safety and equivalence to certain previously marketed devices; clinical evidence of safety and effectiveness is not usually required.

Clinical endpoint. (see also *Endpoint*). "A characteristic or variable that reflects how a patient [or consumer] feels, functions, or survives." (Biomarkers Definitions Working Group, 2001)

Clinical phenotype. The observable physical and biochemical characteristics of an individual with a specific genetic makeup (see also *Phenotype, Phenotyping*). (http://www.ncbi.nlm.nih.gov/bookshelf/br.fcgi?book=gene&part=glossary#IX-T)

Clinical trial. A medical study involving human participants that follows a defined protocol to answer specified questions, for example, about the safety and efficacy of a medical product.

Phase I trials initiate the study of candidate drugs in humans. Such trials typically assess the safety and tolerability of a drug, routes of administration and safe dose ranges, and the way the body processes the drug (e.g., how it is absorbed, distributed, metabolized, and excreted). They usually involve less than 100 individuals, often healthy volunteers.

Phase II trials continue the assessment of a drug's safety and dosing but also begin to test efficacy in people with the target disease. These studies may include a range of controls on potential bias, including use of a control group that receives standard treatment or a placebo, the random assignment of research participants to the experimental and control groups, and the concealment (blinding) from participants and researchers of a participant's assignment.

Phase III trials are expanded investigations of safety and efficacy that are intended to allow a fuller assessment of a drug's benefits and harms and to provide information sufficient to prepare labeling or instructions for the use of the drug. These studies may involve thousands of research participants and multiple sites.

Phase IV studies occur after a product is approved for marketing and are highly variable in their design. They are sometimes required by FDA but may be voluntarily undertaken by manufacturers. They are typically intended to provide further information about outcomes in clinical practice, e.g., in broader populations or over longer periods than studied in the trials used to support FDA approval.

Combination product. "A product that 1) is comprised of two or more regulated components, i.e., drug/device, biologic/device, drug/biologic, or drug/device/biologic, that are physically, chemically, or otherwise combined or mixed and produced as a single entity; 2) is comprised of two or more separate products packaged together in a single package or as a unit and comprised of drug and device products, device and biological products, or biological and drug products; or 3) is packaged separately that according to its investigational plan or proposed labeling is intended for use only with an approved individually specified drug, device, or biological product where both are required to achieve the intended use, indication, or effect and where upon approval of the proposed product the labeling of the approved product would need to be changed, e.g., to reflect a change in intended use, dosage form, strength, route of administration, or significant change in dose." (21 CFR 3.2(e))

Companion diagnostic test. As defined by FDA, a diagnostic test developed for use with a particular therapeutic product to inform treatment, including determining which patients are appropriate candidates for the therapy and tailoring decisions about medications.

Comparative effectiveness analysis. A systematic evaluation of the evidence on the outcomes of different drugs or other options for treating, preventing, or diagnosing a medical condition

Compound library. A collection of small organic molecules organized in a format that facilitates drug discovery and biomedical research, also known as a chemical library. The compounds may be derived from natural sources or synthesized in the laboratory. (http://www.griffith.edu.au/science/queensland-compound-library/about-us)

Computational biology. See *Bioinformatics*.

Custom device. As defined in 21 USC § 360j(b), "a device that:

(1) Necessarily deviates from devices generally available or from an applicable performance standard or premarket approval requirement in order to comply with the order of an individual physician or dentist;

(2) Is not generally available to, or generally used by, other physicians or dentists;

(3) Is not generally available in finished form for purchase or for dispensing upon prescription;

(4) Is not offered for commercial distribution through labeling or advertising; and

(5) Is intended for use by an individual patient named in the order of a physician or dentist, and is to be made in a specific form for that patient, or is intended to meet the special needs of the physician or dentist in the course of professional practice."

Data exclusivity. A period of time during which sponsors of innovative drugs have the exclusive use of the safety and effectiveness data they submitted to obtain FDA approval. (Glover, 2007)

Differentiation. Development of immature, unspecialized cells (see *Pluripotent stem cell*) into mature, specialized cells (see also *Stem cell*). (http://www.cancer.gov/dictionary/?CdrID=46477)

DNA modification. Chemical changes to the DNA such as methylation (see below) that frequently affect gene transcription (see below) and, thereby, gene expression (see below). (http://themedicalbiochemistrypage.org/dna.html#modification)

DNA sequencing. Determining the exact order of the base sequence in a segment of DNA, which carries the information that cells use to assemble proteins and RNA (see also *Nucleotide*). In exome sequencing (see *Exome*), only the coding regions of the genome are analyzed. (http://www.genome. gov/glossary.cfm?key=DNA%20sequencing)

Dose-comparison concurrent control. In a clinical trial, "at least two doses of the drug are compared." (21 CFR 314.126)

Drugs. As defined in 21 USC 321(g)(1): "(A) articles recognized in the official United States Pharmacopoeia, official Homoeopathic Pharmacopoeia of the United States, or official National Formulary, or any supplement to any of them; and (B) articles intended for use in the diagnosis, cure, mitigation, treatment, or prevention of disease in man or other animals; and (C) articles (other than food) intended to affect the structure or any function of the body of man or other animals; and (D) articles intended for use as a component of any article specified in clause (A), (B), or (C)."

Effectiveness. The achievement of desired results in actual clinical practice.

Efficacy. The achievement of desired results in controlled clinical studies.

Endpoint. "A characteristic or variable that reflects how a patient [or consumer] feels, functions, or survives." (Biomarkers Definitions Working Group, 2001)

Epigenetic. Regulation of gene expression (see below) that occurs without altering the structure of the gene. (Feero et al., 2010)

Etiology. Cause or origin of a disease.

Exome. Analogous to genome (see below), the complete set of DNA sequences in a cell that are expressed as proteins. The exome comprises less than 5 percent of the genome.

Formulary. "A continually updated list of medications and related information, representing the clinical judgment of physicians, pharmacists, and other experts in the diagnosis, prophylaxis, or treatment of disease and promotion of health." (http://www.ashp.org/DocLibrary/BestPractices/ FormGdlPTCommFormSyst.aspx)

Gene. The basic physical and functional unit of heredity. A gene is a segment of DNA located in a specific position on a particular chromosome. In each gene, the ordered sequence of chemical groups in DNA, called nucleotides (see below), provides a blueprint used by the cell to synthesize a specific functional product, such as a protein. (Feero et al., 2010) (http://www.ncbi. nlm.nih.gov/bookshelf/br.fcgi?book=gene&part=glossary#IX-T)

Gene expression. The process by which the information encoded in the DNA sequence of a gene produces a functional molecule, such as a protein or RNA, that operates in the cell. Gene expression encompasses both

gene transcription and gene translation (see below). (http://ghr.nlm.nih.
gov/glossary=geneexpression)

Gene expression profile. An indicator of the numbers and amounts of all
messenger RNAs made in various cell types. This information can be obtained using microarray technology (see below). A gene expression profile
may be used to find and diagnose a disease or condition and to see how well
the body responds to treatment. Gene expression profiles may be used in
personalized medicine. (http://www.cancer.gov/dictionary/?CdrID=386201

Gene mapping. The process of establishing the locations of genes on the
chromosomes and the distances between them. Early gene maps used linkage analysis, a technique that correlates coinheritance of traits with the
physical closeness of their genes on chromosomes. More recently, scientists
have used recombinant DNA techniques to establish the actual physical
locations of genes on the chromosomes. (http://www.genome.gov/glossary/
index.cfm?id=74)

Gene product. RNA or protein produced as a result of gene expression (see
above). The amount of gene product is used to measure gene activity, which
may be correlated in some cases with disease (see *Gene expression profile*).
(http://ghr.nlm.nih.gov/glossary=geneproduct)

Gene transfer. "The insertion of genetic material into a cell." (http://www.
cancer.gov/dictionary/?CdrID=270852)

Gene transcription. The process by which cells synthesize a messenger RNA
(mRNA) molecule based on, and complementary to, the sequence of DNA
in a gene. The mRNA is subsequently translated (see *Translation*) into protein. (http://ghr.nlm.nih.gov/glossary=transcription)

Genetic polymorphism. See *Polymorphism*.

Genetic test. "A genetic test is the analysis of human DNA, RNA, chromosomes, proteins, or certain metabolites in order to detect alterations related
to a heritable disorder. This can be accomplished by directly examining the
DNA or RNA that makes up a gene (direct testing), looking at markers
co-inherited with a disease-causing gene (linkage testing), assaying certain
metabolites (biochemical testing), or examining the chromosomes (cytogenetic testing)." (http://www.ncbi.nlm.nih.gov/projects/GeneTests/static/
concepts/primer/primerwhatistest.shtm)

Genetics. The study of genes and heredity.

Genome. The entire set of genetic instructions found in a cell. The human
genome consists of 23 pairs of chromosomes in the cell nucleus and a small
chromosome found in the mitochondria of cells.

Genome-wide association studies. "A study that compares the complete DNA of people with a disease or condition to the DNA of people without the disease or condition. These studies find the genes involved in a disease, and may help prevent, diagnose, and treat the disease. Also called GWAS, WGA study, and whole genome association study." (http://www.cancer.gov/dictionary/?CdrID=636779)

Genomics. The study of the complete genetic material of an organism.

Genotype. "The genetic constitution of an organism or cell, or the genetic sequence at a particular location in the genome" (see *Allele*). (Feero et al., 2010) (http://www.ncbi.nlm.nih.gov/bookshelf/br.fcgi?book=gene&part=glossary#IX-T)

Genotyping. Testing to identify specific genetic sequences (see *Allele*) in individuals—for example, to determine whether a person with type A blood (see *Phenotype*) bears one of two possible genotypes: AO (see *Heterozygous*) or AA (see *Homozygous*). (http://www.ncbi.nlm.nih.gov/bookshelf/br.fcgi?book=gene&part=glossary#IX-T)

Germline. Cells that produce egg or sperm cells. The genetic sequences in parental germline cells are inherited by offspring. (http://www.ncbi.nlm.nih.gov/bookshelf/br.fcgi?book=gene&part=glossary#IX-T)

Glycosylation. Attachment of a carbohydrate group to a protein molecule during its synthesis (co-translationally) or immediately afterward (see also *Posttranslational modification*) to produce a glycoprotein. "Glycoproteins on cell surfaces are important for communication between cells, for maintaining cell structure and for self-recognition by the immune system." (http://themedicalbiochemistrypage.org/glycoproteins.html# mechanism)

Haplotype. A set of DNA polymorphisms (versions of DNA sequences) that are often inherited together. These polymorphisms may be a combination of alleles (see above) or single-nucleotide polymorphisms (see below), all of which are found on the same chromosome (Feero et al., 2010).

Harm. A hurtful or adverse outcome of an action or event, whether temporary or permanent.

Heterozygous. The inheritance of different forms of a particular gene from each parent (see *Allele*). A heterozygous genotype contrasts with a homozygous (see below) genotype, in which both alleles are identical. (http://www.genome.gov/glossary/index.cfm?id=101)

High-throughput screening. A method of drug discovery that permits the simultaneous testing of large numbers of compounds (see *Compound library*) against a particular target. This process typically employs modern robotics, sophisticated control software, advanced liquid handling, and sensitive detection methods. Those compounds that prove to be "hits" can be used as the starting point for a drug discovery effort; they are then refined through medicinal chemistry and lower-throughput assays before entering the clinic. (http://www.htscreening.org/)

Histone. "A protein that provides structural support to a chromosome. In order for very long DNA molecules to fit into the cell nucleus, they wrap around complexes of histone proteins, giving the chromosome a more compact shape. Some variants of histones are associated with the regulation of gene expression." (http://www.genome.gov/glossary/index.cfm?id=102)

Historical control. In a clinical trial, "the results of treatment with the test drug are compared with experience historically derived from the adequately documented natural history of the disease or condition, or from the results of active treatment, in comparable patients or populations." (21 CFR 314.126)

Homozygous. The inheritance of identical forms (see *Allele*) of a particular gene from each parent (see also *Heterozygous*). (http://www.genome.gov/glossary/index.cfm?id=105)

Humanitarian Device Exemption. An application required to obtain FDA approval to market a Humanitarian Use Device; similar to a Premarket Approval application except that evidence of efficacy is not required.

Humanitarian Use Device. A "medical device intended to benefit patients in the treatment or diagnosis of a disease or condition that affects or is manifested in fewer than 4,000 individuals in the United States per year." (21 CFR 814.102(a)(5))

Incidence. The number of new cases of a disease or condition during a defined period in a specified population, or the rate at which new events occur in a defined population. In contrast, prevalence (see below) refers to all cases of a disease or condition existing in the population at a given time. (http://ghr.nlm.nih.gov/glossary=incidence)

In vitro diagnostic (IVD) devices. IVD devices include reagents, instruments, and systems for use in diagnosing diseases or assessing health. They are used in collecting, preparing, or examining human biological specimens and may be regulated by the FDA as devices and as biologic products.

Investigational Device Exemption application. An application to the FDA to approve the legal shipment of a device to be used in a clinical trial when the device has not been approved or cleared for marketing.

Investigational New Drug application. An application to the FDA to approve the legal shipment of a drug to be used in a clinical trial when the drug has not yet been approved for marketing.

Kinase. An enzyme that attaches phosphate groups (see *Phosphorylation*) to other molecules, which often causes the target molecule to become active. Kinases are part of many cell processes and are the targets of some cancer treatments. (http://ghr.nlm.nih.gov/glossary=kinase) (http://www.cancer.gov/dictionary/?CdrID=641114)

Label. As defined in Section 510k of the Food, Drug, and Cosmetic Act, a "display of written, printed, or graphic matter upon the immediate container of a drug or other product." Labels often are included within product packaging rather than on the actual product.

Lysosome. A membrane-enclosed compartment within a cell containing enzymes that break down excess or worn-out cell components and also destroy invading viruses and bacteria. If the cell is damaged beyond repair, lysosomes can help it to self-destruct. (http://ghr.nlm.nih.gov/glossary=lysosome)

Market exclusivity. As provided for by the Orphan Drug Act, a 7-year period during which the sponsor of an orphan drug has exclusive rights to market the drug for the orphan indication.

Mass spectrometry. A technique used to identify chemicals in a substance by their mass and charge. Mass spectrometers are instruments that weigh molecules and measure how much of a compound is present in a mixture. In tandem mass spectrometry, two mass spectrometers are used in series to sort and weigh the molecules in a sample, then break up the molecules (i.e., breaking proteins into amino acids), and sort and weigh their components. (http://www.medterms.com/script/main/art.asp?articlekey=25328) (http://www.medterms.com/script/main/art.asp?articlekey=25329)

Medical device. "An instrument, apparatus, implement, machine, contrivance, implant, in vitro reagent, or other similar or related article, including a component, part, or accessory, which is

- recognized in the official National Formulary, or the United States Pharmacopoeia, or any supplement of them,
- intended for use in the diagnosis of disease or other conditions, or in the cure, mitigation, treatment, or prevention of disease, in man or other animals, or
- intended to affect the structure or any function of the body of man or other animals, and

which does not achieve any of its primary intended purposes through chemical action within or on the body of man of other animals and which is not dependent upon being metabolized for the achievement of its primary intended purposes." (21 USC 321(h))

Metabolomics. The study of the metabolome, "the entire complement of metabolites that are generated in an organism, tissue, or cell type." (NRC, 2007, p. 14)

Methylation. The attachment of methyl groups to DNA at cytosine bases. Methylation is correlated with reduced transcription of genes. (http://www.ncbi.nlm.nih.gov/bookshelf/br.fcgi?book=gene&part=glossary#IX-T)

Microarray technology. A technique used to study the expression of many genes at once. It employs a "gene chip"—a solid surface on which thousands of known gene sequences are immobilized in specific locations. When a sample containing DNA or RNA is placed in contact with the gene chip, base pairing between the expressed sequences in the sample and complementary sequences on the gene chip produces light, which allows the expressed sequences in the sample to be identified. (http://www.genome.gov/glossary/index.cfm?id=125) (http://ghr.nlm.nih.gov/glossary=microarraytechnology)

Microfluidic device. "An instrument that uses very small amounts of fluid on a microchip to do certain laboratory tests. A microfluidic device may use body fluids or solutions containing cells or cell parts to diagnose diseases. Also called lab-on-a-chip." (http://www.cancer.gov/dictionary/?CdrID=561603)

MicroRNAs (miRNAs). Small, noncoding RNAs with a broad spectrum of functions, including posttranscriptional regulation of gene expression. (http://www.nature.com/ng/journal/v38/n6s/full/ng1794.html) (http://www.ncbi.nlm.nih.gov/pmc/articles/PMC2605651/)

Modifier gene. A secondary gene that influences the expression of a primary gene that in turn controls a physical trait. (http://www.biochem.northwestern.edu/holmgren/Glossary/Definitions/Def-M/modifier_gene.html)

Monoclonal antibody. An antibody (see above) made in the laboratory to bind specifically to a single type of cell or molecule. Monoclonal antibodies are used to destroy cancer cells directly and to carry toxic substances into tumors. (http://www.cancer.gov/dictionary/)

Mouse model. A laboratory mouse that possesses physical and/or genetic characteristics of a human disease or disorder and is used for medical research on that condition. Mouse models may have natural mutations similar to disease-associated human mutations, or they may be created by transferring new genes into mice or by inactivating existing genes (see *Animal model*). (http://www.genome.gov/glossary.cfm?key=mouse%20model)

Mutation. A change in a DNA sequence that may or may not affect a physical trait or phenotype (see below). Mutations that occur in eggs or sperm can be passed on to offspring, unlike mutations that occur in body cells (Feero et al., 2010). (http://www.genome.gov/glossary/index.cfm?id=134)

Neglected disease. A label often applied to certain tropical infections that are overwhelmingly concentrated in the world's poorest countries and for which there are inadequate incentives for drug development or inadequate mechanisms to make existing treatments widely available.

New Drug Application. Form used by drug sponsors to request FDA approval to market a new pharmaceutical in the United States based on information about its safety and effectiveness and other requirements.

No treatment concurrent control. In a clinical trial, "the test drug is compared with no treatment." (21 CFR 314.126)

Noninferiority trials. Clinical trials that involve comparison of an investigational product with an active treatment. They seek to demonstrate "that any difference between the two treatments is small enough to allow a conclusion that the new drug has at least some effect or, in many cases, an effect that is not too much smaller than the active control." (http://www.fda.gov/downloads/Drugs/GuidanceComplianceRegulatoryInformation/Guidances/ucm070951.pdf)

Nucleotide. The basic chemical building block of RNA and DNA, which are long chains of nucleotides. A nucleotide consists of a sugar molecule attached to a phosphate group and a nitrogen-containing base. In DNA, each nucleotide contains one of four bases: adenine (A), cytosine (C), guanine (G), and thymine (T). The DNA base sequence carries the information a cell needs to assemble protein and RNA molecules. (http://www.genome.gov/glossary/index.cfm?id=143) (http://www.genome.gov/glossary/index.cfm?id=51)

Off-label use. See *Unlabeled use.*

Personalized medicine. An approach to clinical decision making that uses information about an individual's genetic profile and other characteristics to guide decisions on disease prevention, diagnosis, and treatment. (http://www.genome.gov/glossary/index.cfm?id=150)

Pharmacogenetics. See *Pharmacogenomics.*

Pharmacogenomics. The study of how a person's genes affect the way he or she responds to drugs. (http://www.cancer.gov/dictionary/?CdrID=631052)

Phase I, II, III trials. See *Clinical trial.*

Phenotype. An organism's observable characteristics or traits, such as coloration, size, or the presence or absence of disease. A phenotypic trait may be influenced by genes (genotype), the environment, or both. (http://www.genome.gov/glossary/index.cfm?id=152)

Phenotyping. Diagnostic testing in order to infer the genotype (see above) of an individual based on his or her phenotype (see above). (http://www.ncbi.nlm.nih.gov/bookshelf/br.fcgi?book=gene&part=glossary#IX-T)

Phosphorylation. The attachment of a phosphate group to a protein by an enzyme known as a kinase (see above). Posttranslational phosphorylation, one of the most common protein modifications that occurs in animal cells, often serves to regulate the protein's biological activity (see also *Posttranslational modification*). (http://themedicalbiochemistrypage.org/protein-modifications.html# phosphorylation)

Placebo. "An inactive substance or treatment that looks the same as, and is given the same way as, an active drug or treatment being tested. The effects of the active drug or treatment are compared to the effects of the placebo." (http://www.cancer.gov/dictionary/?CdrID=46688)

Placebo concurrent control. In a clinical trial, the "test drug is compared with an inactive preparation designed to resemble the test drug as far as possible." (21 CFR 314.126)

Pluripotent stem cell. "A cell that is able to develop into many different types of cells or tissues in the body" (see also *Stem cell, Differentiation*). (http://www.cancer.gov/dictionary/?CdrID=44797)

Polymorphism. Variations in the sequence of a particular gene. The most common of these involve differences in one nucleotide among the thousands that can comprise a gene; these are known as single-nucleotide polymorphisms (see below). Some polymorphisms involve long stretches of DNA that differ between versions of the same gene. (http://www.genome.gov/glossary/index.cfm?id=160)

Postmarket. Evaluations, activities, and decisions that occur after regulatory approval, clearance, or registration of a medical product for marketing.

Posttranslational modification. Enzyme-mediated alterations of newly translated proteins, such as the addition of chemical groups including acetyl (see *Acetylation*), carbohydrates (see *Glycosylation*), methyl (see *Methylation*), or phosphate (see *Phosphorylation*). (http://walsh.med.harvard.edu/pubs/PDFs_2/PTM_review.pdf)

Preclinical studies. Investigations of toxicity, pharmacological activity, and other characteristics of a promising drug candidate that occurs prior to research with human participants.

Premarket Approval application. Form used by medical device sponsors to request FDA approval to market certain complex medical devices in the United States based on information about its safety and effectiveness and other requirements.

Prevalence. The number of diagnosed cases of a particular condition or disease existing in a specified population at a given time. It is distinct from incidence, which is the number of *new* cases of the disease arising in the population over a given time period. (http://ghr.nlm.nih.gov/glossary= prevalence)

Proteomics. The study of the proteome, the "entire protein complement in a given cell, tissue or organism." (http://www.nature.com/nature/insights/ 6928.html)

Rare disease. In the Orphan Drug Act, a disease or condition that affects fewer than 200,000 people in the United States (21 USC 360bb).

Receptor. "A molecule inside or on the surface of a cell that binds to a specific substance and causes a specific physiologic effect in the cell." (http://ghr.nlm.nih.gov/glossary=receptor)

Registry. A system for collecting uniform information about a class of individuals or patients who have in common a disease, injury, condition, medical procedure or product, or similar characteristic.

Regulatory science. "The development and use of new tools, standards and approaches to more efficiently develop products and to more effectively evaluate product safety, efficacy and quality." (http://www.fda.gov/News Events/Newsroom/PressAnnouncements/ucm201706.html)

Risk. A potential harm or the potential for an action or event to cause harm.

Safe. A relative term; "There is reasonable assurance that a device is safe when it can be determined, based upon valid scientific evidence, that the probable benefits to health from use of the device for its intended uses and conditions of use, when accompanied by adequate directions and warnings against unsafe use, outweigh any probable risks" (21 CFR 860.7(d)(1)).

Sequencing. See *DNA sequencing.*

Signature molecule. "A biological molecule found in blood, other body fluids, or tissues that is a sign of a normal or abnormal process, or of a condition or disease. A signature molecule may be used to see how well the body responds to a treatment for a disease or condition. Also called biomarker and molecular marker." (http://www.cancer.gov/dictionary/?CdrID=579633)

Single-nucleotide polymorphism (SNP). Variant gene sequence that differs by only a single nucleotide. These polymorphisms (see above) occur frequently throughout the human genome; certain SNPs correlate with disease, drug response, and other inherited traits (phenotype; see above). (http://www.genome.gov/glossary/index.cfm?id=185)

Small interfering RNA (siRNA). Short RNA fragment that regulates gene expression and thereby serves as an important mechanism for regulating protein levels in cells. (NRC, 2009, p. 33)

Splicing. Process by which noncoding regions are removed from the RNA transcript of a gene and coding regions are joined together to generate mature messenger RNA (mRNA). (http://www.ncbi.nlm.nih.gov/bookshelf/br.fcgi?book=gene&part=glossary#IX-B)

Stem cell. "A cell with the potential to form many of the different cell types found in the body. When stem cells divide, they can form more stem cells or other cells that perform specialized functions. Embryonic stem cells have the potential to form a complete individual, whereas adult stem cells can only form certain types of specialized cells. Stem cells continue to divide as long as the individual remains alive." (http://www.genome.gov/glossary/index.cfm?id=188)

Stem cell transplant. "A method of replacing immature blood-forming cells in the bone marrow that have been destroyed by drugs, radiation, or disease. Stem cells are injected into the patient and make healthy blood cells. A stem cell transplant may be autologous (using a patient's own stem cells that were saved before treatment), allogeneic (using stem cells donated by someone who is not an identical twin), or syngeneic (using stem cells donated by an identical twin)." (http://www.cancer.gov/dictionary/?CdrID=46695)

Surrogate endpoint (see also *Endpoint*). "A biomarker that is intended to substitute for a clinical endpoint . . . a surrogate endpoint is expected to predict clinical benefit (or harm or lack of benefit or harm) based on epidemiologic, therapeutic, pathophysiologic, or other scientific evidence. (Biomarkers Definition Working Group, 2001)

Surveillance. "The ongoing, systematic collection, analysis, interpretation, and dissemination of data regarding a health-related event for use in public health action to reduce morbidity and mortality and to improve health" (Guidelines Working Group, 2001).

Systems biology. "The science of discovering, modeling, understanding, and ultimately engineering at the molecular level the dynamic relationships between the biological molecules that define living organisms." (http://www.systemsbiology.org/Systems_Biology_in_Depth)

Tissue bank. See *Biorepository*.

Tissue engineering. "The process of creating living, functional tissues to repair or replace tissue or organ function lost due to age, disease, damage, or congenital defects." This field is also known as regenerative medicine. (http://www.nih.gov/about/researchresultsforthepublic/Regen.pdf)

Translation. The process by which cells turn instructions from mRNA transcribed from a gene (see *Transcription*) into chains of amino acids that fold into proteins. (http://ghr.nlm.nih.gov/glossary=translation)

Translational bioinformatics. "A field of science in which biology, computer science, and information technology merge into a single discipline to analyze biological information using computers and statistical techniques" (see also *Bioinformatics*). (http://www.translationalbioinformatics.org/)

Translational research. Research that includes two areas of translation. One is the process of applying discoveries generated during research in the laboratory, and in preclinical studies, to the development of trials and studies in humans. The second area concerns research aimed at enhancing the adoption of best practices in the community. (http://grants.nih.gov/Grants/glossary.html)

Tumor marker. A substance present in or produced by a tumor, or by the host in response to a tumor, that can be used for differentiating cancerous from normal tissue. Markers are used in diagnosis, staging, and prognosis of cancer; monitoring effects of therapy; detecting recurrence; localizing tumors; and screening in general populations (see also *Biomarker*). (http://ghr.nlm.nih.gov/glossary=tumormarkers)

Unlabeled use. Use of a drug or medical device for a purpose, patient group, or other use that is not specifically approved by the Food and Drug Administration for use as indicated on the product's label. Such use by physicians is considered part of the practice of medicine, which FDA—by statute—does not regulate. Sometimes described as "off-label" use.

Additional Glossary References

Biomarkers Definitions Working Group. 2001. Biomarkers and surrogate endpoints: Preferred definitions and conceptual framework. *Clinical Pharmacology and Therapeutics* 69(3):89-95.

Feero, W. G., A. E. Guttmacher, and F. S. Collins. 2010. Genomic medicine—an updated primer. *New England Journal of Medicine* 362(21): 2001-2011.

Glover, G. J. 2007. The influence of market exclusivity on drug availability and medical innovations. *AAPS Journal* 9(3):34. http://www.aapsj.org/articles/aapsj0903/aapsj0903034/aapsj0903034.pdf (accessed August 20, 2010).

Guidelines Working Group, Center for Disease Control and Prevention. 2001. Updated guidelines for Evaluating Public Health Surveillance Systems. *MMWR* 50(RR13):1-35. (http://www.cdc.gov/mmwr/preview/mmwrhtml/rr5013a1.html).

NRC. (National Research Council). 2000. *Bioinformatics: Converting Data to Knowledge: Workshop Summary.* Washington, DC: National Academy Press.

NRC. 2007. *The New Science of Metagenomics: Revealing the Secrets of Our Microbial Planet.* Washington, DC: The National Academies Press.

NRC. 2009. *A New Biology for the 21st Century.* Washington, DC: The National Academies Press.

ABBREVIATIONS

ACMG	American College of Medical Genetics
AHRQ	Agency for Healthcare Research and Quality
ANDA	Abbreviated New Drug Application
ATSDR	Agency for Toxic Substances and Disease Registry
BLA	Biologics License Application
CAN	Cures Acceleration Network
CBER	Center for Biologics Evaluation and Research
CDC	Centers for Disease Control and Prevention
CDER	Center for Drug Evaluation and Research
CDRH	Center for Devices and Radiological Health
CFF	Cystic Fibrosis Foundation
CLIA	Clinical Laboratory Improvement Amendments of 1988
CML	chronic myelogenous leukemia
CMS	Centers for Medicare and Medicaid Services
COG	Children's Oncology Group
C-Path	Critical path Institute
CTSA	Clinical and Translational Science Awards
CTX	cerebrotendinous xanthomtosis
EMEA	European Medicines Agency
FDA	Food and Drug Administration
FEV1	forced expiratory volume
FMF	familial Mediterranean fever
FOP	fibrodysplasia ossificans progressiva

GAO	Government Accountability Office
GenTAC	National Registry of Genetically Triggered Thoracic Aortic Aneurysms and Cardiovascular Conditions
HDE	Humanitarian Device Exemption
HHS	U.S. Department of Health and Human Services
ICD	International Classification of Diseases
ICD	implantable cardioverter defibrillator
IDE	Investigational Device Exemption
IND	Investigational New Drug
IOM	Institute of Medicine
IRB	Institutional Review Board
MedPAC	Medicare Payment Advisory Commission
NAGS	N-acetylglutamate synthase
NCGC	NIH Chemical Genomics Center
NCI	National Cancer Institute
NDA	New Drug Application
NHLBI	National Heart, Lung, and Blood Institute
NIH	National Institutes of Health
NORD	National Organization for Rare Disorders
OMIM	Online Mendelian Inheritance in Man
OOPD	Office of Orphan Products Development
ORDR	Office of Rare Diseases Research
PHS	Public Health Service
PMA	Premarket Approval application
RAID	Rapid Access to Interventional Development
RDCRN	Rare Diseases Clinical Research Network
REMS	Risk Evaluation and Mitigation Strategy
SEER	Surveillance, Epidemiology, and End Results
SSDI	Social Security Disability Insurance
TRND	Therapeutics for Rare and Neglected Diseases
VEPTR	Vertical Expandable Prosthetic Titanium Rib
WHO	World Health Organization

PUBLIC LAWS

P.L. 94-295	Medical Device Amendments of 1976
P.L. 97-414	Orphan Drug Act of 1983
P.L. 98-417	Drug Price Competition and Patent Term Restoration Act of 1984
P.L. 101-629	Safe Medical Devices Act of 1990
P.L. 102-571	Prescription Drug User Fee Act of 1992
P.L. 105-115	FDA Modernization Act of 1997
P.L. 108-155	Pediatric Research Equity Act of 2003
P.L. 110-85	Best Pharmaceuticals for Children Act of 2007 (Food and Drug Administration Amendments Act of 2007)
P.L. 110-233	Genetic Information Nondiscrimation Act of 2008
P.L. 111-80	Agriculture, Rural Development, Food and Drug Administration, and Related Agencies Appropriations Act of 2010
P.L. 111-148	Patient Protection and Affordable Care Act of 2010

E

Rare Diseases Clinical Research Network

The Rare Diseases Clinical Research Network, which is funded by the National Institutes of Health, includes 19 research consortia, each studying several related conditions as listed below. Each consortium involves patient groups as active participants. Information, including links to each consortium, can be found online at http://rarediseasesnetwork.epi.usf.edu/.

Angelman, Rett, and Prader-Willi Syndromes Consortium
Angelman syndrome
Rett syndrome
Prader-Willi syndrome

Autonomic Rare Diseases Clinical Research Consortium
Multiple system atrophy (MSA)
Baroreflex failure
Autoimmune autonomic neuropathy
Pure autonomic failure (PAF)
Hypovolemic postural tachycardia syndrome (hPOTS)
Dopamine beta hydroxylase deficiency (DBHD)

Brain Vascular Malformation Consortium
Familial cavernous malformations (CCM)
    Common Hispanic mutation
Sturge-Weber syndrome (SWS)
    Leptomeningeal angiomatosis
Hereditary hemorrhagic telangiectasia (HHT)
    Brain arteriovenous malformation (BAVM)

Chronic Graft Versus Host Disease Consortium (cGVHD)
Cutaneous sclerosis
Bronchiolitis obliterans
Late acute graft versus host disease
Chronic graft versus host disease

CINCH: Clinical Investigation of Neurologic Channelopathies
Andersen-Tawil syndrome
Episodic ataxias
Nondystrophic myotonic disorders

Clinical Research Consortium for Spinocerebellar Ataxias
Spinocerebellar ataxia:
SCA 1
SCA 2
SCA 3
SCA 6

Dystonia Coalition
Cervical dystonia
Blepharospasm
Spasmodic dysphonia
Craniofacial dystonia
Limb dystonia

Genetic Disorders of Mucociliary Clearance
Primary ciliary dyskinesia (PCD)
Cystic fibrosis
Pseudohypoaldosteronism (PHA)

Inherited Neuropathies Consortium
Charcot-Marie-Tooth disease (CMT) including CMT1, the dominantly
    inherited demyelinating neuropathies
CMT2, the dominantly inherited axonal neuropathies
CMT4, the recessively inherited neuropathies

Lysosomal Disease Network
Aspartylglucosaminuria
Wolman disease
Cystinosis
Danon disease
Fabry disease

Farber disease
Fucosidosis
Gaucher disease
GM1-gangliosidosis types I/II/III
GM2-gangliosidosis
alpha-Mannosidosis types I / II
Beta-Mannosidosis
Metachromatic leukodystrophy
Sialidosis types I / II
Mucolipidosis type IV
Scheie syndrome
Hunter syndrome
Sanfilippo syndrome A
Sanfilippo syndrome B
Sanfilippo syndrome C
Sanfilippo syndrome D
Galactosialidosis types I / II
Krabbe disease
Sandhoff disease
Vogt-Spielmeyer disease
Hurler syndrome
Niemann-Pick disease
I-cell disease
Pseudo-Hurler polydystrophy
Morquio syndrome
Maroteaux-Lamy syndrome
Sly syndrome
Mucopolysaccharidosis type IX
Multiple sulfatase deficiency
Tay-Sachs disease
Pompe disease
Batten disease, late infantile
Northern epilepsy
Pycnodysostosis
Schindler disease
Sialuria, Salla disease

NEPTUNE: Nephrotic Syndrome Rare Disease Clinical Research Network
Focal and segmental glomerulosclerosis (FSGS)
Minimal change disease (MCD)
Membranous nephropathy (MN)

North American Mitochondrial Diseases Consortium
AID: aminoglycoside-induced deafness
Alpers syndrome
CoQ deficiency
CPEO: chronic progressive external ophthalmoplegia
DAD: diabetes and deafness
Encephalopathy
Encephalomyopathy
FBSN: familial bilateral striatal necrosis
Hepatocerebral disease
KSS: Kearns-Sayre syndrome
Leigh syndrome
Leukoencephalopathy
LHON: Leber's hereditary optic neuropathy
MELAS: mitochondrial encephalopathy lactic acidosis with stroke-like
    episodes
MERRF: Myoclonus epilepsy ragged-red fibers
MILS: maternally inherited Leigh syndrome
MNGIE: Mitochondrial neurogastrointestinal encephalomyopathy
Mitochondrial DNA depletion syndrome
Multiple deletions of mitochondrial DNA
NARP: Neuropathy, ataxia and retinitis pigmentosa syndrome
Pearson syndrome
SANDO: Sensory ataxia neuropathy dysarthria ophthalmoplegia
Complex I deficiency
Complex II (SDH) deficiency
Complex III deficiency
Complex IV deficiency
Complex V deficiency
Multiple respiratory chain enzyme deficiencies

Porphyria Consortium
Acute intermittent porphyria
Hereditary coproporphyria
Variegate porphyria
Aminolevulinate dehydratase deficiency porphyria
Porphyria cutanea tarda
Hepatoerythropoietic porphyria
Congenital porphyria
Erythropoietic protoporphyria and X-linked protoporphyria

Primary Immune Deficiency Treatment Consortium
Severe combined immunodeficiency (SCID)

Wiskott-Aldrich syndrome (WAS)
Chronic granulomatous disease (CGD)

Rare Kidney Stone Consortium
Primary hyperoxaluria
Cystinuria
APRT deficiency (Dihydroxyadeninuria)
Dent's disease

Salivary Gland Carcinomas Consortium
Mucoepidermoid carcinoma (MEC)
Adenoid cystic carcinoma (ACC)
Adenocarcinoma (salivary duct carcinoma) (ACC)

STAIR: Sterol and Isoprenoid Diseases Consortium
Cerebrotendinous xanthomatosis
Mevalonic aciduria
Hyperimmunoglobulinemia D with periodic fever syndrome
Niemann-Pick disease type C
Sitosterolemia
Sjögren-Larsson syndrome
Smith-Lemli-Opitz syndrome

Urea Cycle Disorders Consortium
N-Acetylglutamate synthase (NAGS) deficiency
Carbamylphosphate synthetase (CPS) deficiency
Ornithine transcarbamylase (OTC) deficiency
Argininosuccinate synthetase deficiency (citrullinemia I)
Citrin deficiency (citrullinemia II)
Argininosuccinate lyase deficiency (argininosuccinic aciduria)
Arginase deficiency (hyperargininemia)
Ornithine translocase deficiency (HHH) syndrome

Vasculitis Clinical Research Consortium
Wegener's granulomatosis (WG)
Microscopic polyangiitis (MPA)
Churg-Strauss syndrome (CSS)
Polyarteritis nodosa (PAN)
Takayasu's arteritis (TAK)
Giant cell (temporal) arteritis (GCA)

F

Advocacy Group Approaches to Accelerating Research and Product Development: Illustrative Examples

Many rare disease advocacy organizations focus their resources on assisting patients and families. Others focus on research to understand the disease process and develop diagnostic tools, preventive interventions, or treatments. Some have significant commitments in both areas.

As illustrated by the example of the Progeria Research Foundation in Chapter 1 (Box 1-3), a focused organizational approach can, under some circumstances, contribute to progress in a relatively short period even for an extremely rare condition. Creating that focused organizational approach takes human and financial resources. Although the number of rare conditions for which there are advocacy groups has grown, a great many rare conditions lack research-focused advocacy organizations. Moreover, many existing rare diseases advocacy organizations have very limited funds to support research and are still developing the expertise and experience to support a focused research effort.

The groups represented in this appendix were not selected because they are typical but because their work illustrates different elements and emphases of organizational research strategies. To some degree, new and established groups learn from and build on the experience of others, including some advocacy groups that focus on more common conditions. For example, the Myelin Repair Foundation, which supports research to develop treatments for multiple sclerosis, notes on its website that more than 60 academic, advocacy, and other organizations have contacted it for information about its Advanced Research Collaboration, or ARC, model (http://www.myelinrepair.org/about/). The foundation stresses several features of its strategy, including a comprehensive plan to guide activities; an emphasis on real-time sharing of scientific discoveries among experts; and partnerships with industry. Another often-cited group, FasterCures, seeks to encourage innovation and efficiency in medical research generally and to promote the diffusion of successful strategies (http://www.fastercures.org/index.cfm/OurPrograms/Overview). Among rare diseases organizations, the Cystic Fibrosis Foundation has, in many respects, led the way in developing and implementing a systematic research strategy that is tailored to evolving research progress and scientific and technological opportunities.

Two umbrella organizations, the National Organization for Rare Disorders and the Genetic Alliance, provide assistance to organizations trying to develop and implement research strategies. Advocacy groups with a focus on rare diseases research can also benefit from various initiatives of the Office of Rare Diseases Research at the National Institutes of Health (NIH) and the Office of Orphan Product Development at the Food and Drug Administration.

Rare diseases advocacy organizations that support research and development vary in their approaches and emphases. Their research objectives and the strategies for attaining them may be influenced by a number of factors, including their financial resources, the existence of effective treatments, and the experiences, priorities, and expertise of the group's founders. Other factors that may shape a group's research directions include whether or not a disease's cause is known; how well the disease process is understood; what research, if any, is being undertaken by other public, nonprofit, or commercial entities and what niche the advocacy organization is best equipped to fill; whether it is critical to recruit new scientists into the research area; and how challenging it is to recruit patients and families to participate in research.

Organizational strategies may be highly focused on one segment along the spectrum from basic to clinical research or they may span the spectrum. As research progresses, strategies may shift from an emphasis on identifying the cause and genetic and molecular basis of a disease to identifying and testing promising therapies and securing FDA approval.

Groups vary significantly in their resources. For the organizations used as illustrative examples in this appendix, Table F-1 shows major differences. The years and definitions may not be completely consistent for the figures cited in the table, but they give a sense of the substantial range in organizational resources and the concentration of organizations in the lower end of the range. (Two groups with spending higher than that of most of the groups in the table are the Multiple Myeloma Research Foundation at around $13 million and MDA, formerly the Muscular Dystrophy Association, at around $39 million for 2009 according to their 2009 annual reports.)

The examples below illustrate different components of research strate-

TABLE F-1 Spending on Research or Research Grants for Selected Advocacy Organizations, 2008

Organization	Spending (millions of dollars)
Scleroderma Research Foundation	1.2
Friedreich's Ataxia Research Alliance	1.3
International Rett Syndrome Foundation	1.7
Alpha 1 Foundation (research and detection)	3.7
Spinal Muscular Atrophy Foundation	3.9
Cystic Fibrosis Foundation	71.6

SOURCE: For Cystic Fibrosis Foundation and Scleroderma Research Foundation, 2008 financial statement. For Alpha 1 Foundation and Friedreich's Ataxia Research Alliance, 2009 annual report. For other organizations, IRS form 990 for 2008 as posted on Guidestar.org. (Figures are from Part I, line 13, or Line 10 on the 990-EZ.) Amounts reported do not include fundraising, salaries, or other expenses.

gies that various organizations have developed, often based on a systematic assessment of the gaps in knowledge or resources and the contributions that organizations like theirs can make to bridge those gaps. Not featured but central to organizational research strategies for rare and common diseases alike are three strategic elements: raising funds, political advocacy, and engaging patients, families, and communities in these and other aspects of an organization's work.

The examples of elements of research strategies for the following organizations are excerpted from materials on each group's website; they thus may be worded to attract donors and inspire the community of patients, families, researchers, and other supporters. The accuracy of the excerpted materials has not been checked, and their use does not constitute a recommendation or endorsement. The formatting (e.g., font size, text highlighting) has been altered for consistency, and graphics and some details (as indicated) have been omitted.

EXAMPLE 1
LANDSCAPE ANALYSIS: INTERNATIONAL
RETT SYNDROME FOUNDATION

As part of an effort to understand in detail the environment of research on Rett syndrome, the International Rett Syndrome Foundation (IRSF) undertook a landscape analysis, which in this case involved a detailed examination of the focus of research funding by NIH and private entities. The group has recently applied the same analytic strategy to frontotemporal dementia. Rett syndrome (RTT) is a developmental disorder that is caused by mutations in a gene on the X chromosome; research to identify other possible genetic contributors is ongoing. The condition, which is usually seen in girls, can create problems with learning, speech, mood, sensation, movement, breathing, cardiac function, and digestion.

Landscape Analysis: Executive Summary
(This text is used with permission and excerpted from
http://www.rettsyndrome.org/ dmdocuments/
IRSF_LANDSCAPE%20ANALYSIS_2008-1.pdf.)

Purpose and Format of the Rett Syndrome Landscape Analysis

The Rett syndrome Landscape Analysis is designed to capture a coherent picture of research funding on Rett syndrome in the context of a basic research to clinical research continuum. This analysis was done to review and place into perspective the type of research funding provided by federal and private agencies, explore the overall pattern of research spending, determine where the bottlenecks lie and facilitate targeted funding for these areas.

Overall, the purpose of this landscape analysis is to help identify existing resources and anticipate the future needs of the research community, with a specific emphasis on translational research.

Top-Line Summary of Landscape Analysis Results

The MeCP2 gene considered responsible for the majority of cases of RTT was first identified in 1999 (Amir et al., Nat Genet. 1999). 272 RTT-related grants disbursed by 8 public (including 8 NIH institutes) and 5 private institutions over this past decade and representing $107.5 MM, were categorized using the *Biomedical Research Classification Scheme* specifically developed for this analysis. Each grant was mapped along a continuum from basic and etiologic research, through the stages of drug development and the clinical evaluation of treatments. The scheme was also designed to codify a wide range of accompanying healthcare related areas including reagents, technologies and methodologies that complement and facilitate this process. This exercise was undertaken in order to develop a snapshot of RTT research spending over the past decade and permit a detailed analysis of the research funded in this field.

Public agencies contributed 77% of all funds, 72% from the NIH alone; the US funded 88% of RTT research. 55% of private grants originated at the IRSF, representing 12.7% of total funding. 82% went toward etiological research in general and 0.5%, or $500K, went toward treatment development, all of which came from the IRSF. Research in this field is significantly under-resourced, even by comparison with related disorders, however basic disease research for RTT is relatively well funded. The majority of resources (53%) went towards the identification or validation of drug targets after which there are few grants. This is a reflection of the lack of RTT programs that have advanced into treatment development and evaluation and is largely due to the complexity of targeting MeCP2 and the number of its target genes.

Conclusions

Analysis of research spending for RTT over the past ten year period revealed a clear bottleneck in the translation of basic research findings into the development of novel therapies to treat the disease. This bottleneck is illustrated by a steep decline in funding beyond the target validation stage of the drug discovery and development process. While it is clear there is still much to be learned regarding the complex biology of MeCP2, this analysis nevertheless underscores a need for future funding to be directed towards specific programs and resources that will help alleviate the current obstacles to translation and facilitate treatment development for RTT.

EXAMPLE 2
DEVELOPING A RESEARCH AGENDA: ALPHA-1 FOUNDATION

The Alpha-1 Foundation was founded in 1995 by three people with Alpha-1 Antitrypsin Deficiency (AAT Deficiency or Alpha-1). Alpha-1 is genetic condition that is highly variable. Some individuals may have no or few symptoms whereas others may develop serious lung or liver disease. As described on its website, the foundation seeks to provide "the leadership and resources that will result in increased research, improved health, worldwide detection, and a cure for Alpha-1." The research section of its website describes the group's research portfolio and grant opportunities, provides information about its patient registry and DNA and tissue bank, and provides links to information about research findings, research centers, scientific meetings, and other resources. It also provides a description of the group's research agenda.

Research Agenda
(This text is used with permission and excerpted from
http://www.alpha-1foundation.org/researchers/?c=02-Research-Agenda.)

The Alpha-1 Foundation has spent considerable time and resources to devise a feasible and relevant research agenda. The process started at the strategic planning level, a formal exercise that the Foundation completed in 2000. This global evaluation of the Foundation's programs and research activities included input from both the existing AAT research network as well as input from a wide range of associated organizations and experts. This strategic planning process included sessions involving focused planning groups, scientists, government representatives of the National Institutes of Health, Food & Drug Administration and written comments from the Center of Disease Control [and Prevention], and input from other Voluntary Health Agencies who are represented on the National Health Council. During the numerous strategic planning sessions, the major research foci were identified as well as gaps in scientific knowledge that needed to be addressed by further research.

The second stage in devising a research agenda involved the Alpha-1 Foundation's Medical and Scientific Advisory Committee (MASAC), the Foundation's primary medical advisory body, to evaluate the research areas identified by the strategic planning process on a regular (annual) basis. In 2001, an ad hoc committee was appointed by MASAC to carefully review the suggested research foci that were identified in the strategic planning process, and place these recommendations within the context of what is feasible to achieve scientifically with current expertise and technology. The ad hoc committee produced the research agenda shown below and it serves as a working document used by the grants award program for prioritizing the relevance of grant applications to the Foundation's overall research goals. The use of the strategic plan and research agenda for evaluation of grant applications is only one use envisioned for the research agenda document. It has also been utilized to identify the most relevant topics for their critical issue workshops.

[**Note:** Some details for the lists below are not included.]

Basic Research: Identifying Targets & Developing Therapeutic Approaches

- Molecular biology of alpha-1 antitrypsin (AAT) expression
- Lung-Focused Research
- Liver-Focused Research
- Technology Development

Clinical Research: Identifying Alphas & Defining the Natural History of AAT Deficiency

- Epidemiology of AAT deficiency
- Modifier genes affecting lung and liver in AAT deficient individuals

- Role of inflammation in the pathogenesis of AAT lung disease
- Establishment of effective clinical outcomes measures in AAT deficiency
- Quality of life, healthcare utilization, and symptom management
- Environmental modifiers of lung and liver disease in AAT deficient individuals
- Clinical manifestations of AAT deficiency other than in the lungs and liver

Translational Research: Evaluating Novel Therapeutic Approaches

- Alpha-1 antitrypsin replacement therapy
- Improving outcomes in lung and liver transplant recipients
- Treatment of pulmonary hyperinflation
- Anti-inflammatory therapy
- Small molecule antiprotease therapy
- Gene therapy
- Chemical chaperone therapy

Ethical, Legal & Social Issues Research: Eliminating Barriers for Alphas

- Newborn testing/screening
- Targeted detection
- Social dimensions of A1ATD
- Equitable distribution of medical therapies

EXAMPLE 3
CREATING A DRUG DEVELOPMENT ARM: CYSTIC FIBROSIS FOUNDATION

The Cystic Fibrosis Foundation (founded in 1955 as the National CF Research Foundation) was one of the earliest advocacy groups to develop and fund a systematic research strategy. Effective symptomatic therapies, some emerging from foundation-funded research, have significantly increased life expectancy for this genetic disease that affects the lungs and digestive system. In 1980, the foundation created a network of academic research centers. In 2000, the foundation created Cystic Fibrosis Research Foundation Therapeutics, a nonprofit research affiliate, to oversee drug discovery and development activities.

Cystic Fibrosis Foundation Therapeutics
(This description is used with permission and excerpted from
http://www.cff.org/research/CFFT/.)

Established in 2000, Cystic Fibrosis Foundation Therapeutics, Inc. (CFFT) is the non-profit drug discovery and development affiliate of the Cystic Fibrosis Foundation. CFFT supports and governs activities related to cystic fibrosis (CF) drug discovery through the many stages of drug development and clinical evaluation.

The CF Foundation provides support to fund CFFT's operations, specifically the Therapeutics Development Program. Sound investment by the Foundation in cutting edge science has built an extensive base of knowledge about this disease. Some of these ideas have already led to innovative new therapies now in the Drug Development Pipeline.

In fact, one way to look at the wide-ranging and diverse science supported by the CF Foundation and its affiliate, CFFT (more than $66 million in 2005), is to think that each study could be a step toward a new CF therapy. Molecular biologists, cell physiologists and immunologists, for example, all ask the same question: How does this study lead to a potential CF therapy or the cure? Seeking the answers drives the research advances forward to improve the lives of individuals with CF.

Therapeutics Development Program

To bridge the gap between what has been learned in the laboratory and the evolution of new therapies, the Therapeutics Development Program was created. This model initiative has the infrastructure in place to support a virtual "pipeline" of CF therapeutics development from the discovery phase through several stages of clinical evaluation.

Despite the increasing age of survival, people with CF continue to need new medications to reduce the effects of their disease until the cure is found. Therefore, the CF Foundation and its affiliate, CFFT, strive to maximize the number of innovative drugs being developed because, on average, only one in five compounds will successfully make it through clinical trials all the way to the patient.

Increasing the number of promising compounds increases the odds of success! Such investment by a voluntary health organization is unprecedented and has already served as a model for others to follow.

How the Program Works

Through the Therapeutics Development Program, CFFT offers matching research awards to scientists, as well as access to a specialized network of CF clinical research centers. These awards provide support for the drug discovery phase through several stages of evaluation to complete the full-length drug development pipeline.

This is a win-win equation—the Therapeutics Development Program provides companies and academia with a powerful new opportunity to have investment capital during the early phases of drug research. And, it ensures the availability of new potential compounds for clinical investigation for the CF community.

Current estimates suggest that it costs more than $800 million to move a drug from its concept stage to the market place. There is a critical need to help provide support to pharmaceutical and biotechnology companies that conduct drug discovery and early-stage clinical evaluation studies in small population diseases such as CF.

Even with incentives, such as the Orphan Drug Tax Credit (that encourages investment in orphan diseases like CF, which affect patient populations of less than 200,000), the fact remains that pharmaceutical companies must first secure the financial resources to invest in these diseases.

Further, with increasing demands being placed on pharmaceutical and biotechnology companies, especially the small "start-ups," investors are often hesitant about making major capital investments for orphan disease-classified drugs. The Therapeutics Development Program attracts researchers to the CF drug development process and shows a level of commitment unrivaled by any other voluntary health organization.

Opportunities Abound

As the understanding of the science of CF increases, there is a correlated growth in the number of opportunities to discover and develop new potentially lifesaving therapies. Today, there are early phase trials underway in CF gene therapy, protein-assist therapy, as well as studies testing anti-infective drugs, and anti-inflammatory drugs. With the increasing number of potential drugs and an innovative network of specialized clinical trial centers to evaluate them, the future for those battling CF has never been brighter.

EXAMPLE 4
ACCESS TO RESEARCH TOOLS:
SPINAL MUSCULAR ATROPHY FOUNDATION

The Spinal Muscular Atrophy Foundation (SMAF), founded by the parents of a child with the condition, began operations in 2003 to help accelerate the development of a cure or treatment for the disease. SMA is an inherited disease that is characterized by muscle atrophy and loss of motor function.

It generally develops in infancy or childhood; different types vary in severity and prognosis. The SMA Foundation works to achieve its mission by encouraging alliances between academia, government, and pharmaceutical and biotechnology companies; increasing government support; and increasing awareness of the disease among government, pharmaceutical and biotechnology companies, and the public. Its website includes information on its research programs and funded projects as well as other resources, including a page with links to various research tools.

Research Tools
(This material is used with permission and excerpted from the upcoming revision of the information at http://www.smafoundation.org/research-tools-portfolio.html.*)*

As part of our mission to accelerate treatments for SMA, the SMA Foundation has engaged in licensing and/or developing animal models and other research tools to make them available as resources for the community. These assays and animal model resources are described below and also include listings of licenses, SMA patents and antibodies, websites for other organizations serving the SMA community, as well as information on the biology and genetics of SMA.

SMN ELISA

The SMN (human), ELISA Kit is a complete kit for the quantitative determination of SMN in cell lysates of human origin. The kit was developed in collaboration between the SMA Foundation and Enzo Life Sciences Inc. The assay is currently validated for the detection of SMN protein levels in human Peripheral Blood Mononuclear Cell (PBMC) lysates. Additional protocols for human and mouse tissues and fluids are currently under development to measure SMN protein. A limited number of SMN ELISA kits are currently available to researchers and request forms may be obtained through the Foundation. The SMA Foundation encourages the sharing of protocols and feedback from using the ELISA kit to make this a more effective tool for the SMA community.

Animal Models

There are several SMA mouse models available. Many of these models are genetically modified to be deficient in mouse SMN protein and also have varying types and amounts of human SMN genes introduced to their genome in an effort to recapitulate a range of disease features and severities seen in patients. The Foundation is actively engaged in developing *in vivo* drug testing platforms in SMA mice and testing experimental therapies in these animals.

- Surveying SMA Therapeutic Candidates at PsychoGenics
  The SMA Foundation and PsychoGenics have developed a standardized platform for *in vivo* drug testing in a severe model of SMA which includes analysis of survival and motor function. Parties interested in having compounds with strong rationale for efficacy in SMA tested in this platform may contact the Foundation at researchtools@smafoundation.org for more information.
- The Jackson Laboratories
  The SMA Foundation has partnered with Regeneron Pharmaceuticals to engineer an SMA Allelic Series of mice that have different copy numbers of chimeric human/mouse SMN2 genes and human SMN2 (designated as lines A-D). These mice have been deposited at Jackson Labs and mice with severe to moderate phenotypes are now available; mice with the mildest phenotypes and combinations of these alleles will be available in late 2010. In addition, conditional SMN rescue allele mice are also in development at Jackson Labs. A table of the SMA allelic series lines is provided below and will be updated as more lines become available.

Licenses

The SMA Foundation has entered into licensing agreements with several Institutions in order to facilitate access to critical research tools, while giving the Inventors and Institutions acknowledgment of key contributions and fair compensation for their intellectual property. The Foundation offers the opportunity to obtain sublicenses for the research and therapeutics development tools listed in the section below. The portfolio is designed to reduce or eliminate barriers for drug discovery efforts and to accelerate the development of a treatment for SMA. For more information, please contact us at researchtools@smafoundation.org.

- University of Wuerzburg
  Certain SMA mouse models deficient in SMN mRNA and protein due to the targeted mutation Smntm1Msd
- The Ohio State University
  Certain SMA mouse models that are deficient in mouse SMN mRNA and protein as above, but including human SMN transgenes

Patents: [**Note:** Links to European Patient Office and U.S. Patent and Trademark Office omitted]

Antibodies:

• For a spreadsheet that gives basic information about antibodies used in SMA research, please click here. Reviews and comments on these antibodies have been gathered from SMA researchers by the SMA Foundation.

• If you have any experience with antibodies used in SMA research, we strongly encourage you to share reviews or comments on their general usefulness and reliability, applications tested and dilution notes. For information on how to provide comments or updates, please email the SMA Foundation at researchtools@smafoundation.org.

Other SMA Community Resources: [**Note:** links to advocacy organizations omitted]

Other Clinical Resources on SMA:

• National Institute of Neurological Disorders and Stroke (NINDS) Information Page on SMA
• MedlinePlus Information on SMA
• GeneClinics Clinical Review of SMA
• Genetic Testing Resources from GeneTests
• Columbia University Medical Center Spinal Muscular Atrophy Clinical Research Center
• Treat-NMD Clinical Research Initiatives in Europe

Scientific Literature Resources:

• SMA Foundation Bibliography at http://www.smafoundation.org/bibliography

EXAMPLE 5
FRIEDREICH'S ATAXIA RESEARCH ALLIANCE

The Friedreich's Ataxia Research Alliance (FARA) raises funds for scientific research on the disease with a focus on translational and clinical research and on national and international public-private collaborations and partnerships. It also maintains a patient registry and encourages collaboration and information sharing through scientific conferences and meetings. Friedreich's ataxia (FA) is a debilitating, life-shortening degenerative neuromuscular disorder that causes loss of coordination and strength in all four limbs necessitating the use of a wheelchair. Symptoms develop in children or adults and affect about 1 in 50,000 people in the United States. Although symptoms vary, it often leads to diminished vision, hearing and speech, diabetes, scoliosis, and cardiomyopathy. FA ultimately leads to early death.

Scientific Conference Program
(This material is used with permission and excerpted from http://www.curefa.org/conference.html.)

FARA has organized and supported a number of scientific conferences to keep the field informed of research progress and build collaborations and synergistic connections between FA researchers. FARA's International Scientific Conference on Friedreich's Ataxia has grown over its three iterations demonstrating the remarkable research advances into the underlying mechanisms of FA and increased interest within the scientific research community.

Upcoming Conference

4th International Friedreich's Ataxia Scientific Conference
Dates: May 5th – May 7th, 2011
Location: Institute of Genetics and Molecular and Cellular Biology
     IGBMC—Strasbourg, France
Information coming on the preliminary agenda, program sessions,
     abstracts, registration, sponsorship.
Abstracts will be due December 1, 2011

Conference History

On the day following FARA's incorporation, the new organization submitted a grant application to the National Institutes of Health (NIH) for the first International Scientific Conference on Friedreich's Ataxia convened April 1999.

1999—1st FARA International Conference (3 days)
     80 scientists from around the world
2003—2nd FARA International Conference (5 days)
     100 scientists from 12 countries
2006—3rd FARA International Conference (3 days)
     150 scientists from 12 countries

[**Note:** The web page also has research abstracts from the meetings.]

In the interim time between its International Conferences on Friedreich's Ataxia, FARA helped support the Ataxia Investigators Meeting held in 2006 and 2008.

Summit Meetings

FARA has also convened summit meetings to focus on significant areas of FA research such as cardiology and mitochondrial function. Such meetings facilitate in-depth discussions among experts and advance a specific research need.

Cardiac Summit

During the Cardiac Summit, held in 2007, leading cardiologists and researchers gathered to discuss FA related cardiology issues. One of the primary outcomes of this meeting was the documentation of gaps in knowledge regarding cardiac disease in FA and the assignment of research teams to begin work in these areas. A full list of outcomes can be found in the right hand column. To further support these efforts, FARA and the American Heart Association have entered a partnership agreement to co-fund grants.

[**Note:** A second Cardiac Summit was held on June 11, 2010.]

Mitochondrial Summit

FARA also co-sponsored a Mitochondrial Summit with the Muscular Dystrophy Association, on May 20-21, 2008, to share and discuss approaches, insights, and mechanisms that suggest new therapeutics for mitochondrial neurodegenerative diseases.

Therapeutics Symposium

More than 100 FA researchers and our advocacy partners from around the world gathered July 15-17, 2009 for the FA Therapeutics Symposium in Philadelphia, PA. Presentations and discussions highlighted:

• progress in the development of previously identified therapeutic candidates, such as HDACI and TAT-Frataxin results from clinical trials including the Phase I study of A0001 and Phase III of Idebenone;
• recent discoveries that point to new therapies;
• advancements in new cell models and drug discovery and development assays; and
• clinical research including biomarker studies and new clinical outcome measures.

EXAMPLE 6
FUNDING RESEARCH FELLOWSHIPS:
SCLERODERMA RESEARCH FOUNDATION

The Scleroderma Research Foundation (SRF) was created in 1987 by a woman diagnosed with the condition who set out to raise awareness of the condition and stimulate research on a little-studied disease. The organization's website describes a research strategy that emphasizes scientific collaboration and establishment of clinical research centers to support both research and training. One element of its research strategy is attracting promising new investigators to study this complex, variable, and often debilitating and even life-threatening disease. Scleroderma is generally characterized as a rheumatic disease of the connective tissue that produces fibrosis and inflammation. Although collectively it is not uncommon, some forms qualify as rare.

Fellowship Program
(This material is used with permission and excerpted from http://www.srfcure.org/about-us; http://sclerodermaresearch.org/ research/fellowship-program; *and* http://www.srfcure.org/research/ research-fellowship-grants/post-doctoral-fellowship-guidelines.)

. . . Knowing that future discovery will come from the next generation of scientists, the SRF continues to provide grants to young investigators. Postdoctoral fellowship grants allow researchers to enter the field of scleroderma research and work alongside established investigators. As an indicator of success, several SRF-funded fellows are now dedicating their early careers to the field of scleroderma research. . . .

The Scleroderma Research Foundation's Postdoctoral Fellowship program funds grants aimed at focusing talented young investigators on specific research questions in the nation's top laboratories. It has become a central element to the overall research effort, leveraging the momentum of SRF core research projects and bringing bright young scientists to scleroderma research. The SRF endeavors to support their interest in dedicating their early careers to scleroderma research—ideally providing the tools, relationships and knowledge that will allow them to become the next generation of leaders in the field. The SRF has funded Postdoctoral Fellows in the laboratories of nationally respected senior scientists. . . .

Application Guidelines

The Scleroderma Research Foundation is dedicated to bringing talented early-career scientists to scleroderma research. The Scleroderma Research Foundation Fellows Program aims to attract outstanding postdoctoral fellows with strong records of accomplishment, who have a clear sense of direction and/or novel idea they wish to develop in the field of scleroderma research. In particular, the SRF encourages exploration of new approaches and hypotheses on the pathogenesis of scleroderma.

Up to two, two-year postdoctoral fellowships in scleroderma research will be awarded, with a stipend of $35,000-$55,000 to support the candidate. Funding support from the SRF is in the form of a grant.

Mission of the Scleroderma Research Foundation

In its mission to find a cure for scleroderma, the Scleroderma Research Foundation seeks to advance research by: promoting collaboration and cross-institutional cooperation among scientists in a variety of disciplines; attracting promising new scientists to scleroderma research; maintaining scleroderma Centers of Excellence; and bringing new technology and thinking to the field of scleroderma research.

Eligibility Requirements

- U.S. citizen or permanent resident
- Completion of Ph.D. or M.D. prior to appointment

Sponsorship

Before submitting a fellowship application, the applicant must identify a sponsoring institution and an individual who will serve as a sponsor and will supervise the training and research experience. The sponsoring institution may be private or public non-profit.

The applicant's sponsor should be an active investigator in the area of the proposed research who will directly supervise the candidate's research. The sponsor must document the availability of staff, research support, and facilities for high-quality research training.

[**Note:** Sections on Accountability, Scientific Conduct and IRB Approval, Application Procedure, and Submission Deadline omitted.]

Review Considerations

Completed applications will be evaluated by the SRF Scientific Advisory Board. Fellows will be selected on the basis of previous achievements, the commitment of the applicant, sponsor and sponsoring institution to scleroderma research, the scientific and technical merit of the research proposal, and the relevance of the proposal to the SRF's ongoing research program.

G

Committee and Staff Biographies

Thomas F. Boat, M.D. (*Chair*), is Executive Associate Dean, University of Cincinnati College of Medicine and CEO of UC Physicians. He is immediate past Director of the Children's Hospital Research Foundation and past Chairman of the College's Department of Pediatrics. He also was physician-in-chief of Children's Hospital Medical Center of Cincinnati. A pediatric pulmonologist by training, Dr. Boat worked early in his career to define the pathophysiology of airway dysfunction and develop more effective therapies for chronic lung diseases of childhood, such as cystic fibrosis. More recently he has worked at local and national levels to improve research efforts, subspecialty training, and clinical care in pediatrics. Dr. Boat previously served as chairman of the Department of Pediatrics at the University of North Carolina, Chapel Hill and co-director of the Cystic Fibrosis Center at Rainbow Babies and Children's Hospital in Cleveland. He is Immediate Past Board President of the Association of Accreditation of Human Research Protection Programs, Inc. He has also served as Chair of the American Board of Pediatrics and President of the Society for Pediatric Research as well as the American Pediatric Society. Dr. Boat is a member of the Institute of Medicine and has served as member or chair of a number of IOM and National Research Council committees.

Peter C. Adamson, M.D., is Chief of the Division of Clinical Pharmacology and Therapeutics and Director of Clinical and Translational Research at the Children's Hospital of Philadelphia (CHOP). For 8 years Dr. Adamson led the National Cancer Institute's Children's Oncology Group (COG) Developmental Therapeutics Program, and currently he is co-Director of the University of Pennsylvania–CHOP Clinical Translational Science Award (CTSA). Dr. Adamson was recruited from the National Cancer Institute (NCI) where he was an Investigator in the Pharmacology and Experimental Therapeutics Section of the Pediatric Oncology Branch. He was a member of the IOM committee on shortening the timeline for new cancer treatments and co-edited the report *Making Better Cancer Drugs for Children* (2005).

Carolyn Asbury, Sc.M.P.H., Ph.D., is a Senior Consultant at the Dana Foundation (a New York-based non-profit that supports translational and clinical research in neuroscience, immunology, and neuroimmunology) and is also an adjunct Senior Fellow, Leonard Davis Institute of Health Economics at the University of Pennsylvania. She has served as Vice Chair and Chair of the Board of the National Organization for Rare Disorders, is a member of the Board of the U.S. Pharmacopeia, and is a Trustee of the College of Physicians of Philadelphia. Dr. Asbury has a master's degree in public health and a doctorate in health systems business. She served as an advisor on market exclusivity, tax credit, and regulatory provisions of the 1983 Orphan Drug Act and subsequently authored the book *Orphan Drugs: Medical versus Market Value*. She has also authored several journal articles and book chapters on orphan drug issues and policies. Prior to her role at Dana, she was Senior Program Officer at the Robert Wood Johnson Foundation and then Director of the Health and Human Services Program at the Pew Charitable Trusts.

Paul Citron, M.S.E.E., retired in 2003 as Vice President of Technology Policy and Academic Relations at Medtronic, Inc., where he was previously Vice President of Science and Technology. He had responsibility for corporate-wide assessment and coordination of technology and for establishing and prioritization of corporate research. Currently he is adjunct professor at the Jacobs School of Engineering, University of California San Diego and an advisor to the Harvard-MIT Division of Health Sciences and Technology. He is also an advisor to several firms in the biotechnology sector. Mr. Citron has a B.S. and M.S. in electrical engineering. He was elected a Founding Fellow of the American Institute of Medical and Biological Engineering. He has authored numerous publications and holds eight U.S. medical device patents. He is a member of the National Academy of Engineering (NAE) and serves on the advisory group of the NAE's Center for Engineering, Ethics, and Society. He served on the IOM committee on postmarket surveillance of pediatric medical devices.

Peter B. Corr, Ph.D., is a Founder and General Partner of Celtic Therapeutics LLLP, a private equity firm focused on the development of innovative therapeutics, the development of alliances that advance solutions for diseases of the developing world, and global advocacy for biomedical innovation. Dr. Corr retired from Pfizer Inc. at the end of 2006, where he served as Senior Vice President for science and technology. Before that, he served as Executive Vice President of Pfizer Global Research and Development and President of Worldwide Development. Prior to joining Pfizer in 2000, Dr. Corr was President of pharmaceutical research and development at Warner Lambert/Parke Davis (until the merger with Pfizer), and he previously served as Senior Vice President of discovery research at Monsanto/Searle. Dr. Corr also spent 18 years as a researcher in molecular biology and pharmacology at Washington University in St. Louis, Missouri, where he was a professor of medicine (cardiology) and a professor of pharmacology and molecular biology. Dr. Corr serves on the Board of Governors of the New York Academy of Sciences, the Board of Regents of Georgetown University, and several other nonprofit and for-profit boards. He is also a member of the IOM Forum on Drug Discovery, Development, and Translation and served on the IOM committee on conflict of interest in medical research, education, and practice.

Michael DeBaun, M.D., is Director of the Sickle Cell Medical Treatment and Education Center at St. Louis Children's Hospital and Professor of Pediatrics, Biostatistics, and Neurology, Washington University in St. Louis. Dr. DeBaun's research has focused on understanding the etiology, pathogenesis, and management of cerebrovascular injury in children with sickle cell disease. He was among the first clinical investigators to carefully document the epidemiology, cognitive and clinical significance of silent cerebral infarcts in children with sickle cell anemia and to demonstrate that both size and location of cerebral infarcts result in specific cognitive loss in children. These studies subsequently led to the basis of the first international clinical trial in sickle cell disease, Silent Cerebral Infarct Multi-Center Trial. In oncology, Dr. DeBaun has focused on understanding the epidemiology, optimal management and molecular basis for overgrowth syndromes associated with cancer in children, specifically Beckwith Wiedemann Syndrome (BWS). Dr. DeBaun established an international BWS registry. The clinical work has been coupled with molecular genetic analysis documenting phenotype and epigenotype correlations in BWS. Dr. DeBaun and his colleagues were the first to describe the association between in vitro fertilization (IVF), congenital malformation syndromes, and epigenotype mutations in children born after IVF.

Harry Dietz, M.D., is Victor A. McKusick Professor of Genetics and Medicine in the Institute of Genetic Medicine and the Departments of Pediatrics, Medicine, and Molecular Biology and Genetics, Johns Hopkins University

School of Medicine. He is Director of the University's William S. Smilow Center for Marfan Syndrome Research and Investigator, Howard Hughes Medical Institute. Dr. Dietz studies how blood vessel walls develop and are maintained with a focus on processes that contribute to inherited forms of cardiovascular disease. His work on Marfan syndrome, a rare and potentially fatal connective tissue disease, has led him from discovery of the molecular basis of the disease to a current clinical trial of a surprising potential treatment: a medication used to treat high blood pressure. He has received awards from the Society for Pediatric Research, the American Society of Human Genetics, and the National Marfan Foundation. Dr. Dietz is a member of the Institute of Medicine.

Ellen J. Flannery, J.D., is a partner at Covington & Burling LLP, Washington, DC. She advises clients regarding the regulation of medical devices, pharmaceuticals, and biological products, as well as on product liability law. She has chaired the American Bar Association (ABA) Section of Science & Technology Law and the ABA Coordinating Group on Bioethics and the Law. Ms. Flannery has been counsel in cases involving the scope of the Food and Drug Administration's legal authority and has taught Food and Drug Law seminars at Boston University, University of Maryland, and University of Virginia Law Schools. She serves on the editorial boards of the *Guide to Medical Device Regulation* and the *Food and Drug Administration Enforcement Manual* and has published a number of articles related to medical device regulation. She served on the IOM committee on postmarket surveillance of pediatric medical devices.

Pat Furlong, R.N., B.S.N., is the Founding President and CEO of Parent Project Muscular Dystrophy (PPMD), the largest nonprofit organization in the United States solely focused on Duchenne muscular dystrophy (Duchenne). Its mission is to improve the treatment, quality of life, and long-term outlook for all individuals affected by Duchenne through research, advocacy, education, and compassion. Ms. Furlong is the mother of two sons who lost their battle with Duchenne in their teenage years. She is on the board of the Genetic Alliance and the Muscular Dystrophy Coordinating Committee at the U.S. Department of Health and Human Services, and she is also a committee member on the Collaboration in Education and Test Translation Program, which was developed by the NIH Office of Rare Diseases to promote the development and clinical and research use of tests for rare genetic diseases. She serves on the data safety monitoring board for both the Rare Diseases Clinical Research Network and Cooperative International Neuromuscular Research Group and on the Steering Committee for TREAT-NMD.

Marlene Haffner, M.D., M.P.H., is a consultant who has served as Executive Director of Regulatory Affairs at Amgen and as Director, Office of Orphan Products Development at the U.S. Food and Drug Administration from 1987 to 2006. She held the rank of Rear Admiral in the U.S. Public Health Service (PHS) and serves on the faculty of F. Edward Hébert School of Medicine, Uniformed Services University of the Health Sciences. She began her career in the PHS with service on the Navaho Reservation. Her medical training is in internal medicine, dermatology, and hematology. Dr. Haffner is an expert on rare disease research and treatment and international orphan product legislation. She has received awards or honors from the National Organization of Rare Disorders and the National Hemophilia Foundation. She served on the IOM Forum on Drug Discovery, Development, and Translation.

Haiden Huskamp, Ph.D., is a Professor of Health Care Policy in the Department of Health Care Policy at Harvard Medical School. Her research focuses on prescription drug policy and the economics of the pharmaceutical industry, mental health policy, and the financing and utilization of end-of-life care. Dr. Huskamp has also developed a body of research on the impact of pharmacy management tools used to control drug costs. She recently completed a Career Development Award from the National Institute of Mental Health focused on the economics of psychotropic medications. She served on the IOM committee on pediatric palliative care.

Anthony So, M.D., M.P.A., is Professor of the Practice of Public Policy Studies and Director, Program on Global Health and Technology Access at Duke University's Terry Sanford Institute of Public Policy. Current projects include an NIH-funded study to conceptualize a technology trust in genomics, a study of U.S. tissue biobanking practices, a study on innovation and access to health technologies in developing countries, and a World Health Organization/World Alliance on Patient Safety report on research and development for health technologies combating antimicrobial resistance. Previously, Dr. So served as Associate Director of the Rockefeller Foundation's Health Equity program, where he co-founded a program on intellectual property rights. Earlier, he served as Senior Advisor to the Administrator at the Agency for Health Care Policy and Research, U.S. Department of Health and Human Services and as a White House Fellow. A general internist by training, he also has an M.P.A. and completed a fellowship in the Robert Wood Johnson Clinical Scholars Program. He serves on the Advisory Board for TropIKA, a new web-based research and policy portal from the Special Programme for Research and Training in Tropical Diseases.

Robert D. Steiner, M.D., is Credit Unions for Kids Professor of Pediatric Research, Vice Chair for Research in Pediatrics, and, Faculty: Program in Molecular and Cellular Biosciences, Pediatrics, and Molecular and Medical Genetics at the Child Development and Rehabilitation Center/Doernbecher Children's Hospital, Oregon Health & Science University (OHSU), in Portland. Dr. Steiner is a pediatrician and medical geneticist who specializes in inborn errors of metabolism, along with clinical and research interests in cholesterol disorders, osteogenesis imperfecta, and autism. Dr. Steiner has led and participated in clinical research and clinical trials in many rare disorders and has conducted research with funding from NIH, industry, and private foundations under OHSU contract terms that protect data access and publication rights. He is board-certified in pediatrics and both clinical genetics and clinical biochemical genetics.

Nancy S. Sung, Ph.D., is a Senior Program Officer with the Burroughs Wellcome Fund (BWF). She oversees BWF's Interfaces in Science Programs and Clinical Scientist Awards in Translational Research. Dr. Sung has also focused on building collaboration among other private foundations, government agencies, and professional societies who share BWF's interests in strengthening training and career pathways for researchers in the clinical research as well as for physical and computational scientists entering biology areas. She is founding board chair of the Health Research Alliance, a consortium of 40 foundations and public charities. Her research has focused on gene regulation in Epstein-Barr virus and its link to nasopharyngeal carcinoma. She was a member of the IOM Clinical Research Roundtable and is currently a member of the IOM Forum on Drug Discovery, Development, and Translation. She chaired a Forum recent workshop on the topic of drug development for rare diseases.

Study Staff

Marilyn J. Field, Ph.D. (*Study Director*), is a senior program officer at the Institute of Medicine (IOM). Her recent projects at IOM have examined conflicts of interest in medical research, education, and practice and the safety of medical devices for children. Among earlier projects, she has directed three studies of the development and use of clinical practice guidelines, two studies of palliative and end-of-life care, and Congressionally requested studies of employment-based health insurance and Medicare coverage of preventive services. Past positions include Associate Director of the Physician Payment Review Commission, Executive Director for Health Benefits Management at the Blue Cross and Blue Shield Association, and Assistant Professor of Public Administration at the Maxwell School of Citizenship and Public Affairs, Syracuse University. Her doctorate in political science is from the University of Michigan, Ann Arbor.

Claire F. Giammaria, M.P.H. (from August 2010), is a research associate for the Board on Health Sciences Policy. Before joining the Institute of Medicine, she was the research associate for the Technology and Liberty Program at the ACLU's Washington Legislative Office where she primarily worked on issues concerning genetics and privacy. Ms. Giammaria received her master's degree from the Department of Health Management and Policy of the University of Michigan, Ann Arbor, and a certificate in public health genetics. Ms. Giammaria received her B.A. in biology from Grinnell College.

Erin S. Hammers, M.P.H. (until May 2010), was a research associate on the Board on Health Sciences Policy at the Institute of Medicine. She completed her master's of public health degree at Columbia University with a focus on socio-medical sciences and health promotion. Ms. Hammers is now a student at Georgetown University Law Center, pursuing her J.D.

Robin E. Parsell is a senior program assistant for the Board on Health Sciences Policy. Her recent project at the IOM examined the conflict of interest in medical research, education, and practice. Before joining the Institute of Medicine, she gained 3 years of community-based preparatory research experience with special populations as a project director at the Johns Hopkins University Center on Aging and Health and other applied research experience at the Pennsylvania State University. Ms. Parsell graduated with a B.S. in biology (focus in molecular genetics and biochemistry) and a certificate in gerontology from the University of Alabama at Birmingham.

Index

A

Abbreviated New Drug Application (ANDA), 76, 89, 93
AbioCor Implantable Replacement Heart, 218 n.12, 221
Abiomed, 218 n.12
Acceleration of discovery research (*see also* Integrated national strategy)
  advocacy group approaches, 371-386
  barriers to, 18
  biomarkers as surrogate endpoints and, 8
  opportunities for, 6-7
  patient registries and, 8
  task force on, 14, 242, 247-248
Access to orphan drugs (*see also* Coverage and reimbursement)
  advocacy groups and, 83 n.4, 200
  company assistance programs, 83 n.4, 198-200
Acetylation, 116, 117, 345, 357
Achondrogenesis type 1A, 127
Acne rosacea, 318
Acromegaly, 45 n.3, 328, 330
Activa Dystonia Therapy, 221
Acute hyperammonemia, 96
Acute intermittent porphyria, 368
Acute lymphoblastic leukemia, 298-299, 329, 330, 338, 339

Acute lymphocytic leukemia, 48 n.5
Acute myeloid leukemia, 48 n.5, 131
Acute promyelocytic leukemia, 325
Acute respiratory distress syndrome (adult), 131
Adalimumab (Humira), 304 n.31, 340, 42
Adenocarcinoma salivary duct carcinoma, 369
Adenoid cystic carcinoma, 369
Adenosine deaminase deficiency, 300 n.20
Advanced Medical Technology Association, 237-238
Advanced Research Collaboration model, 127, 141, 371
Advancing Regulatory Science Initiative, 102, 103
Advocacy groups (*see also specific groups*)
  activities of, 2, 21, 28, 29, 70, 71
  consolidation of, 70-71
  educating clinicians, 66
  research strategies, 71-72, 137-138, 168, 371-386
  resource differences, 372-373
Aetna, 225
Agency for Healthcare Research and Quality, 10, 133, 193, 203
Agency for Toxic Substances and Disease Registry, 46, 54